Diagnosis and Treatment of Osteoporosis

Diagnosis and Treatment of Osteoporosis

A Case-Based Approach

Ronald C. Hamdy, MD, FRCP, MTh.
Professor of Medicine, Cecil Cox Quillen Chair of Excellence in Geriatric Medicine, Johnson City, TN, United States
Director, Osteoporosis Center, Johnson City, TN, United States

ELSEVIER

Elsevier
Radarweg 29, PO Box 211, 1000 AE Amsterdam, Netherlands
125 London Wall, London EC2Y 5AS, United Kingdom
50 Hampshire Street, 5th Floor, Cambridge, MA 02139, United States

Copyright © 2024 Elsevier Inc. All rights are reserved, including those for text and data mining, AI training, and similar technologies.

Publisher's note: Elsevier takes a neutral position with respect to territorial disputes or jurisdictional claims in its published content, including in maps and institutional affiliations.

No part of this publication may be reproduced or transmitted in any form or by any means, electronic or mechanical, including photocopying, recording, or any information storage and retrieval system, without permission in writing from the publisher. Details on how to seek permission, further information about the Publisher's permissions policies and our arrangements with organizations such as the Copyright Clearance Center and the Copyright Licensing Agency, can be found at our website: www.elsevier.com/permissions.

This book and the individual contributions contained in it are protected under copyright by the Publisher (other than as may be noted herein).

Notices
Knowledge and best practice in this field are constantly changing. As new research and experience broaden our understanding, changes in research methods, professional practices, or medical treatment may become necessary.

Practitioners and researchers must always rely on their own experience and knowledge in evaluating and using any information, methods, compounds, or experiments described herein. In using such information or methods they should be mindful of their own safety and the safety of others, including parties for whom they have a professional responsibility.

To the fullest extent of the law, neither the Publisher nor the authors, contributors, or editors, assume any liability for any injury and/or damage to persons or property as a matter of products liability, negligence or otherwise, or from any use or operation of any methods, products, instructions, or ideas contained in the material herein.

ISBN: 978-0-323-99550-4

For information on all Elsevier publications
visit our website at https://www.elsevier.com/books-and-journals

Publisher: Stacy Masucci
Acquisitions Editor: Elizabeth Brown
Editorial Project Manager: Samantha Allard
Production Project Manager: Selvaraj Raviraj
Cover Designer: Matthew Limbert

Typeset by STRAIVE, India

ELSEVIER Book Aid International Working together to grow libraries in developing countries
www.elsevier.com • www.bookaid.org

Contents

SECTION 1

The diagnosis of osteoporosis

CHAPTER 1

Clinical diagnosis: Fragility hip fracture

Learning objectives

- Osteoporosis is a silent, asymptomatic disease until a fracture is sustained.
- Fragility fractures are diagnostic of osteoporosis, regardless of densitometric findings, but after excluding localized bone diseases.
- All fractures sustained, regardless of whether they are fragility or nonfragility fractures, increase the risk of subsequent fractures.
- Most fractures are preceded by a fall, but most falls do not result in fractures.
- The usefulness and limitations of hip protectors.

The case study

Reason for seeking medical help

- MT, 69 years old, sustained a right hip fragility fracture after tripping over her granddaughter's toy in the bedroom and falling on the carpet. She underwent surgery and recovered well.

Past medical and surgical history

- No relevant past medical or surgical history, no history of fractures, falls, or renal calculi.
- Natural menopause at age 50 years, no hormonal replacement therapy.
- Menarche at age 13 years, regular menstrual periods.
- Three children aged 38, 36, and 29 years, all in good health.

Lifestyle

- Active physical lifestyle: works as a part-time dietitian in a nursing home.
- For most of her adult life, she has been swimming at least 1 h a day, 5 days a week.
- Good appetite, states that she eats a well-balanced diet, and her daily calcium intake is "good."
- No cigarette smoking, no excessive sodium intake, two cups of hot black tea with milk, and one cup of coffee with milk daily. No soda drinks.

Diagnosis and Treatment of Osteoporosis. https://doi.org/10.1016/B978-0-323-99550-4.00028-9
Copyright © 2024 Elsevier Inc. All rights are reserved, including those for text and data mining, AI training, and similar technologies.

Medications

- None.

Family history

- Negative for osteoporosis, fractures, and renal calculi.

Clinical examination

- Weight 130 pounds, height 66″, no height loss and no kyphosis.
- No significant clinical findings: alert, oriented, appears cognitively intact. No clinical evidence of orthostatic hypotension: lying BP 124/72; standing BP 128/70, no arrhythmias, no carotid stenosis, no sensitive carotid sinus, no vertebrobasilar insufficiency, no arrhythmias, no involuntary movements, no evidence of localizing neurologic diseases. Good coordination of movements, cerebellar functions intact, tendon reflexes present, equal on both sides, plantar responses downgoing on both sides. No evidence of visual impairment.

Laboratory results

- MT recently had the following laboratory tests done as part of her annual physical examination: comprehensive metabolic panel (CMP), complete blood count (CBC), serum vitamin D, and serum thyroid stimulating hormone (TSH): all within normal limits.

DXA and/or radiologic results

- Plain X-ray: total right hip replacement, post right femoral neck fracture, good placement.

Multiple choice questions

1. ***In MT's case, the final complete diagnosis of her bone health status is:***
   A. Osteoporosis.
   B. Status posthip fracture.
   C. Osteoporosis, status posthip fracture.
   D. Osteoporosis, status postfragility hip fracture.
   E. Probable osteoporosis, status postfragility hip fracture.
   Correct answer: D
   Comment:
   Fragility fractures are diagnostic of osteoporosis even in the absence of densitometric evidence of osteoporosis, provided other metabolic bone diseases have been excluded.[1–4] MT has sustained a fragility hip fracture, i.e., a fracture that occurred in the absence of significant trauma: she tripped over her granddaughter's toy and fell on the carpet. The

magnitude of this trauma is not expected to result in a fracture in most healthy people. The final diagnosis of MT's bone status is therefore "osteoporosis, status postfragility right hip fracture" or "established osteoporosis." There is no need for further diagnostic tests, including a DXA scan, to confirm the diagnosis of osteoporosis. A DXA scan, however, is needed to establish the patient's baseline bone mineral density and evaluate her response (or lack thereof) to any prescribed medication.

Once a fragility fracture has occurred the risk of subsequent fragility fractures is substantially increased, hence the importance of including the term: "fragility fracture" with the diagnosis. A study conducted on 377,561 female Medicare beneficiaries who sustained a fracture shows that the cumulative risk of subsequent fractures was 10%, 18%, and 31% at 1, 2, and 5 years postindex fracture, respectively.[5,6] The risk of subsequent fractures is increased even in patients who sustain traumatic fractures.[7]

There is, therefore, some urgency to initiate medical management for osteoporosis in these patients, especially as medications are now available to significantly reduce the risk of patients sustaining further fragility fractures. Conversely, the longer the patient is left untreated, the more likely she is to sustain another fragility or traumatic fracture.

Fragility fractures occur most commonly in the vertebrae and are also diagnostic of osteoporosis after excluding secondary causes of localized osteoporosis. There are 2 types of vertebral compression fractures:

(a) "Clinical vertebral compression fractures" are usually associated with severe disabling pain of sudden onset. These are discussed in a separate case.

(b) Silent vertebral compression fractures are also referred to as "morphometric vertebral compression fractures." Unlike clinical vertebral compression fractures they are not associated with severe pain and are often asymptomatic, accidentally discovered while performing imaging studies for some other reason. The main clinical manifestations are loss of height, arm span exceeding body height, kyphosis, a reduced space between the lower ribs and pelvic cavity, and a protuberant abdomen. In severe cases the lower ribs lie close to and may overlap the pelvic bones. Morphologic vertebral compression fractures are discussed in a separate case.

2. ***Match the following:***

i. Fragility fractures.
ii. Pathologic fractures.
iii. Traumatic fractures.
iv. i and ii.
v. All of the above.

With:

A. Associated with a relatively good prognosis.
B. Associated with a poor prognosis.
C. Have a bimodal age distribution: common among young and older patients.
D. The result of trauma that would not be expected to result in a fracture.
E. Associated with an increased risk of further fractures

Correct answers: A. iii; B. iv; C. iii; D. iv; E. v

Comment:

There are essentially four main types of fractures:

(a) *Posttrauma fractures.*

These fractures are the result of the fractured bone having been subjected to significant mechanical trauma. The trauma is of such magnitude that it disrupts the mechanical structural integrity of the bone and results in a fracture. Any bone exposed to such trauma, even a "normal" bone, is likely to fracture. However, as mentioned earlier, once a fracture is sustained, other fractures are likely to occur subsequently.

Traumatic fractures have a bimodal distribution: more common in younger and older individuals. Whereas the prognosis is good in younger individuals, it is often poor in older patients, probably because of other underlying pathologies.

(b) *Fragility fractures.*

These fractures, also known as low trauma, atraumatic, low impact, or low energy fractures, are the result of the inherent physical mechanical weakness of osteoporotic bones. The bones are structurally impaired, mechanically weak, and unable to maintain their mechanical integrity: they fracture after sustaining minimal trauma that ordinarily would not be expected to lead to a fracture. Fragility fractures also may occur spontaneously, in the absence of trauma: atraumatic fractures.

In an attempt to standardize the definition of fragility fractures, they have been defined as fractures occurring after a fall from a height that does not exceed the body height such as occurs when the patient is walking and trips over an object that she had not seen. There is nevertheless controversy as to the impact of falling on a carpeted versus noncarpeted area, on the pavement as opposed to a wooden floor, and falling in a frozen outdoors parking spot as opposed to inside a garage.

Fragility fractures also can occur while the patient tries to get out of a chair or turns around while standing: the torque force exerted on the upper femur may be of sufficient magnitude to induce a fracture. In severe cases, they may occur while the patient is lifted out of her bed or is turned in bed by attendants.

(c) *Pathologic fractures.*

Pathologic fractures are the result of an underlying localized bone pathology such as multiple myeloma or neoplastic deposits that may interfere with the integrity of the bone and may be responsible for the fracture.

(d) *Fissure or insufficiency fractures.*

Stress fissure fractures extend from one surface into the bone, but not through it, unless displaced. They are often the result of an excessive workload on the bone as may occur when a person who has been leading a sedentary lifestyle decides—without adequate preparation—to undertake taxing physical exercises. These fractures are often referred to as stress fractures and are discussed in a separate case study.

3. ***Factors predisposing to osteoporosis in MT's case include:***
   A. Status postnatural menopause.
   B. No postmenopause hormonal replacement therapy.
   C. Caucasian ethnicity.
   D. A and B.
   E. A, B, and C.

   Correct answer: E

   Comment:

   The menopause is a major factor predisposing to a reduced bone mass, increased bone fragility, and osteoporosis. The cessation of estrogen production at the menopause is associated with an increased rate of bone resorption. As the rate of bone formation is not increased, the bone mass tends to decrease, and the patient develops osteoporosis.

   Osteoporosis is essentially asymptomatic until a fragility fracture occurs. Unfortunately by this time, the bone mass is significantly reduced, and once the patient develops a fragility fracture, she is more likely to sustain other fragility fractures. The National Bone Health Alliance Working Group recommends postmenopausal women and men aged 50years and older be treated for osteoporosis if their 10-year fracture risk is or exceeds 3% for the hip or 20% (major) fracture[8]. This issue is further discussed in a different section.

4. ***Factors reducing the likelihood that MT has osteoporosis include:***
   A. She has been swimming about an hour, 5days a week for most of her adult life.
   B. Her stated daily calcium intake exceeds the minimum recommended daily allowance.
   C. She does not smoke cigarettes.
   D. A and C.
   E. A, B, and C.

   Correct answer: C

   Comment:

   Cigarette smoking increases the risk of developing osteoporosis.[9] Unlike most physical exercises, however, swimming has not been shown to significantly increase the bone mineral density.[10] Patients also often overestimate their daily calcium intake, and it is important to inquire in detail about the source and amount of their calcium intake. On further questioning, MT stated that her main source of calcium intake is a 4-oz cup of yogurt (150mg) she often has for breakfast with some fresh fruit. She also has some milk with her cup of coffee mid-morning and a cup of tea, also with milk, in the afternoon. She does not like cheese. Clearly, her daily calcium intake is well below the 1200mg daily recommended. The calcium content of select foods is listed separately.

5. ***The following is correct:***
   A. Most fragility fractures are preceded by falls.
   B. Most falls are followed by fractures.
   C. Once a patient has sustained a fracture, the risk of subsequent fractures is increased.

D. A and C.
E. A, B, and C.

Correct answer: D

Comment:

Although some fragility fractures occur spontaneously, in the absence of any type of trauma, most fractures are preceded by falls. Fortunately, most falls are not preceded by fractures. This gives clinicians a unique opportunity to reduce the risk of fractures, especially fragility fractures, by identifying patients likely to sustain falls, identifying the causes of the falls and managing them, prior to the patient sustaining another fall. Susceptibility to falls should be an integral part of the evaluation of patients for osteoporosis, especially older patients. About one-third of community-dwelling people 65 years of age and older experience repeated falls; many more experience near falls, which are precursors of falls.[11,12] Falls and fractures are discussed in separate case studies.

6. ***Causes of repeated falls in older people include:***
   A. Intrinsic causes, such as diseases interfering with posture, balance, and steadiness.
   B. Extrinsic causes—hazardous environment.
   C. Inadequate perception of the environment.
   D. Impaired cognitive functions.
   E. All of the above.

Correct answer: E

Comments:

Causes of falls can be grouped into four different groups: First, falls resulting from some pathology such as orthostatic hypotension, arrhythmias, peripheral neuropathy, Parkinson's disease, and inappropriate foot wear. Second, falls due to a hazardous environment as is the case with the present patient who tripped on her grandchild's toy. Visual impairment may also aggravate the hazardous environment. Third, a number of medications, and alcoholic drinks, may increase the risk of falls by inducing unsteadiness. Fourth, cognitive impairment also may cause the patient to engage in potentially hazardous activities that may result in a fall. Abuse also can be an underlying cause of falls, albeit a difficult one to address. Signs of abuse include bruises of various ages, especially on the medial aspects of the humerus. Anxiety and depression are also likely to induce unsteadiness and repeated falls.

7. ***Intrinsic causes of falls include:***
   A. Diabetes mellitus.
   B. Arrhythmias.
   C. Vertebrobasilar insufficiency.
   D. Foot problems.
   E. All of the above.

Correct answer: E

Comments:

Several intrinsic factors increase the fall risk of patients with diabetes mellitus, including the associated polyuria, frequent trips to the toilet, peripheral neuropathy, and autonomic neuropathy which may lead to orthostatic hypotension. Visual acuity is also often impaired in older patients with diabetes mellitus. Arrhythmias, by reducing the stroke volume and cardiac output, may lead to unsteadiness and a fall. Similarly, vertebrobasilar insufficiency, as seen sometimes in patients with cervical spondylosis, increases the risk of unsteadiness and falls especially when the patient turns her head and further increases the magnitude of vertebrobasilar insufficiency and cerebellar ischemia. A number of foot problems and inappropriate footwear may interfere with balance and increase the risk of falls. Common intrinsic causes of falls are listed in a different case study.

8. ***Extrinsic causes of repeated falls in older people include:***
   A. Inadequate lightning.
   B. Small decorative rugs and clutter.
   C. Bifocal eye glasses.
   D. A and C.
   E. A, B, and C.

Correct answer: E

Comments:

Often environmental factors, extrinsic to the patient, are responsible for falls. This may occur when the patient relocates to a new environment or spends one or more nights in an unfamiliar surrounding as often happens when the patient stays a couple of days with her son and family or is transferred to a nursing home or other living accommodation. Not being familiar with the layout, the patient may trip over trailing electric wires or various objects she had not seen, as has occurred in the present case study.

Inadequate lightning and glare can interfere with visual acuity and may lead to repeated falls. Similarly, bifocal lenses may lead to repeated falls because the lower part of the lens which is meant to sharpen near vision is the part used to visualize the area immediately around the feet and the patient may not be able to clearly visualize obstacles or irregularities in the carpet or a small rug. As a general rule, especially for older people, it is best to have two sets of eyeglasses: one for reading and near vision and another for distant vision.

Older people are often fond of keeping small decorative rugs at the foot of the bed, entrance to rooms, and on paths they use to go from one place in their living accommodation to another. Often these small rugs are frayed and the older person may trip over such obstacles. Inadequate footwear also may lead to imbalance, unsteadiness, and repeated falls.

Common extrinsic causes of falls are discussed further in different case studies.

9. ***Main medications increasing the risk of falls include:***
   A. Hypnotics.
   B. Anxiolytics.
   C. Hypotensives.
   D. A and B.
   E. A, B, and C.

Correct answer: E

Comment:

A number of medications may lead to repeated falls especially medications that cloud the sensorium or induce drowsiness. Hypnotics, including over-the-counter hypnotics obtained without prescription, are particularly likely to induce repeated falls as they have a longer half-life than most prescription hypnotics. To complicate matters, it is not uncommon for patients to refrain from telling their treating clinician that they are taking over-the-counter hypnotics.

Anxiolytics increase the risk of falls by a similar mechanism as hypnotics. Hypotensives also may induce falls by reducing the cardiac output and cerebral blood flow, especially if the patient also has orthostasis. In older hypertensive patients the optimum blood pressure is usually higher than in the younger population. Alcoholic drinks also increase the risk of falls by interfering with the patient's sensorium, steadiness, and executive functions.

10. ***Hip protectors:***
    A. Significantly reduce the risk of hip fractures.
    B. Patients often forget to wear them.
    C. Patients do not like to wear them.
    D. A, B, and C.
    E. B and C.

Correct answer: D

Comments:

Hip protectors reduce the risk of hip fractures, provided the patient wears them. Nowadays most hip protectors are relatively small, nonintrusive, comfortable to wear, and not allergenic. Patients nevertheless need to be reminded that hip protectors are effective only if they are worn.

Unfortunately, most patients tend to take the hip protector off while getting ready to go to bed. When they wake up some time later, because of an urge to empty their urinary bladder, they tend to postpone getting out of bed until such a time that the urge to micturate becomes quite significant. At this stage, they quickly get up out of bed and try to reach the toilet as rapidly as possible. In the process they forget the wear the hip protector, may develop orthostatic hypotension, fall on their way to the toilet, and sustain a fragility fracture.

Patients need to be reminded to get out of bed slowly and ideally sit on the bed for a few seconds while transitioning from the supine to the standing position to ensure they do not become orthostatic before walking to the toilet. They also should allow sometime to put the hip protector. Alternatively, they may elect to wear the hip protector all day and night.

Case summary

Analysis of data

Factors predisposing to bone demineralization/osteoporosis

- Caucasian ethnicity.
- Status postmenopause, no hormonal replacement therapy.
- Low daily calcium intake, even though MT, a certified dietician, states that she is getting an adequate amount of calcium through her diet.

Factors reducing the risk of bone demineralization/osteoporosis

- Negative family history of osteoporosis.
- Physically active lifestyle.
- Well balanced diet, except for the low calcium intake.
- No cigarette smoking.
- No excessive alcohol, sodium, or caffeine intake.

Factors increasing risk of falls/fractures

- Objects inadvertently placed in the patient's path: MT tripped over her granddaughter's toy which had been inadvertently left on the carpet in her path.

Factors reducing the risk of falls/fractures

- Good cognitive functions.
- Physically active life style.

Diagnosis

- Osteoporosis, status postfragility hip fracture.

Management recommendations

Treatment(s)

- Antiresorptive or osteoanabolic medication. This is discussed in other cases.
- Calcium supplements if the patient is unable to get minimum recommended daily calcium intake from food: 1200mg daily for women 50years old and older and men 70years old and older.

Diagnostic test(s)

- No laboratory tests needed at this stage. MT had a few laboratory tests done recently.
- Baseline DXA scan, not needed to establish the diagnosis, but needed to evaluate response to treatment.

Lifestyle

- Encourage the patient to walk and undertake light weight-bearing exercises at least three times a week to increase bone mass and also muscle mass. Caution must be taken not to put too much stress on the rest of the skeleton. Free weight exercises should be avoided because of the risk of self-injury.
- Follow-up office visit depending on the medication prescribed for osteoporosis.

Rehabilitation

- Physical therapy and, if need be, occupational therapy to ensure patient is physically independent.

DXA and radiological

- Repeat DXA scan in 2years' time to evaluate the bone mass and effect of prescribed therapy (Fig. 1).

Key points

- Fragility fractures are diagnostic of osteoporosis and should be treated, regardless of the BMD and T-scores. In these patients there is no need for a DXA scan to confirm the diagnosis of osteoporosis. The DXA scans are nevertheless needed to allow evaluation of the patient's progress or lack thereof.
- Identifying the reason(s) for the patient's falls is important. Although the etiology is often multifactorial, reversible cause(s) may be identified. Referral to a dedicated "Falls Clinic" may be appropriate if the cause(s) of the repeated falls cannot be readily identified.
- Causes of falls can be classified in the following groups:
  a. Intrinsic factors.
  b. Extrinsic factors.
  c. Inadequate perception of the environment.
  d. Medications.
  e. Impaired cognitive functions.
  f. Abuse.

Often the causes of repeated falls in older people are multifactorial.

- Hip protectors are useful to reduce the risk of fractures, but to be effective they must be worn by the patient at the time of the fall.

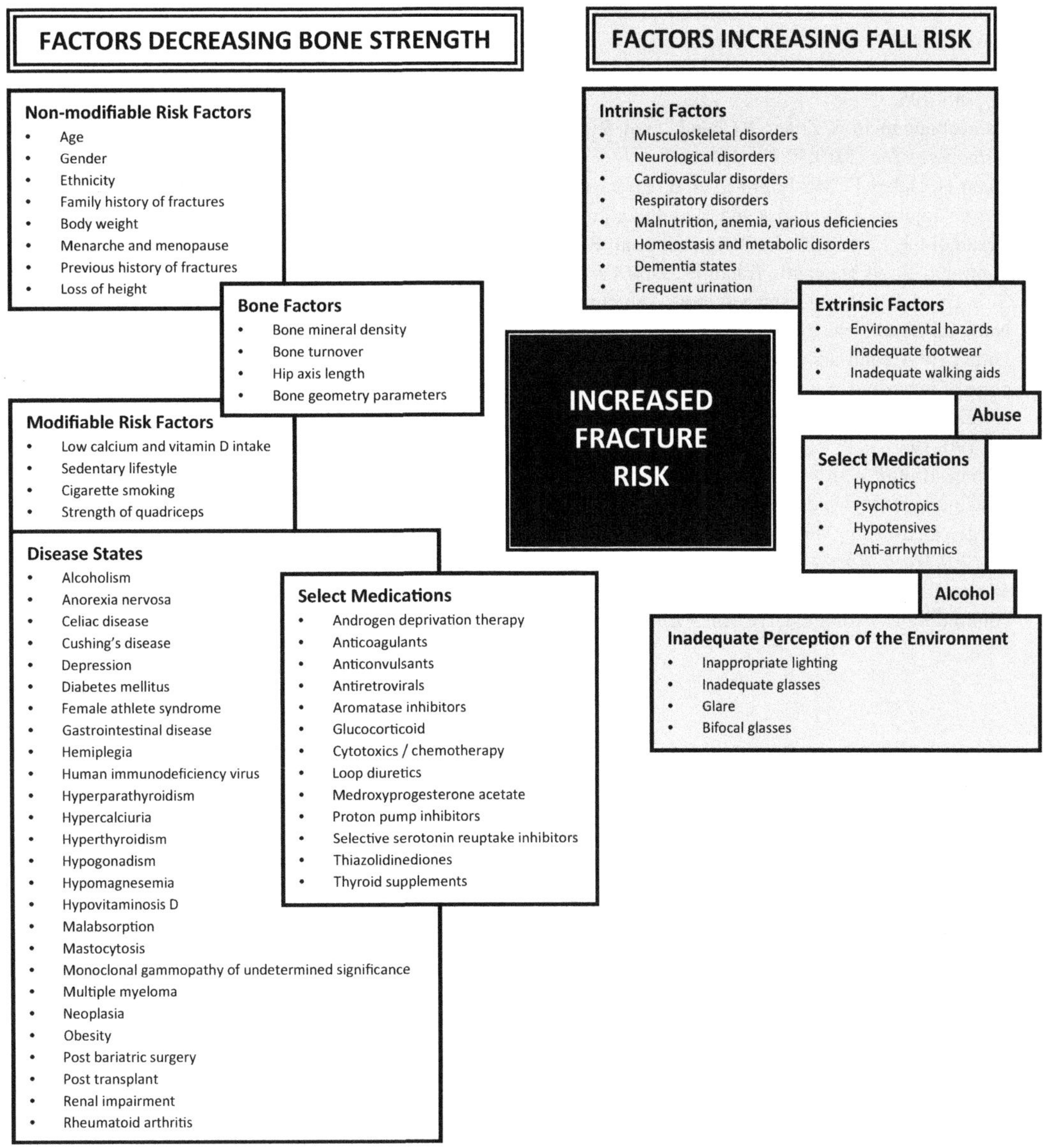

Fig. 1
Factors affecting fracture risk.

References

1. Camacho PM, Petak SM, Binkley N, et al. American Association of Clinical Endocrinologists/American College of Endocrinology Clinical Practice Guidelines for the diagnosis and treatment of postmenopausal osteoporosis – 2020 update. *Endocr Pract*. 2020;26(Suppl. 1):1–46.
2. Siris ES, Boonen S, Mitchell PJ, et al. What's in a name? What constitutes the clinical diagnosis of osteoporosis? *Osteoporos Int*. 2012;23(8):2093–2097.

3. Kanis J, Melton 3rd LJ, Christiansen C, et al. The diagnosis of osteoporosis. *J Bone Miner Res*. 1994;9 (8):1137–1141.
4. NIH Consensus Development Panel on Osteoporosis Prevention. Diagnosis and therapy. *JAMA*. 2001;285 (6):785–795.
5. Balasubramanian A, Zhang J, Chen L, et al. Risk of subsequent fracture after prior fracture among older women. *Osteoporos Int*. 2019;30:79–92.
6. Blain H, Dabas F, Mekhinini S, et al. Effectiveness of a programme delivered in a falls clinic in preventing serious injuries in high-risk older adults: a pre- and post-intervention study. *Maturitas*. 2019;122:80–86.
7. Crandall CJ, Larson JC, LaCroix AZ, et al. Risk of subsequent fractures in postmenopausal women after nontraumatic vs traumatic fractures. *JAMA Intern Med*. 2021;181(8):1055–1063.
8. Siris ES, Adler R, Bilezikian J, et al. The clinical diagnosis of osteoporosis: a position statement from the National Bone Health Alliance Working Group. *Osteoporos Int*. 2014;25:1439–1443.
9. Dimai HP, Chandran M, FRAX(®)Position Development Conference Members. Official positions for FRAX® clinical regarding smoking from joint official positions Development Conference of the International Society for Clinical Densitometry and International Osteoporosis Foundation on FRAX®. *J Clin Densitom*. 2011;14 (3):190–193.
10. Gomez-Bruton A, Montero-Marín J, González-Agüero A, et al. Swimming and peak bone mineral density: a systematic review and meta-analysis. *J Sports Sci*. 2018;36(4):365–377.
11. Bergen G, Stevens MR, Burns ER. Falls and fall injuries among adults aged ≥65 years — United States, 2014. *MMWR Morb Mortal Wkly Rep*. 2016;65:993–998.
12. O'Loughlin JL, Robitaille Y, Boivin JF, et al. Incidence of and risk factors for falls and injurious falls among the community-dwelling elderly. *Am J Epidemiol*. 1993;137(3):342–354.

CHAPTER 2

Clinical diagnosis: Fragility fracture long bones☆

Learning objectives

- A fragility fracture, per se, is diagnostic of osteoporosis and increases the risk of further fractures.
- The impact of hazardous environments leading to falls and fractures.
- The integration of medical history, clinical findings, densitometric results, FRAX results, and NOF recommendations to develop a management plan tailored to individual patients.

The case study

Reason for seeking medical help

- MG is a 57-year-old Caucasian woman. Her daughter is concerned she may have osteoporosis because about 6 months ago she sustained a fracture of the right distal radius after tripping over a small rug in her bedroom, falling onto the bed and then sliding onto the floor. She recovered very well, resuming full function of her right wrist and hand. She was given an appointment at the bone clinic but did not go because she did not feel there was anything wrong with her bones, especially as she recovered so well after the fracture. She feels very well, has not lost any height, and leads a socially active lifestyle. She is essentially asymptomatic.

Past medical and surgical history

- Right Colles' fracture about 6 months ago, excellent recovery.
- She has not sustained any fall and did not experience "near-falls."
- Natural menopause at age 51 years, no hormonal replacement therapy.
- Menarche at age 12 years, regular menstrual periods.
- Three children aged 36, 33, and 30 years, all in good health.

☆ MG is a 57-year-old Caucasian woman, who sustained a distal radius fracture.

Diagnosis and Treatment of Osteoporosis. https://doi.org/10.1016/B978-0-323-99550-4.00026-5
Copyright © 2024 Elsevier Inc. All rights are reserved, including those for text and data mining, AI training, and similar technologies.

Lifestyle

- Independent, lives with her husband, and drives her own car. Both enjoy traveling.
- Sedentary lifestyle, except for swimming for about an hour, three to four times a week.
- Works as a receptionist in a dentist's office.
- Good appetite, healthy, well-balanced diet.
- Daily calcium intake from food estimated to be about 1200 mg.
- No cigarette smoking, no recreational drugs, no caffeine, no soft drinks, low sodium intake.
- Occasional glass of wine with dinner, once or twice a week.

Medication(s)

- No medication prescribed or over the counter.

Family history

- Negative for osteoporosis.
- Mother and father alive and well.

Clinical examination

- Weight 135 pounds, height 65″ no kyphosis.
- Vision good, has bifocal eyeglasses.
- Hearing good; no hearing aids.
- Lying BP 125/82; standing BP 128/81, no orthostasis.
- No clinical evidence of carotid sinus sensitivity, carotid stenosis, or vertebrobasilar insufficiency. Passive movement of the neck does not induce any pain that may suggest cervical spondylosis.
- Gums healthy. She visits her dentist every 6 months.
- No other significant clinical findings.
- Get-up-and-Go test completed in 5 s.

Laboratory result(s)

About 2 weeks before her visit she had a number of laboratory tests done as part of her annual examination. All results were within normal limits, including complete blood count (CBC), comprehensive metabolic panel (CMP), serum vitamin D, parathyroid hormone (PTH), and thyroid stimulating hormone (TSH).

DXA and radiological result(s)

- Lowest T-score −1.8 in the upper four lumbar vertebrae.
- Vertebral fracture assessment: no evidence of vertebral compression fracture.
- FRAX scores (MG's probability of sustaining a hip or major fracture in the next 10 years): 1.2% for the risk of hip fracture and 12% for the risk of a major fracture, respectively. These thresholds do not reach the level recommended by the National Osteoporosis Foundation to initiate treatment to increase BMD and reduce the risk of fractures.

Multiple choice questions

1. ***In MG's case, factors increasing the risk of low bone mass and osteoporosis include:***
   A. Status postmenopause.
   B. No hormonal replacement therapy.
   C. Sedentary lifestyle.
   D. Caucasian ethnicity.
   E. All of the above.
   Correct answer: E
   Comment:
   All the listed factors increase the risk of low bone mass and osteoporosis. Fragility fractures of the distal radius occur much earlier than fractures of the hip and are often due to underlying abnormalities of bone mass and bone architecture.[1] They offer a unique and ideal opportunity to evaluate, diagnose, and treat fragile bones and reduce the risk of subsequent fractures.
2. ***In MG's case, factors reducing the risk of osteoporosis include:***
   A. The regular swimming exercises she undertakes.
   B. A negative family history for osteoporosis.
   C. No cigarette smoking.
   D. Low sodium and caffeine intake.
   E. B, C, and D.
   Correct answer: E
   Comment:
   Unlike most other physical exercises, it is debatable whether swimming has the same protective effects on the skeleton. Cigarette smoking increases the risk of low bone mass and osteoporosis.[2] It is, however, debatable whether this is due to the cigarette smoking per se or whether it is due to the lifestyle many smokers adopt, including sedentary lifestyles and low level or lack of physical activities.

Excessive caffeine and sodium intake induces a negative calcium balance by increasing the renal calcium loss which may trigger the release of parathyroid hormone and stimulate the osteoclasts to increase bone resorption in an attempt to mobilize calcium from the bones to the circulation, thus leading to a low bone mass and possibly osteoporosis. Many soft drinks also contain phosphates which may interfere with the intestinal absorption of calcium.

3. ***In MG's case, factors increasing the risk of falls (and hence fractures) include:***
   A. The fall she sustained 6months ago that resulted in a fragility fracture of the radius.
   B. The bifocal glasses she wears.
   C. Small rug(s) in her bedroom, if still present.
   D. All of the above.
   E. None of the above.

   Correct answer: D

   Comment:

   All of the above increase the risk of falls and therefore fractures. The fall she sustained about 6 months ago also increases the risk of sustaining further fractures. Although most fractures are preceded by falls, most falls do not result in fractures. This gives clinicians a unique opportunity to identify patients who are at risk of sustaining falls.

   Bifocal eyeglasses are sometimes responsible for repeated falls because the area immediately around the patient's feet is perceived through the lower lenses which are meant to be used for near vision, such as reading. As a result, while wearing bifocal glasses the patient may misjudge the proximity and size of obstacles in her path, may stumble over them and fall. This is particularly likely to happen when the patient is going up or down the stairs. It is safer for older people who need reading glasses to have two sets of eyeglasses: one for distant vision and one for near vision. Similarly, small rugs on the floor should be avoided as they increase the risk of falling.

   A sedentary lifestyle also increases the risk of muscle wasting which further increases the risk of falls and therefore fractures.

4. ***In MG's case, factors reducing the risk of falls (and hence fractures) include:***
   A. No history of falls and no near-falls.
   B. No clinical evidence of vertebrobasilar insufficiency.
   C. No clinical evidence of carotid stenosis or carotid sinus sensitivity.
   D. B and C.
   E. A, B, and C.

   Correct answer: E

   Comment:

   About 6months ago, MG sustained a fall that led to a fragility fracture. A number of pathologies may increase the risk of falling including carotid stenosis, a sensitive carotid sinus, vertebrobasilar insufficiency, and any pathology increasing the risk of light-headedness, dizziness, unsteadiness, and falls. Clinically carotid stenosis is suspected when the pulsations of one carotid artery are weaker than those of the contralateral side. Auscultation may reveal the presence of an ejection systolic murmur.

Vertebrobasilar insufficiency often presents with bouts of dizziness that may be clinically reproduced by passively moving the patient's head. It is often due to cervical spondylosis which causes the cervical vertebrae to become malaligned with the potential of interfering with the cerebral blood flow as the vertebral artery cruises inside the transverse process of the cervical vertebrae before joining the contralateral artery to form the basilar artery which perfuses the cerebellum where posture, equilibrium, and balance are coordinated. A sensitive carotid sinus should be considered if the patient's heart rate slows, or stops, when gentle pressure is applied on the carotid sinus. MG has none of the previously mentioned symptoms.

5. ***In MG's case:***
   A. The FRAX scores reach the threshold recommended by the NOF to initiate pharmacologic treatment.
   B. The clinical diagnosis of osteoporosis (based on the patient sustaining a fragility fracture) overrides the densitometric diagnosis.
   C. She should be offered pharmacologic treatment for osteoporosis.
   D. The NOF guidelines are overridden by the presence of a fragility fracture.
   E. B, C, and D.

   Correct answer: E

   Comment:

   The FRAX scores (1.2% and 12% for the 10-year probability of sustaining a hip or major fracture, respectively) do not reach the threshold recommended by the National Osteoporosis Foundation to initiate pharmacologic treatment (3% and 20% for the probability of sustaining a hip or major fracture, respectively).

   The presence of fragility fractures, however, overrides the T-scores, FRAX scores, and NOF recommendations as these fractures are, per se, diagnostic of osteoporosis and warrant pharmacologic treatment after excluding localized bone diseases.[3–5] In fact, in these patients DXA scans are not needed to make a diagnosis of osteoporosis or osteopenia but, as previously noted, are needed to establish a baseline against which the patient's progress, or lack of progress, may be noted.

   One of the major deficiencies of the FRAX algorithm is that falls are not taken into consideration in the permutation to calculate the fracture risk. In these patients therefore, FRAX scores underestimate the real risk of fractures. Once a fracture is sustained the risk of sustaining further fractures is increased.

6. ***The final diagnosis is:***
   A. Osteoporosis.
   B. Osteopenia.
   C. Status postfragility fracture of the distal radius.
   D. A and C.
   E. B and C.

   Correct answer: D

Comment:

The presence of a fragility fracture is, per se, diagnostic of osteoporosis and an indication that pharmacologic treatment, supported by a healthy lifestyle, should be prescribed and individualized for each patient. In these instances, a DXA scan is required not to confirm the diagnosis, but to establish a baseline against which the patient's progress, or lack of progress, can be assessed.

7. ***The following assessments are recommended:***
   A. An assessment of cognitive functions such as the Mini Mental Status Examination (MMSE) or Montreal Cognitive Assessment (MoCA).
   B. A depression scale.
   C. A falls risk assessment.
   D. A comprehensive nutrition evaluation.
   E. None of the above.

   Correct answer: E

   Comment:

   At this stage there is no indication for any of the listed assessment scales. MG is independent, actively employed, and drives her own car safely. She sustained a single fall which could be attributed to the bifocal eyeglasses she had acquired only a few days before the fall. Since then, she has not experienced any other falls or near-falls. There is therefore no need for any of the previously mentioned assessments to be done at this stage.

8. ***Pharmacologic management recommendations include:***
   A. A selective estrogen receptor modulator: raloxifene.
   B. A bisphosphonate: alendronate, risedronate, ibandronate, or zoledronic acid.
   C. A RANK-Ligand antagonist: denosumab.
   D. An osteoanabolic medication: teriparatide, abaloparatide, or romosozumab.
   E. A, B, or C.

   Correct answer: A, B, or C

   Comment:

   The presence of a fragility fracture is diagnostic of osteoporosis and overrides the densitometric diagnosis. In MG's case, the fracture of her right wrist is a fragility fracture because it is the result of trauma that ordinarily would not be expected to result in a fracture: she tripped over a rug in her bedroom and fell on the bed and then slid on the carpet.

   MG should be treated pharmacologically for osteoporosis as soon as possible, even though the DXA scan shows evidence of only osteopenia, not osteoporosis and even though the FRAX scores do not reach the threshold recommended by the NOF to initiate treatment in patients with osteopenia.

   There is some urgency to prescribe a medication to increase the bone mass. Patients who sustain fragility fractures are likely to sustain more fractures. The morbidity and mortality associated with fractures are substantial, even after the fracture itself has healed well.

At this stage, given the age of the patient (57 years), the magnitude of bone loss, as well as the cost of the medication, most clinicians would prescribe first an antiresorptive medication and observe the patients' response to treatment. A weak or lack of response will trigger a series of tests to identify possible causes of secondary osteoporosis. This issue is discussed in a different case study.

9. ***Nonpharmacologic recommended management includes:***
   A. Engage in resistive and aerobic exercises.
   B. Ensure an adequate daily calcium and vitamin D intake.
   C. Take calcium and vitamin D supplements.
   D. A and B.
   E. A, B, and C.

   Correct answer: A

   Comment:

   A combination of aerobic and resistive exercises has been shown to increase bone mass. Given that MG enjoys water exercises, she may be offered the opportunity of performing resistive exercises while in the pool, such as, for instance, walking in the shallow end of the pool while wearing flippers. Overcoming the resistance to the flippers in the water is a form of resistive exercise. Unfortunately exercise-induced increases in bone mass decrease if the person stops exercising regularly.

   Given that MG's daily dietary calcium and vitamin D intake is within the recommended limits, there is no need for calcium supplementation.

10. ***The following follow-up is recommended:***
    A. Repeat DXA scan in 1 year.
    B. Repeat DXA scan in 2 years.
    C. Repeat DXA scan in 5 years.
    D. Repeat the FRAX score in 6 months.
    E. None of the above.

    Correct answer: B

    Comment:

    Once pharmacologic management is initiated it is useful to repeat the DXA scans to monitor the patient's response (or lack of response) to treatment. Although patients' compliance is quite good in clinical trials, in real life, compliance, especially with the intake of oral bisphosphonates, is low and frequently patients do not adhere to the directions on how to take oral bisphosphonates: while fasting, with 6 oz of water and to refrain from eating, taking any medication, and drinking any fluid but water for 30 min (alendronate and risedronate) or 60min (ibandronate) after taking the medication. Patients need to be motivated. Without reinforcements they may discontinue taking the medication or may not take it exactly as directed. Compliance with denosumab is better than with oral bisphosphonates. This is discussed further in the chapter on denosumab.

    Repeating the DXA scan more often than every other year is unlikely to yield significant changes, i.e., changes exceeding the Least Significant Change (LSC) and may actually backfire and encourage discontinuation of the antiresorptive medication if the patient erroneously feels the lack of increase in BMD is due to lack of effect.

On the other hand, a positive change exceeding the LSC will encourage the patient to continue with the medication. A smaller change or a negative change in BMD will alert the treating clinician that the patient may have stopped taking the medication or may have stopped adhering to the prescribed regimen or may have secondary osteoporosis.

It is not recommended to repeat the FRAX score once pharmacologic treatment is initiated because the patient's age influences so much the fracture risk, as calculated by the FRAX permutation, that any change in BMD/T-score is likely to be obscured by the patient's age. Similarly, some of the medication-induced changes in trabecular bone thickness may not be captured by DXA scans.

Not being able to monitor the patient's response to treatment with the FRAX algorithm is a drawback as patients who have been motivated to take their medication based on the FRAX score are no longer able to assess their progress or lack of progress.

Case summary

Analysis of data

Factors predisposing to bone demineralization/osteoporosis

- Status postnatural menopause, no hormonal replacement therapy.
- Sedentary lifestyle.

Factors reducing risk of bone demineralization/osteoporosis

- Good, well-balanced diet.
- No excessive sodium and caffeine intake.
- No excessive phosphate intake.
- Moderate alcohol intake.
- No cigarette smoking.

Factors increasing risk of falls/fractures

- Bifocal eyeglasses.
- Possible hazardous environment such as small rugs in the bedroom.

Factors reducing risk of falls/fractures

- None.

Diagnosis

- Osteoporosis, as evidenced by the fragility fracture of the right distal radius.
- The presence of a fragility fracture, per se, justifies the diagnosis of osteoporosis and overrides the results of bone densitometry, FRAX scores, and National Osteoporosis

Foundation recommendations as to when therapy for osteoporosis should be initiated. The fact that the fracture has healed well suggests MG should respond well to antiresorptive therapy after secondary causes of osteoporosis have been ruled out.

Management recommendations

Medical management

- Antiresorptive medication.
- Lifestyle changes, including active lifestyle, adequate, well-balanced diet, and physical exercises.

Further diagnostic test(s)

- None at this stage. She has been adequately investigated for secondary osteoporosis.

If, however, there is concern the patient may not adhere to the medication prescribed, the changes in blood levels of bone markers before starting the medication and 6 to 8 weeks later would confirm whether she is taking the medication as directed, whether it is absorbed, and whether it is working. Markers of bone resorption, such as serum cross-linked C-telopeptide of type I collagen (CTx), can be assayed if she is prescribed antiresorptive medication. Similarly, markers of bone formation such as Procollagen Type I Intact N-terminal Propeptide (P1NP) or bone-specific alkaline phosphatase isoenzyme can be used to monitor the changes in markers of bone formation, and hence the rates of bone formation. There is no need for any of these tests if the patient is prescribed parenterally administered medication. Biomarkers are discussed separately.

Key points

- Osteopenia and osteoporosis are silent diseases until a fracture is sustained.
- The densitometric diagnosis of osteopenia is overridden by the presence of fragility fractures. Once a fragility fracture is sustained, the final diagnosis is osteoporosis regardless of the densitometric diagnosis, provided secondary causes of bone demineralization have been excluded.
- Patients with osteopenia who have sustained fragility fractures need pharmacologic treatment for their low bone mass unless there are contraindications.
- The FRAX permutation does not consider repeated falls and therefore underestimates the probability of sustaining fractures in patients who experience near-falls and falls.

References

1. Shoji MM, Ingall EM, Rozental TD. Upper extremity fragility fractures. *J Hand Surg Am.* 2021;46(2):126–132. https://doi.org/10.1016/j.jhsa.2020.07.010.
2. Tarantino U, Cariati I, Greggi C, et al. Skeletal system biology and smoke damage: from basic science to medical clinic. *Int J Mol Sci.* 2021;22(12):6629. https://doi.org/10.3390/ijms22126629. Published 21 June 2021.

3. Robinson WA, Carlson BC, Poppendeck H, et al. Osteoporosis-related vertebral fragility fractures: a review and Analysis of the American Orthopaedic Association's own the bone database. *Spine (Phila Pa 1976)*. 2020;45(8): E430–E438. https://doi.org/10.1097/BRS.0000000000003324.
4. Siris ES, Adler R, Bilezikian J, et al. The clinical diagnosis of osteoporosis: a position statement from the National Bone Health Alliance Working Group. *Osteoporos Int*. 2014;25(5):1439–1443. https://doi.org/10.1007/s00198-014-2655-z.
5. Camacho PM, Petak SM, Binkley N, et al. American Association of Clinical Endocrinologists and American College of endocrinology, clinical practice guidelines for the diagnosis and treatment of postmenopausal osteoporosis. *Endocr Pract*. 2017;23(3):383.

CHAPTER 3

Clinical diagnosis: Acute vertebral fragility fracture☆

Learning objectives

- Fragility vertebral fractures are diagnostic of osteoporosis.
- The presentation and management of acute symptomatic (clinical) and asymptomatic (morphometric) vertebral compression fractures are different.
- The usefulness and limitations of vertebral augmentation procedures.

The case study

Reason for seeking medical help

- CD presents with sudden onset of severe constant mid-back pain, with no radiation. She ranks the pain as 8 on a scale of 1–10. It started spontaneously 4 days ago while watching TV, is resistant to acetaminophen and ibuprofen, and only partly relieved by lying down, local heat, and hydrocodone/acetaminophen tablets. She has not noticed any localized muscle weakness or sensory deficit. She is ambulant, continent of urine, and has good sphincteric control. She appears to be cognitively intact.

Past medical and surgical history

- Natural menopause at age 48 years, no hormonal replacement therapy.
- Lost about 2 in. in height since her early forties.
- Bilateral hip replacement because of osteoarthritis.

Lifestyle

- Daily dietary calcium intake about 1200 mg.
- No excessive sodium or caffeine intake.

☆ CD, 74-year-old Caucasian woman, developed sudden, severe mid-back pain while watching TV.

Diagnosis and Treatment of Osteoporosis. https://doi.org/10.1016/B978-0-323-99550-4.00012-5
Copyright © 2024 Elsevier Inc. All rights are reserved, including those for text and data mining, AI training, and similar technologies.

- No cigarette smoking.
- No alcoholic drinks.
- Sedentary lifestyle.

Medication(s)

- Hydrocodone/acetaminophen tablets as required every 4h, started 3 days ago. She is, however, reluctant to continue taking this medication as she is concerned about habituation and addiction.
- Multiple vitamins/minerals supplement.

Family history

- Mother sustained fragility hip fracture.

Clinical examination

- Cognitively intact.
- Moderate kyphosis.
- Weight 132 pounds, height 60″, during early adulthood she was about 65″.
- Point tenderness on the vertebral spines in the lower thoracic vertebrae region and localized adjacent paravertebral muscle spasms.
- Limited range of motion of lumbar vertebrae because of pain.
- No localizing neurological lesions.

Multiple choice questions

1. ***In CD's case, the clinical presentation is suggestive of:***
   A. Intervertebral disc prolapse.
   B. Paget's disease of bone.
   C. Vertebral compression fracture (VCF).
   D. All the above.
   E. None of the above.
   Correct answer: C
   Comment:
   The clinical presentation is characteristic of a fragility vertebral compression fracture (VCF): it occurred suddenly; in the absence of trauma; is severe, localized, and associated with point tenderness on the vertebral spines and adjacent paravertebral muscle spasm.
   Sometimes osteoporotic VCFs are precipitated by trying to lift or push a heavy object and need to be differentiated from prolapsed intervertebral discs. The loss of height and kyphosis are suggestive of VCFs. The pain associated with disc prolapse often radiates to

the legs, while that associated with Paget's disease of bone is usually low grade and worse when the patient lies in a warm bed.

2. ***Fragility vertebral compression fractures (VCF):***
   A. Most are asymptomatic.
   B. Are diagnostic of osteoporosis regardless of the T-scores.
   C. Are associated with significant mortality and morbidity.
   D. B and C.
   E. A, B, and C.

   Correct answer: D

   Comment:

   Fragility fractures occur most commonly in the vertebrae and are also diagnostic of osteoporosis after excluding secondary causes of localized osteoporosis. There are two types of vertebral compression fractures:

   (a) "Clinical vertebral compression fractures" are associated with sudden onset of severe, often disabling pain.

   (b) "Silent vertebral compression fractures" are also referred to as "morphometric vertebral compression fractures." Unlike clinical vertebral compression fractures, they are not associated with severe pain and are often totally asymptomatic, accidentally discovered while performing imaging studies for some other reason.

   The main clinical manifestations are loss of height, arm span exceeding body height, kyphosis, a reduced space between the lower ribs and pelvic cavity, and a protuberant abdomen.

   Diagnosing osteoporosis on the basis of discovering one (or more) vertebral compression fracture while the patient is being investigated for a different pathology is often referred to as an "opportunistic" diagnosis of osteoporosis.

3. ***Vertebral Fracture Assessment (VFA) by bone densitometry:***
   A. Visualizes the vertebrae laterally between T8 and S1.
   B. The lateral contour of each vertebra can be visualized.
   C. Is useful to diagnose VCFs.
   D. A, B, and C.
   E. B and C.

   Correct answer: E

   Comment:

   VFA allows visualization of the thoracolumbar vertebrae, usually from T4 to the sacrum. The contour of each vertebra can be clearly visualized by altering the brightness and contrast of the screen. VFA is useful to determine the type (wedge, biconcave, or crush) and degree (mild, moderate, and severe) of VCFs either visually or by using markers to highlight the anterior, posterior, and midpoint heights of suspected vertebrae: a difference of 20% or more between these heights is diagnostic of VCF.[1] Osteoporosis, however, still remains underdiagnosed and undertreated even though its diagnosis now is relatively simple and effective and relatively safe medications are available. Osteoporosis is a major public health issue.[2]

A number of guidelines are also available to help clinicians develop a therapeutic management strategy tailored to the needs and status of the individual patient.[3]

4. ***CD's DXA and VFA scans:***

DXA and VFA scan results:

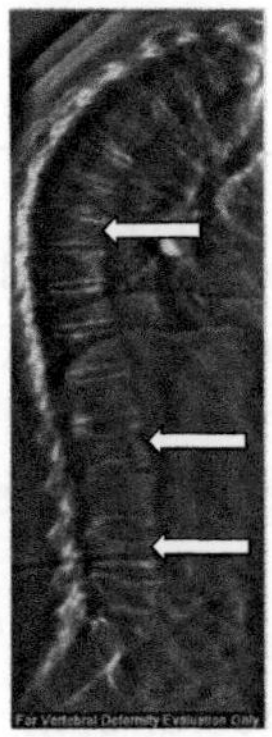

LUMBAR VERTEBRAE- AP DATA:			
	Area	**BMD**	**T-scores**
L1	12.65	0.649	-2.8
L2	11.80	1.012	-0.2
L3	15.55	0.720	-2.5

Neither hip could be scanned because of bilateral hip replacement.

A. L1-L4 T-score is normal.
B. L1-L4 T-score is artificially elevated because of VCFs.
C. Suggestive of L2, L4, and T9 vertebral compression fractures.
D. L2 and L4 should be excluded from the final analysis.
E. B, C, and D.

Correct answer: E

Comment:

Densitometric evidence of VCFs includes a smaller surface area of the affected vertebra compared to the vertebra immediately above, a higher BMD compared to the vertebra immediately below, and a difference in T-scores of more than 1.0 when compared to the adjacent vertebrae.

Normally the surface area and BMD of each vertebra increase from L1 to L4. When a vertebra is compressed, its surface area is reduced, and as the bone mineral content remains unchanged, its density appears to be higher than the vertebra below. Compressed vertebrae should be excluded before analyzing the scan. There nevertheless should be at least 2 evaluable vertebrae.[4]

5. ***The following can be useful to relieve pain associated with VCFs:***

A. Analgesics and nonsteroidal antiinflammatory drugs.
B. Narcotics.
C. Calcitonin.
D. Any of the above.
E. None of the above.

Correct answer: D

Comment:

Pain management is the prime goal of managing patients with acute symptomatic VCFs to avoid triggering a vicious cycle: pain leading to reduced physical activity, muscle wasting, unsteadiness, and increased risk of falls and subsequently fractures. All the listed modalities are useful to reduce pain associated with VCFs. The analgesic effect of calcitonin is mediated through endorphins.[5]

Narcotics may be indicated. There is, however, evidence to suggest that the addition of codeine to a combination of acetaminophen and ibuprofen does not increase the analgesic potency of the latter as evidenced by a randomized double-blind controlled trial on 131 subjects undergoing surgical removal of an impacted third molar tooth. Pain was assessed by a visual analogue scale.[6] Another randomized controlled trial on 416 patients presenting to emergency departments with acute extremity pain showed neither statistically nor clinically significant differences in pain reduction 2h after a single dose treatment with one of 4 regimens: ibuprofen and acetaminophen, oxycodone and acetaminophen, hydrocodone and acetaminophen, or codeine and acetaminophen.[7]

Notwithstanding, as the pain associated with an acute VCF is usually, spontaneously, at least partly, relieved within 4–6weeks of the fracture, it is seldom necessary to continue with narcotics for longer periods. The adverse effects of narcotics, especially in older people, are well known and include cognitive impairment, delirium, depression, constipation, unsteadiness, repeated falls, accidents, injuries, peripheral edema, respiratory depression, hypoventilation, apnea, hypoxia, somnolence, nausea, vomiting, dizziness, pruritus, urine retention, and urinary incontinence.[8–11]

6. ***The following are useful modalities to relieve pain associated with VCFs:***
   A. Back braces.
   B. Transcutaneous nerve stimulation.
   C. Gentle massage and heat application.
   D. All the above.
   E. None of the above.

Correct answer: D

Comment:

Back braces are often effective at alleviating the pain. However, by providing support they reduce muscle tone and may lead to muscle wasting if worn for prolonged periods. Most patients like back braces because of the support and comfort they provide.

Transcutaneous nerve stimulation is effective at reducing the pain. Gentle superficial massage (effleurage), local heat, and menthol-based or lidocaine ointments are soothing adjunct comforting measures. A number of plant-based ointments are also commercially available over the counter. Their evidence-based efficacy has not been thoroughly evaluated. Deep massage is better avoided as it may jeopardize the fragile integrity of the vertebrae.

7. ***Match the following:***
   (a) Acetaminophen.
   (b) Nonsteroidal antiinflammatory medications.

(c) Narcotics.
(d) All the above.
(e) None of the above.
A. Nephrotoxicity.
B. Hepatic toxicity.
C. Constipation.
D. Increased fall risk.
E. Upper GI adverse effects.

Correct answers: A (b); B (a); C (c); D (c); E (b)

Comments:

Constipation, impaired cognitive functions, drowsiness, and repeated falls are the main adverse effects of narcotics in older patients. Gastric irritation and upper gastrointestinal irritation are often seen in patients taking nonsteroidal antiinflammatory drugs. NSAIDs also should be avoided or administered in reduced doses, and for short periods of time to patients with impaired renal functions. The need for analgesia should be regularly evaluated as the pain is often limited to 4–6 weeks after the fracture is sustained.

8. ***Match the following:***
(a) Kyphoplasty.
(b) Vertebroplasty.
(c) Both.
(d) Neither.
A. A cavity is created in the compressed vertebral body.
B. Biological cement is injected under high pressure into affected vertebra.
C. If successful it is usually associated with almost immediate complete pain relief.
D. Activities of daily living can be resumed almost immediately after the procedure.
E. The risks of biological cement extravasation are higher.

Correct answers: A: (a); B: (b); C: (c); D: (c); E: (b)

Comment:

Kyphoplasty and vertebroplasty are vertebral augmentation procedures during which biological cement (usually polymethylmethacrylate) is introduced in the compressed vertebral body. During vertebroplasty, the cement is introduced under high pressure. During kyphoplasty, a cavity is first created in the vertebral body by a balloon tamp and then cement is introduced under low pressure into that cavity. The pressure required to administer biological cement is lower with kyphoplasty than with vertebroplasty and therefore the risk of extravasation is less. Kyphoplasty may restore some height loss.[12] When successful, these procedures are associated with almost immediate pain relief with the patient able to resume her daily activities.[13]

9. ***The following is/are true concerning vertebral augmentation procedures:***
   A. Long-term pain relief is well established.
   B. Success rate is higher if done soon after the fracture occurred.
   C. Risk of adjacent VCFs is significantly higher after the procedure.
   D. A and B.
   E. A, B, and C.

   Correct answer: B

   Comments:

   Whereas, when successful, the acute pain relief is almost immediate and remarkable, the long-term pain relief of vertebral augmentation procedures is still questionable.[13–17] The success rate, however, is higher if the procedure is done soon after the fracture.

   A concern about injecting biological cement in a compressed vertebra is the increased mechanical stress on adjacent vertebrae and increased risk of adjacent vertebral fractures and biological cement extravasation. On the other hand, the mechanical stress imposed by a compressed vertebra on the adjacent vertebrae and the inherent increased fragility of adjacent vertebrae also must be considered.

   The two main indications for vertebral augmentation procedures are: first, pain relief and improvement of the patient's functional status; and second, vertebral body stabilization. As in most patients, the pain improves spontaneously; the effects of vertebral augmentation, per se, on pain are difficult to assess.[3,14]

   Notwithstanding, neither vertebroplasty, nor kyphoplasty is at present recommended as first-line treatment in patients with painful vertebral compression fractures because of the unclear benefit on pain and the potential increased risk of fractures developing in adjacent vertebrae.[3]

10. ***The goals of vertebral augmentation procedures include:***
    A. Pain control.
    B. Improving the patient's functional status.
    C. Vertebral body stabilization.
    D. A and B.
    E. A, B, and C.

    Correct answer: E

    Comments:

    Vertebral augmentation is an image-guided, minimally invasive procedure during which bone cement, such as polymethylmethacrylate, is injected in the compressed vertebra to manage painful fractures not responding to conservative medical therapy. Secondary goals include stabilizing the affected vertebral body and preventing future fractures.[14]

Case summary

Analysis of data

Factors predisposing to bone demineralization/osteoporosis in CD's case

- Status postmenopause, no HRT.
- Positive family history: mother sustained fragility hip fracture.
- Sedentary lifestyle.
- Caucasian race.

Factors reducing risk of bone demineralization/osteoporosis in CD's case

- Good daily calcium intake.
- No excessive sodium, caffeine, alcohol intake and no cigarette smoking.

Factors increasing risk of falls/fractures

- Vertebral compression fracture.
- Height loss and kyphosis.
- Intake of narcotics.

Factors reducing risk of falls/fractures

- None.

Diagnosis

- Osteoporosis, acute vertebral compression fracture.

Management recommendations

Treatment recommendation(s)

- Antiresorptive or osteoanabolic therapy for osteoporosis.
- Pain control.

Diagnostic test(s)

- Rule out secondary causes of osteoporosis and osteolytic deposits.

Rehabilitation

- Vertebral augmentation procedures may be considered in some select patients.

Key points

- Fragility vertebral compression fractures (VCF) are diagnostic of osteoporosis unless they are secondary to diseases associated with localized osteolytic deposits such as multiple myeloma, hemangiomas, and osteolytic deposits.
- When symptomatic, VCF present with sudden severe back pain. Most are, however, asymptomatic and discovered during imaging studies for unrelated conditions.
- Diagnosis of vertebral compression fractures can be established radiologically or by Vertebral Fracture assessment (VFA) during bone densitometry.
- Pain management is important and may include narcotics. Ancillary modalities are available.
- Calcitonin is sometimes prescribed for its analgesic effect mediated through the release of endorphins.
- Unless complicated by other pathologies the severe pain associated with VCF lasts about 4–6 weeks.
- The underlying osteoporotic condition must be treated.

Diagnosis of acute vertebral compression fractures

- ***Clinical diagnosis:***
  - Acute back pain, sudden onset, localized, no specific radiation.
  - Point tenderness along spine of affected vertebra(e) and adjacent paravertebral muscle spasm.
  - Limited range of flexion and extension of affected and adjacent vertebrae because of pain.
  - Loss of height.
  - Kyphosis.
  - Most vertebral compression fractures are asymptomatic and accidentally discovered during imaging studies, often performed for reasons not related to osteoporosis. These are known as "morphometric" vertebral compression fractures and are discussed in the next case study.
- ***Radiological diagnosis:***
  Plain X-rays or other imaging studies of the vertebrae reveal the characteristic radiological features of compressed vertebra(e).
- ***On PA lumbar vertebrae DXA scan, features suggestive of a VCF include:***
  - A smaller surface area that is out of line with adjacent vertebrae: normally the surface area of the vertebrae gradually increases from L1 to L4, although occasionally L4 has the same surface area or may even appear smaller than L3. The surface area of a compressed vertebra is smaller than expected.
  - A Bone Mineral Density (BMD) out of line with adjacent vertebrae: normally the BMD increases from L1 to L4. After a vertebral compression fracture is sustained, the BMD of the compressed vertebra is higher than the vertebra immediately below the compressed vertebra.

- A T-score that is out of line and more than 1.0 higher or lower than the adjacent vertebrae.

- ***On a lateral vertebral X-ray or Vertebral Fracture Assessment (VFA) during bone densitometry, VCF may be identified by:***
  - Visual inspection: noting the shape of the suspected vertebra and comparing it to adjacent ones.
  - Morphometry: markers are placed on the superior and inferior anterior, midpoint, and posterior ends of the suspected vertebra. The ratio between the anterior, midpoint, and posterior heights is calculated. If it exceeds 20% it is suggestive of a vertebral compression fracture. Depending on the densitometer, this ratio is calculated during VFA either automatically or once markers are placed on the suspected vertebra.
- ***Types of vertebral compression fractures:***
  - Wedge, if the difference of 20% or more is between the anterior and posterior heights of the affected vertebra.
  - Biconcave, if the difference of 20% or more is between the midpoint and anterior or posterior heights of the affected vertebra.
  - Crush, if the difference of 20% or more is between one vertebra and adjacent ones: immediately above or below the affected vertebra.
- ***Vertebral compression fractures can be rated as:***
  - Mild: the difference between the heights is between 20% and 25%. These are often ignored as they are easily confused with vertebral deformities. This is further discussed later.
  - Moderate: the difference between the heights is between 25% and 35%.
  - Severe: the difference between the heights exceeds 35%.
- ***When the vertebral compression fracture is rated as "mild,"*** **i.e.,** ***a difference between 20 and 25% between the vertebral heights, it should be differentiated from:***
  - A "vertebral deformity" in which case:
    - More than one vertebra is usually affected.
    - The BMD of the deformed vertebra is not in line with other adjacent vertebrae, i.e. it is lower than the vertebra immediately below and higher than the vertebra immediately above, as opposed to the BMD of a compressed vertebra which tends to be higher than the one immediately below it.
    - The T-score of the deformed vertebra is in line with other adjacent vertebrae, i.e., the difference between T-scores of individual vertebrae does not exceed 1.0.
  - A Schmorl's nodule is the result of the intervertebral disc partly invaginating the adjacent vertebral plates. In that case the intervertebral disc space is usually narrower than other intervertebral disc spaces

Consequences of vertebral compression fractures

- Clinical consequences:
  - Acute and chronic pain, limited range of movement, and immobilization with all their consequences. Although the severe acute pain typically is relieved within 4–6 weeks. Often it is followed by a lower grade chronic pain that may interfere with daily activities and the patient's mobility.
  - When several vertebrae are compressed:
    - Decreased height and kyphosis the patient cannot be corrected by standing upright.
    - Reduced pulmonary functions.
    - Abdominal discomfort.
    - Loss of independence.
    - Loss of self-esteem and depression.
- Increased risk of subsequent fragility fractures, vertebral, and others.[18]
- 20% increased 5-year mortality (Table 1).[13]

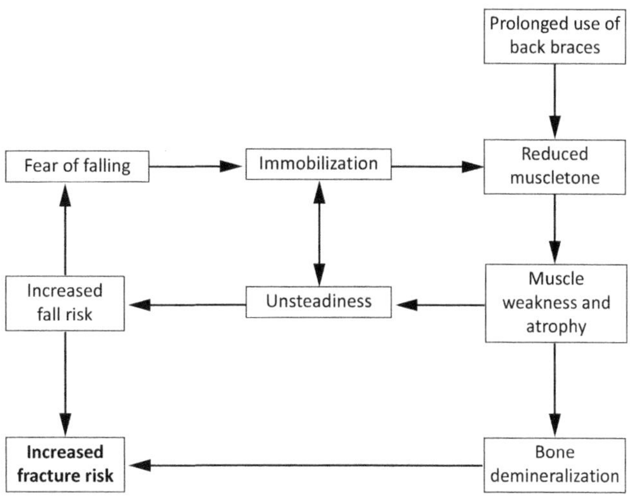

Table 1 Vertebral augmentation procedures.

Procedure	Vertebroplasty	Kyphoplasty
Cavity created in body of vertebra	No	Yes
Cement injected in vertebral body under	High pressure	Low pressure
Risk of cement extravasation	High	Low
Acute pain relief	Immediate	Immediate
Long-term pain relief	Undetermined	Undetermined
Complication rate	Higher	Lower

The vicious cycle of immobilization, muscle weakness, bone demineralization, and increased fracture risk.

References

1. Genant HK, Jergas M, Palermo L, et al. Comparison of semiquantitative visual and quantitative morphometric assessment of prevalent and incident vertebral fractures in osteoporosis The Study of Osteoporotic Fractures Research Group. *J Bone Miner Res.* 1996;11(7):984–996. https://doi.org/10.1002/jbmr.5650110716.
2. Haffner MR, Delman CM, Wick JB, et al. Osteoporosis is undertreated after low-energy vertebral compression fractures. *J Am Acad Orthop Surg.* 2021;29(17):741–747. https://doi.org/10.5435/JAAOS-D-20-01132.
3. Camacho PM, Petak SM, Binkley N, et al. American Association of Clinical Endocrinologists, American College of Endocrinology Clinical Practice Guidelines for the diagnosis and treatment of postmenopausal osteoporosis – 2020 update. *Endocr Pract.* 2020;26(Suppl. 1):1–46. https://doi.org/10.4158/GL-2020-0524SUPPL.
4. Hamdy RC, Petak SM, Lenchik L, International Society for Clinical Densitometry Position Development Panel and Scientific Advisory Committee. Which central dual X-ray absorptiometry skeletal sites and regions of interest should be used to determine the diagnosis of osteoporosis? *J Clin Densitom.* 2002;5(Suppl):S11–S18. https://doi.org/10.1385/jcd:5:3s:s11.
5. Ofluoglu D, Akyuz G, Unay O, Kayhan O. The effect of calcitonin on beta-endorphin levels in postmenopausal osteoporotic patients with back pain. *Clin Rheumatol.* 2007;26(1):44–49. https://doi.org/10.1007/s10067-006-0228-z.
6. Best AD, De Silva RK, Thomson WM, Tong DC, Cameron CM, De Silva HL. Efficacy of codeine when added to paracetamol (acetaminophen) and ibuprofen for relief of postoperative pain after surgical removal of impacted third molars: a double-blinded randomized control trial. *J Oral Maxillofac Surg.* 2017;75 (10):2063–2069. https://doi.org/10.1016/j.joms.2017.04.045.
7. Chang AK, Bijur PE, Esses D, Barnaby DP, Baer J. Effect of a single dose of oral opioid and nonopioid analgesics on acute extremity pain in the emergency department: a randomized clinical trial. *JAMA.* 2017;318 (17):1661–1667. https://doi.org/10.1001/jama.2017.16190.
8. Pergolizzi JV, Raffa RB, Marcum Z, Colucci S, Ripa SR. Safety of buprenorphine transdermal system in the management of pain in older adults. *Postgrad Med.* 2017;129(1):92–101. https://doi.org/10.1080/00325481.2017.1270699.
9. Swart LM, van der Zanden V, Spies PE, de Rooij SE, van Munster BC. The comparative risk of delirium with different opioids: a systematic review. *Drugs Aging.* 2017;34(6):437–443. https://doi.org/10.1007/s40266-017-0455-9.
10. Viscusi ER, Ding L, Itri LM. The efficacy and safety of the fentanyl iontophoretic transdermal system (IONSYS®) in the geriatric population: results of a meta-analysis of phase III and IIIb trials. *Drugs Aging.* 2016;33(12):901–912. https://doi.org/10.1007/s40266-016-0409-7.
11. Allen C, Zarowitz BJ, O'Shea T, Datto C, Olufade T. Clinical and functional characteristics of nursing facility residents with opioid-induced constipation. *Consult Pharm.* 2017;32(5):285–298. https://doi.org/10.4140/TCP.n.2017.285.
12. Pitton MB, Morgen N, Herber S, et al. Height gain of vertebral bodies and stabilization of vertebral geometry over one year after vertebroplasty of osteoporotic vertebral fractures. *Eur Radiol.* 2008;18:608–615. https://doi.org/10.1007/s00330-007-0776-x.
13. Boonen S, Van Meirhaeghe J, Bastian L, et al. Balloon kyphoplasty for the treatment of acute vertebral compression fractures: 2-year results from a randomized trial. *J Bone Miner Res.* 2011;26(7):1627–1637. https://doi.org/10.1002/jbmr.364.
14. Amans MR, Carter NS, Chandra RV, Shah V, Hirsch JA. Vertebral augmentation. *Handb Clin Neurol.* 2021;176:379–394. https://doi.org/10.1016/B978-0-444-64034-5.00017-1.

15. Buchbinder R, Osborne RH, Ebeling PR, et al. A randomized trial of vertebroplasty for painful osteoporotic vertebral fractures. *N Engl J Med.* 2009;361(6):557–568. https://doi.org/10.1056/NEJMoa0900429.
16. Kallmes DF, Comstock BA, Heagerty PJ, et al. A randomized trial of vertebroplasty for osteoporotic spinal fractures [published correction appears in N Engl J Med. 2012 Mar 8;366(10):970]. *N Engl J Med.* 2009;361(6):569–579. https://doi.org/10.1056/NEJMoa0900563.
17. Wardlaw D, Cummings SR, Van Meirhaeghe J, et al. Efficacy and safety of balloon kyphoplasty compared with non-surgical care for vertebral compression fracture (FREE): a randomized controlled trial. *Lancet.* 2009;373(9668):1016–1024. https://doi.org/10.1016/S0140-6736(09)60010-6.
18. Lindsay R, Silverman SL, Cooper C, et al. Risk of new vertebral fracture in the year following a fracture. *JAMA.* 2001;285(3):320–323. https://doi.org/10.1001/jama.285.3.320.

CHAPTER 4

Opportunistic/morphometric diagnosis—Silent vertebral fractures ☆

Learning objectives

- Vertebral Compression Fractures (VCF) are often silent and referred to as "morphometric vertebral compression fractures."
- The radiological appearances of vertebral deformities and VCF.
- In the absence of trauma, and after excluding localized osteolytic lesions, morphometric VCF are diagnostic of osteoporosis and override the densitometric diagnosis.
- The importance of opportunistic imaging studies.

The case study

Reasons for seeking medical help

DK has been recently hospitalized because of left lower lobe pneumonia. In addition to the characteristic features of pneumonia, a plain chest X-ray revealed moderate wedge vertebral compression fracture of T7. She denies recent and remote trauma to her back, but admits to experiencing occasional bouts of mild, vague, ill-defined pain in the mid to lower back, especially after standing for prolonged periods of time or carrying her two-year-old granddaughter.

She grades the pain as 3 on a 1 to 10 scale, with 10 being the worst possible pain. The pain is localized, usually readily relieved by lying down, analgesics (Acetaminophen 650mg), nonsteroidal antiinflammatory drugs (Ibuprofen 200mg), and local heat application. She uses these medications less frequently than once a month. Osteolytic deposits and other causes of localized bone demineralization have been excluded. She states that she lost about 2in. in height since early adulthood.

☆ DK, 71-year-old Caucasian woman, recovering from pneumonia.

Diagnosis and Treatment of Osteoporosis. https://doi.org/10.1016/B978-0-323-99550-4.00007-1
Copyright © 2024 Elsevier Inc. All rights are reserved, including those for text and data mining, AI training, and similar technologies.

Past medical and surgical history

- Surgical menopause: at age of 39 years when she underwent a hysterectomy and bilateral oophorectomy, no hormonal replacement therapy was prescribed.
- Menarche at 12 years, regular menstrual periods.
- She categorically denies any trauma to the back.

Lifestyle

- Sedentary lifestyle.
- Daily dietary calcium intake estimated to be about 1300 mg.
- No cigarette smoking.
- No alcohol abuse: not more than one glass of wine once or twice a week.
- No excessive sodium or caffeine intake.
- Common causes of low body weight have been investigated and ruled out.

Medication(s)

- No regular medications, apart from occasional analgesic and NSAID. Does not use opioids.

Family history

- Negative for osteoporosis.

Clinical examination

- Weight 131 pounds, steady; height 62″.
- Mild kyphosis.
- Slight tenderness along mid and lower thoracic vertebrae with adjacent paravertebral muscle spasm.
- No other significant clinical findings, no neurologic deficits.

Laboratory result(s)

- Complete blood count (CBC) and Comprehensive Metabolic Panel (CMP): no abnormal finding.
- Serum 25-hydroxy-vitamin D: within the normal range (46 ng/mL).
- Serum and urine protein electrophoresis: no abnormality detected.
- Erythrocytic sedimentation rate 3 mm in first hour.

DXA and radiological result(s)

- T-scores: right femoral neck −0.5, right total hip −0.3, left femoral neck −0.8, left total hip −0.7, L1–L4 −1.0.

- Vertebral Fracture Assessment (VFA): moderate wedge compression fracture of T7 (34% for the T7 antero/posterior ratio of vertebral heights).
- FRAX scores: 1.2% and 11% for the 10-year risk of sustaining a hip fracture and major osteoporotic fracture, respectively.

Multiple choice questions

1. ***In DK's case, the vertebral compression fracture identified by vertebral fracture assessment (VFA):***
   A. It is not a true fracture, but vertebral deformity.
   B. It is not relevant because it is essentially asymptomatic.
   C. It is an incidental benign finding and can be ignored.
   D. It increases neither mortality nor morbidity risks.
   E. It is diagnostic of osteoporosis after causes of localized osteolytic lesions have been excluded.

   Correct answer: E

   Comments:

   Although vertebral deformities are common, especially in older patients, they are seldom of the magnitude seen in DK's case: moderate (34%) wedge compression fracture. Deformities also usually affect several vertebrae. It would be unusual for vertebral deformities to be confined to just one vertebra.

   After excluding causes of localized osteoporosis, silent VCFs, also referred to as "morphometric" fragility fractures, are diagnostic of osteoporosis. They are associated with an increased fracture risk of any bone, increased mortality, and significant morbidity,[1–3] including chronic back pain, loss of height, kyphosis, protuberant abdomen, decreased pulmonary function, sleep disturbances, loss of independence, loss of self-esteem, depression, and cognitive impairment. Nerve entrapment and paraplegia, on the other hand, are rare. The 5-year mortality postvertebral fractures are increased by about 20%.[2] Within 12months of a VCF, 19% of untreated patients are expected to sustain another vertebral fracture.[2] The presence of these fractures therefore—even though essentially asymptomatic—emphasizes the urgency of addressing the underlying osteoporosis.[4] Abdominal CT scans can be used to identify patients with previously undetected fractures who are at risk of further fractures.[5]

2. ***Match the following:***
   (a) Morphometric VCF.
   (b) Clinical or acute VCF.
   (c) Both.
   (d) Neither.
      A. Usually associated with acute severe localized pain.
      B. Painless when it occurs.
      C. Leads to height loss.

D. Usually associated with spinal cord compression.
E. Usually discovered during imaging studies for an unrelated condition.

Correct answers: A (b); B (a); C (c); D (d); E (a).

Comments:

Morphometric VCFs are asymptomatic fractures, discovered when imaging studies are conducted for some unrelated medical condition. Clinical VCFs occur spontaneously or after sustaining trauma that ordinarily would not be expected to lead to a fracture. Both are considered fragility fractures and diagnostic of osteoporosis, regardless of the bone density, but after causes of localized bone demineralization have been ruled out. Both lead to height loss. Spinal cord compression may complicate traumatic vertebral fractures, but seldom occurs in patients with osteoporotic VCFs.

Although morphometric VCFs are not associated with the typical acute pain experienced by patients sustaining clinical VCFs, they are often associated with gradually worsening low-grade back pain and kyphosis. The pain is usually at least partly relieved by lying down and analgesics. Heat and gentle massage are useful ancillary aids to relieve pain.

The pain associated with clinical VCFs is acute and severe, usually self-limited, and relieved spontaneously, within 4–6 weeks after the incident. It nevertheless may be replaced by low-grade pain worsened by standing and exertion and relieved by lying down.

The densitometric diagnosis (normal bone density in DK's case) is overridden by the presence of fragility fractures, including morphometric VCFs. After ruling out common causes of localized bone demineralization,[6] the presence of VCFs in the absence of significant trauma establishes the fracture as a fragility fracture and therefore the final diagnosis is osteoporosis, even if the T-score is not within the osteoporotic range and even if the fracture risk as calculated by the FRAX algorithm does not reach the threshold recommended by the National Osteoporosis Foundation to initiate pharmacologic treatment for osteoporosis.[4]

If the workup of the patient reveals pathologies that may be responsible for the vertebral compression fracture such as, for instance, multiple myeloma or osteolytic deposits, the diagnosis would be "pathological vertebral compression fracture." Unfortunately, although osteoporosis is a major health issue that affects the day-to-day quality of life, it remains largely undetected, underdiagnosed, and undertreated.[7–9]

3. ***Morphometric VCFs:***
   A. Most often due to an underlying pathology such as multiple myeloma.
   B. Vertebral augmentation procedures should be considered.
   C. Lumbar vertebrae are affected more than thoracic vertebrae.
   D. All of the above.
   E. None of the above.

Correct answer: E

Comments:

The commonest cause of morphometric VCFs is osteoporosis. There is no need for vertebral augmentation procedures as the main goal of this procedure is to relieve pain associated with clinical VCF and the results are best when performed soon after the fracture. The short- and especially long-term efficacy of vertebral augmentation procedures has been questioned and is further discussed in the case study on "Acute vertebral compression fractures."

4. ***Vertebral Fracture Assessment:***
   A. The presence of morphometric vertebral compression fractures is diagnostic of osteoporosis and overrides the densitometric diagnosis.
   B. The exposure to radiation is about the same as a plain X-ray of the thoracolumbar vertebrae.
   C. Depending on the densitometer used, the patient can remain supine during the VFA imaging study.
   D. A and C.
   E. B and C.

   Correct answer: D

   Comments:

   By identifying a VCF in a patient with osteopenia who denies trauma to her back, VFA changes the densitometric diagnosis to osteoporosis, after causes of localized bone demineralization have been excluded. The exposure to radiation resulting from VFA is much less than that resulting from a plain X-ray of the vertebrae. Some densitometers allow for VFA to be done without having to reposition the patient.
5. ***Factors predisposing to osteoporosis in DK's case are:***
   A. Caucasian ethnicity.
   B. Status postmenopause at a young age, and no hormone replacement therapy.
   C. Sedentary lifestyle.
   D. Low body weight.
   E. A, B, C, and D.

   Correct answer: E

   Comments:

   All listed predispose to osteoporosis.
6. ***Clinical signs suggestive of morphometric vertebral compression fractures include:***
   A. Kyphosis.
   B. Reduced space between lower ribs and pelvic cavity.
   C. Increased arm span/height ratio.
   D. Loss of height.
   E. All of the above.

   Correct answer: E

Comments:

All the listed clinical signs are suggestive of multiple vertebral compression fractures, morphometric fractures, if there is no history of back trauma. However, apart from kyphosis and loss of height which can be reliably measured and quantified, the reproducibility of measuring the arm span and the space between the lower ribs and pelvic cavity is such that, unless excessive, it cannot be used reliably for diagnostic purposes.

7. ***Loss of height in older patients can be due to:***
   A. The patient assuming a stooped position.
   B. A reduced volume of the intervertebral disc.
   C. Vertebral compression fractures.
   D. Buckling of the knees.
   E. All of the above.

   Correct answer: E

   Comments:

   Loss of height is a very common finding in older people and is usually multifactorial. Older people often assume a stooped position to make up for the exaggerated lumbar lordosis and buckling of the knees. In these instances, the patient is able to reduce the thoracic curvature and, at least partly, straighten the kyphotic posture. Old age is often associated with some desiccation and a reduced volume of the intervertebral disc. The intervertebral disc also may invaginate the plates of the adjacent vertebral body: Schmorl's nodules. It is possible that these represent early stages of vertebral compression fractures.

8. ***DK would benefit from the following:***
   A. Estrogen.
   B. Large daily doses of vitamin D and calcium supplements.
   C. Vertebroplasty or kyphoplasty.
   D. A and B.
   E. None of the above.

   Correct answer: E

   Comments:

   Largely based on the results of Women's Health Initiative (WHI) study, estrogen is no longer approved for the treatment of osteoporosis in older postmenopausal women even though this study showed that, compared to placebo, hormonal replacement therapy reduced the risk of osteoporosis and the incidence of hip fractures (36%), clinical vertebral fractures (36%), and other osteoporotic fractures (23%).[10,11] The WHI study, however, also showed that, in older postmenopausal women, HRT is associated with an increased risk of strokes, urinary incontinence, neoplasia, gall bladder diseases, and dementia, including Alzheimer's disease. At present HRT is approved only for the prevention of osteoporosis, provided it is administered soon after the menopause and in the smallest dose, for the shortest period of time.

It has nevertheless been pointed out that the average age of patients enrolled in the WHI study was about 60 years and therefore the findings of this study may not be applicable to younger postmenopausal women.

DK is getting a good daily amount of calcium through food, and her serum vitamin D level is within the normal range. There is therefore no need for either vitamin D or calcium supplementation. She is also not likely to benefit from vertebral augmentation procedures (vertebroplasty or kyphoplasty) as she is not complaining of severe pain: the main indication for these procedures.

9. ***The following are recommended in DK's case:***

   A. Back brace.

   B. Heat pads.

   C. Transcutaneous nerve stimulation.

   D. All of the above.

   E. None of the above.

   Correct answer: E

   Comments:

   Although these measures may be useful for the management of pain associated with acute clinical osteoporotic VCFs, they are not indicated for morphometric VCFs, unless the patient is experiencing pain. The pain experienced by DK is, usually, not of a sufficient magnitude to prescribe transcutaneous nerve stimulation. The long-term use of back braces may be counterproductive as it may lead to muscle atrophy. By increasing the local circulation, heat pads may reduce the muscle spasm and hence pain experienced at the level of the affected vertebra(e).

10. ***The following exercises are recommended in patients who have sustained vertebral compression fractures:***

    A. Sit-ups.

    B. Free weightlifting, as high a weight as can be safely tolerated.

    C. Weighted backpacks.

    D. All of the above.

    E. None of the above.

    Correct answer: E

    Comments:

    In healthy premenopausal women, physical exercise, especially a combination of resistive and aerobic high-impact exercises such as running and rope jumping, increases the bone mineral density of the lumbar vertebrae and femoral necks, with the greatest increases in BMD being in the bones undergoing the greatest biomechanical loading.[12,13]

    Physical exercise selectively affects some bones more than others. For instance, aerobic and resistive exercises selectively affect the lumbar vertebrae more than the proximal femur. Walking, on the other hand, has no significant effect on the lumbar vertebrae but significantly increases the BMD at the hips.[14] Several exercise programs, including balance training, gait training, strength training, and Tai Chi, have been shown to be effective at reducing the risk of falls and, hence, the risk of fractures.[15–21] It also has been shown that the BMD of patients who have sustained strokes associated with hemiplegia or hemiparesis is lower on the paralyzed or paretic side than the healthy side[22] further emphasizing the exercise/bone density relationship.

Sit-ups are not recommended in patients who have sustained vertebral compression fractures because they increase the mechanical load on the vertebrae and may induce further compression of the osteopenic/osteoporotic vertebra and adjacent vertebrae. Reverse sit-ups, on the other hand, are recommended as they strengthen the paravertebral and abdominal muscles without putting undue stress on the vertebrae.

While performing "reverse sit-ups" the patient lies on a firm surface and uses her arms to sit up. Then, while sitting she crosses her arms on her shoulders and slowly extends her back until she is lying horizontally. When performing reverse sit-ups it is recommended that another person be beside the patient, with one hand under the patient's head, in case the patient's muscles give way and she falls back.

Whereas resistive exercises are recommended as part of the physical exercise program to increase muscle bulk and strength as well as bone mineral density, free weightlifting is not recommended because it may be associated with accidents as may happen should the patient feel dizzy and release the free weights. Feeling dizzy while lifting weights is often due to the patient straining which results in an increased intrathoracic pressure, reduced venous return, reduced stroke volume, reduced cardiac output, and reduced cerebral blood flow with the patient feeling dizzy.

Weight machines are much safer than free weights: while exercising on a weight machine, should the patient feel dizzy, she will just let go of the cord fixed to the weights. This may in fact alert the attendees that this person is having problems with the selected weights and a lighter load may be recommended.

Heavy backpacks and jackets laden with weights are not recommended for most patients with osteoporosis as they increase the pressure on the vertebrae and may induce vertebral compression fractures. Heavy handbags may in addition subject the cervical vertebrae to undue physical stress, which may interfere with the vertebrobasilar and cerebral circulation and worsen the extent and degree of dizziness.

Weight bands that can be attached to the wrists and ankles are convenient ways to undertake resistive and aerobic exercises: the patient wears a band on each ankle and each wrist. In order to reduce the risk of putting too much mechanical strain on the rest of the skeleton and especially the vertebral column, light weights, about half a pound each, are recommended. Patients are also more likely to tolerate the half pound on each limb. Many patients wear them all day long, taking them off only at night. In this manner, with every single step they take, they lift 2 pounds. Given that the average person walks 3000–4000 steps a day, the approximate daily weight lifted by having half a pound strapped to each wrist and each ankle is about 6000–8000 pounds each day, performed without needing to go to a gym. After using them for some time most patients get used to wearing these light weights and enjoy being able to alter the weight lifted according to their circumstances that day.

Given the complexity of various exercise programs and the diverse needs and background of patients with osteoporosis, especially older ones, it is advisable to consult a qualified physical therapist or personal trainer, with a special interest in osteoporosis to develop an exercise program tailored to the individual needs of the interested person. Physical exercise programs and related issues are discussed separately.

Case summary

Analysis of data

Factors predisposing to bone demineralization/osteoporosis in DK's case

- Status postmenopause, no HRT.
- Sedentary lifestyle.
- Caucasian ethnicity.
- Low body weight.

Factors reducing risk of bone demineralization/osteoporosis in DK's case

- Good daily dietary calcium intake.
- No excessive sodium, caffeine intake.
- No cigarette smoking.
- Negative family history of osteoporosis/fractures.

Factors increasing risk of falls/fractures

- Kyphosis, vertebral compression fracture.
- Sedentary lifestyle.

Factors reducing risk of falls/fractures

- None.

Diagnosis

- Osteoporosis, morphometric vertebral compression fracture.

Management

Treatment(s)

- Antiresorptive or osteoanabolic medication.

Diagnostic test(s)

- Ensure that causes of localized bone demineralization have been excluded.

Lifestyle changes

- None recommended.

Rehabilitation

- Physical exercises: combination of aerobic and resistive exercises.

Key points

- Morphometric vertebral compression fractures are clinically silent.
- Morphometric vertebral fractures have the same implications as clinical vertebral fractures: they are diagnostic of osteoporosis, are associated with increased mortality and morbidity risks, and an increased risk of subsequent fractures.
- Once localized causes of bone demineralization have been ruled out, the patient should be treated for osteoporosis.
- Vertebral augmentation procedures are not indicated in morphometric vertebral compression fractures.

References

1. Fang J, Franconeri A, Boos J, et al. Opportunistic bone density measurement on abdomen and pelvis computed tomography to predict fracture risk in women aged 50 to 64 years without osteoporosis risk factors. *J Comput Assist Tomogr*. 2018;42(5):798–806.
2. Lindsay R, Silverman SL, Cooper C, et al. Risk of new vertebral fracture in the year following a fracture. *JAMA*. 2001;285(3):320–323. https://doi.org/10.1001/jama.285.3.320.
3. Klotzbuecher CM, Ross PD, Landsman PB, Abbott 3rd TA, Berger M. Patients with prior fractures have an increased risk of future fractures: a summary of the literature and statistical synthesis. *J Bone Miner Res*. 2000;15(4):721–739. https://doi.org/10.1359/jbmr.2000.15.4.721.
4. Camacho PM, Petak SM, Binkley N, et al. American Association of Clinical Endocrinologists, American College of Endocrinology Clinical Practice Guidelines for the diagnosis and treatment of postmenopausal women – 2020 update. *Endocr Pract*. 2020;26(Suppl. 1):1–46.
5. Michalski AS, Besler BA, Burt LA, Boyd SK. Opportunistic CT screening predicts individuals at risk of major osteoporotic fracture. *Osteoporos Int*. 2021;32(8):1639–1649. https://doi.org/10.1007/s00198-021-05863-0.
6. Stein E, Shane E. Secondary osteoporosis. *Endocrinol Metab Clin North Am*. 2003;32(1):115–vii. https://doi.org/10.1016/s0889-8529(02)00062-2.
7. Haffner MR, Delman CM, Wick JB, et al. Osteoporosis is undertreated after low-energy vertebral compression fractures. *J Am Acad Orthop Surg*. 2021;29(17):741–747. https://doi.org/10.5435/JAAOS-D-20-01132.
8. Lems WF, Paccou J, Zhang J, et al. Vertebral fracture: epidemiology, impact and use of DXA vertebral fracture assessment in fracture liaison services. *Osteoporos Int*. 2021;32(3):399–411. https://doi.org/10.1007/s00198-020-05804-3.
9. Che H, Breuil V, Cortet B, et al. Vertebral fractures cascade: potential causes and risk factors. *Osteoporos Int*. 2019;30(3):555–563. https://doi.org/10.1007/s00198-018-4793-1.
10. Rossouw JE, Anderson GL, Prentice RL, et al. Risks and benefits of estrogen plus progestin in healthy postmenopausal women: principal results from the Women's Health Initiative randomized controlled trial. *JAMA*. 2002;288(3):321–333. https://doi.org/10.1001/jama.288.3.321.
11. Anderson GL, Limacher M, Assaf AR, et al. Effects of conjugated equine estrogen in postmenopausal women with hysterectomy: the Women's Health Initiative randomized controlled trial. *JAMA*. 2004;291(14):1701–1712. https://doi.org/10.1001/jama.291.14.1701.
12. Martyn-St James M, Carroll S. Effects of different impact exercise modalities on bone mineral density in premenopausal women: a meta-analysis. *J Bone Miner Metab*. 2010;28(3):251–267.

13. Babatunde OO, Forsyth JJ, Gidlow CJ. A meta-analysis of brief high-impact exercises for enhancing bone health in premenopausal women. *Osteoporos Int*. 2012;23(1):109–119.
14. Howe TE, Shea B, Dawson LJ, et al. Exercise for preventing and treating osteoporosis in postmenopausal women. *Cochrane Database Syst Rev*. 2011;7:CD000333. Published 2011 July 6 https://doi.org/10.1002/14651858.CD000333.pub2.
15. American College of Sports Medicine, Chodzko-Zajko WJ, Proctor DN, et al. American College of Sports Medicine position stand. Exercise and physical activity for older adults. *Med Sci Sports Exerc*. 2009;41(7):1510–1530.
16. Gillespie LD, Robertson MC, Gillespie WJ, et al. Interventions for preventing falls in older people living in the community. *Cochrane Database Syst Rev*. 2012;2012(9):CD007146. Published 2012 September 2012 https://doi.org/10.1002/14651858.CD007146.pub3.
17. Chang JT, Morton SC, Rubenstein LZ, et al. Interventions for the prevention of falls in older adults: systematic review and meta-analysis of randomised clinical trials. *BMJ*. 2004;328(7441):680. https://doi.org/10.1136/bmj.328.7441.680.
18. Tinetti ME, Kumar C. The patient who falls: "It's always a trade-off". *JAMA*. 2010;303(3):258–266. https://doi.org/10.1001/jama.2009.2024.
19. Body JJ, Bergmann P, Boonen S, et al. Non-pharmacological management of osteoporosis: a consensus of the Belgian Bone Club. *Osteoporos Int*. 2011;22(11):2769–2788. https://doi.org/10.1007/s00198-011-1545-x.
20. Smulders E, Weerdesteyn V, Groen BE, et al. Efficacy of a short multidisciplinary fall's prevention program for elderly persons with osteoporosis and a fall history: a randomized controlled trial. *Arch Phys Med Rehabil*. 2010;91(11):1705–1711.
21. Madureira MM, Takayama L, Gallinaro AL, Caparbo VF, Costa RA, Pereira RM. Balance training program is highly effective in improving functional status and reducing the risk of falls in elderly women with osteoporosis: a randomized controlled trial. *Osteoporos Int*. 2007;18(4):419–425.
22. Hamdy RC, Moore SW, Cancellaro VA, Harvill LM. Long-term effects of strokes on bone mass. *Am J Phys Med Rehabil*. 1995;74(5):351–356.

CHAPTER 5

Densitometric diagnosis: DXA scans☆

Learning objectives

- The basic principles of bone densitometry.
- The densitometric diagnostic criteria of osteoporosis and osteopenia.
- Osteoporosis is asymptomatic until a fracture occurs.

The case study

Reason for seeking medical help

- DI, 68-year-old, is asymptomatic and enjoys good health. Given her age, she is referred for a DXA scan to screen her for osteoporosis.

Past medical and surgical history

- No relevant past medical history, no history of fractures, falls, or renal calculi.
- Natural menopause at age 47 years, no hormonal replacement therapy.
- Menarche at age 12 years, regular menstrual periods.
- Four children aged 39, 37, 32, and 30 years, all in good health.

Lifestyle

- Sedentary lifestyle.
- Plays golf at least three times a week.
- Good dietary daily calcium intake: about 1200 mg daily.
- No cigarette smoking, no alcohol intake, no excessive caffeine, no excessive sodium intake.
- Good appetite, well-balanced diet.

☆ DI, asymptomatic, 68-year-old Caucasian woman.

Diagnosis and Treatment of Osteoporosis. https://doi.org/10.1016/B978-0-323-99550-4.00002-2
Copyright © 2024 Elsevier Inc. All rights are reserved, including those for text and data mining, AI training, and similar technologies.

Medications

- Multivitamin tablet daily.

Family history

- Negative for osteoporosis.

Clinical examination

- Weight: 133 pounds, height: 64″, no height loss.
- No significant clinical findings.

Laboratory result(s)

- She recently had the following laboratory tests done as part of her annual clinical examination: comprehensive metabolic panel (CMP), complete blood count (CBC), serum vitamin D, and thyroid stimulating hormone (TSH): all within normal limits.

DXA and radiological result(s)

T-scores: lumbar vertebrae (L1-L4): −2.6, right femoral neck −2.2, right total hip −1.9.

Multiple choice questions

1. ***The diagnosis of osteoporosis can be established by:***
   A. The presence of a fragility fracture.
   B. Bone densitometry: dual X-ray absorptiometry.
   C. Laboratory tests.
   D. A or B.
   E. A, B, or C.
   Correct answer: D
   Comment:
   Osteoporosis is a silent disease until a fracture is sustained. Patients have no warning symptoms and are usually unaware of having osteoporosis until a fragility fracture occurs. This is often the first manifestation of osteoporosis and is diagnostic of osteoporosis.

   A fragility fracture is defined as a fracture occurring after a fall from the standing position or from a height not exceeding body height. Fragility fractures also can be the result of trauma that ordinarily would not be expected to lead to a fracture and are referred to as low trauma, low impact, or low energy fractures. They also can occur spontaneously in the absence of any trauma and are known as atraumatic fractures. In the absence of underlying localized bone pathologies such as neoplastic deposits that may lead to fractures, fragility fractures are diagnostic of osteoporosis regardless of the bone densitometry results.

The diagnosis of osteoporosis also can be established by bone densitometry. During this procedure the bone scanned is exposed to two different X-ray wavelengths, hence the name Dual X-ray Absorptiometry (DXA) or Dual Energy X-ray Absorptiometry (DEXA). The International Society for Clinical Densitometry (ISCD) recommends that the term "DXA" be used. The two waves of X-rays are attenuated to different extents by soft and bone tissue, thus allowing the differentiation of soft from bone tissue and the calculation of the bone mineral content (BMC) and surface area of the bone scanned. The BMC is then divided by the bone surface area to calculate the bone mineral density (BMD).

The patient's BMD is then compared to the mean BMD of an adult healthy reference population. The number of standard deviations the patient's BMD is compared to that of the reference population is expressed as the T-score which is then used to classify subjects according to the World Health Organization guidelines[1] (Fig. 1) into three categories: osteoporosis (T-score −2.5 or lower), osteopenia (T-score less than −1.0, but higher than −2.5), or normal BMD (T-score −1.0 or higher).[1] The patient's BMD may also be compared to that of an age-matched population and the results expressed as Z-scores (Fig. 2).

The densitometric diagnosis is based on the lowest T-score of the femoral neck, total hip, upper 4 lumbar vertebrae (antero-posterior projection only, not lateral), or distal one-third radius of the nondominant arm. Although several sites are considered when the hip is scanned, only the BMD and T-scores of the femoral neck and total hip are considered.[2–6] Similarly, although the BMD and T-scores of various sites of the distal radius are routinely calculated and listed on the computer-generated report, only the one-third (or 33%) distal radius site of the nondominant arm should be considered for diagnostic purposes (Fig. 3).[2–6]

The minimum recommended is to scan one hip and the lumbar vertebrae. There is no consensus as to which hip should be scanned: this is often determined by the physical location of the densitometry table in the scanning room. Many centers, however, routinely scan both hips and the lumbar vertebrae and modern densitometers offer the possibility of scanning both hips simultaneously without having to reposition the patient. There is also

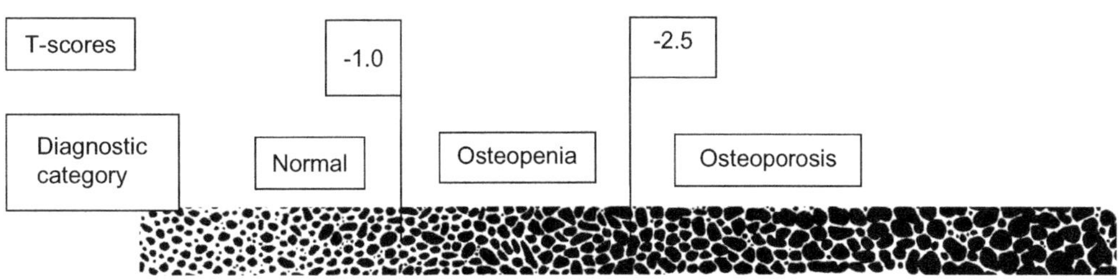

Fig. 1
T-scores and diagnostic classification (MCQ #1).

- $$\text{Bone Mineral Density} = \frac{\text{Bone Mineral Content}}{\text{Surface area of bone scanned}}$$

- $$\text{T-score} = \frac{\text{Patient's BMD} - \text{mean BMD of young healthy reference population}}{\text{Standard deviation of the mean BMD of young healthy reference population}}$$

- $$\text{Z-score} = \frac{\text{Patient's BMD} - \text{mean BMD of age-matched healthy reference population}}{\text{Standard deviation of the mean BMD of age-matched healthy reference population}}$$

Which Reference Population to use when calculating the T-scores:

- International Osteoporosis Foundation recommends using a female Caucasian reference population for both genders.
- National Osteoporosis Foundation (USA) recommends using a male reference population for men and a female reference population for women.
- International Society for Clinical Densitometry recommends using a female Caucasian reference population for both genders but leaves it to the discretion of each Center/Clinician to decide which reference population to use.

Fig. 2
Calculating BMD, T- and *Z*-scores.

evidence to show that when both hips are scanned more patients with osteoporosis will be identified (Fig. 4).[7]

Another advantage of scanning both hips is that it allows monitoring the patient's BMD even after a hip fracture is sustained or the patient undergoes hip replacement surgery. In some centers the Vertebral Fracture Assessment (VFA) is also routinely done. VFA is further discussed in another case.

As long bones are not perfect cylinders and as the BMD is an aerial, not volumetric density calculated by dividing bone mineral content by bone surface area, any change in the bone surface area may affect the results. It is therefore important to ensure that patients having a DXA scan done be positioned exactly according to universal guidelines to ensure meaningful comparison to the reference population and calculation of the T-scores (Fig. 5).

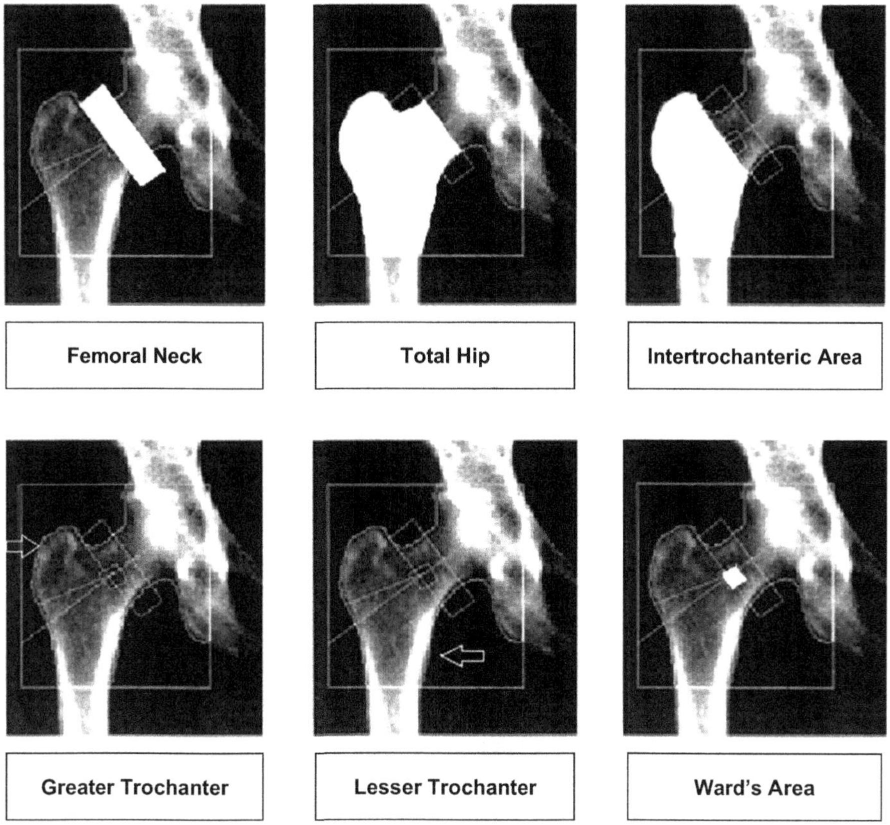

Fig. 3
Anatomical Sites Scanned—Proximal Femur.

Therefore, before accepting the scan results, it is important for the clinicians to review the pictorial scans to ensure the patient has been properly positioned, the regions of interest correctly identified, and the absence of artifacts. The anatomical sites scanned, criteria of well-positioned patients, and some common errors in positioning and analyzing the scans are shown in the accompanying figures.

Given the poor prognosis after a fragility fracture is sustained and given the availability of relatively safe medications that can significantly reduce the risk of fractures, including hip fractures, the challenge is to identify patients at risk of sustaining fractures before these fractures occur. This is particularly relevant as the morbidity and mortality associated with osteoporotic hip fractures are significant: one-year mortality is increased

For diagnostic purposes, the lowest T-score of the femoral neck or total hip areas should be considered, in addition to the upper 4 lumbar vertebrae or distal one-third radius.

- No artifacts.
- Long axis of femur perpendicular to base of box outlining Region of Interest.
- Soft tissue visible lateral to the femur.
- Lesser trochanter is just visible.
- Femoral neck box is positioned according to manufacturer's specifications:
- GE/Lunar: hip axis mid-point
- Hologic: adjacent to greater trochanter

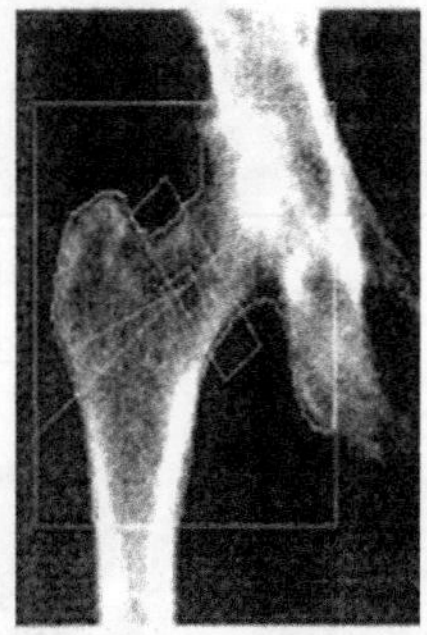

Fig. 4
Characteristics of a well-positioned DXA scan of the proximal femur.

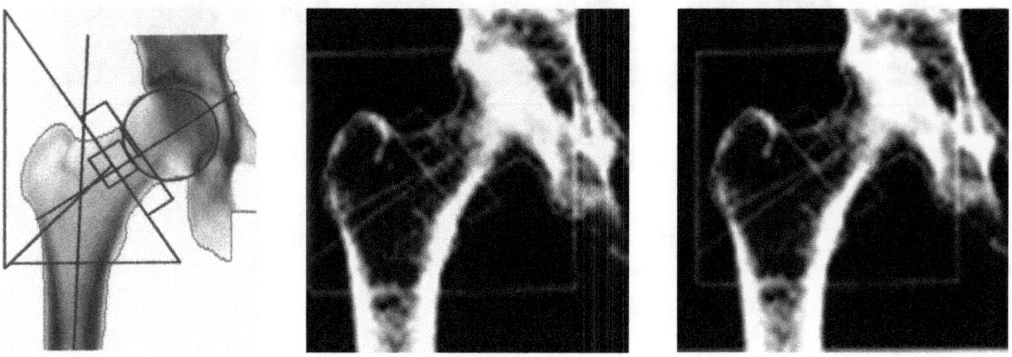

GE Lunar

Fig. 5
Placement of femoral neck box: GE Lunar densitometers place it on the midpoint of the hip axis. Hologic densitometers anchor it to the greater trochanter.

by 8% to 36%, with the rate being higher in men than in women,[8] about 20% of the survivors require long-term institutional care and only about 40% are able to resume their prefracture level of independence.[9] After a fracture is sustained the risk of subsequent fractures is increased by about 2.5-fold, thus triggering a vicious cycle.[10] The health-related quality of life in men with osteoporosis is significantly impaired after sustaining an osteoporotic fracture.[11]

BMD is an important factor, probably the single most important factor, determining fracture risk, but it is not the only one and many other factors modulate the BMD/fracture relationship. Indeed, many patients with a densitometric diagnosis of osteoporosis do not sustain fractures and many patients with osteopenia or even normal BMD sustain fractures, including fragility fractures.[12,13] It has therefore been suggested that the diagnosis of osteoporosis in addition could be made on clinical grounds based on an elevated fracture risk.[14] Notwithstanding, assessing fracture risk should be an integral part of the diagnostic process of osteoporosis as it may be used to develop a management strategy tailored to the circumstances of individual patients and convince patients and attendants of the gravity of fractures. This is further discussed in other cases in this series.

There are no laboratory tests to diagnose osteoporosis. They are used to identify secondary causes of osteoporosis. Markers of bone turnover are sometimes used for diagnostic purposes and to monitor the patient's response to treatment. Laboratory tests are discussed in another case in this series.

2. ***The T-score, not BMD, is used to diagnose osteoporosis because of different densitometers:***
   A. Use different technologies to produce the 2 waves of X-rays.
   B. Use different algorithms to differentiate soft from bone tissue.
   C. Use different anatomical sites.
   D. A and B.
   E. A, B, and C.

   Correct answer: E

   Comment:

   The absolute BMD is different when measured by different densitometers because of all the previously listed reasons. Whereas Hologic densitometers consider the area immediately adjacent to the greater trochanter as being the femoral neck, GE Lunar densitometers consider the femoral neck area at the midpoint of the hip axis. The femoral neck BMD, therefore, is often different when the patient is scanned with GE Lunar or Hologic densitometer (Fig. 6). Therefore the "T-score" rather than the absolute BMD is used to assess the patient's bone status.

   Although it may appear more rational to compare the patient's BMD to that of an age-matched population, the patient's BMD is compared to a reference population in whom the risk of fracture is low, i.e., an adult healthy population, hence the use of the T-score.

   In the USA, the National Osteoporosis Foundation recommends that the young healthy reference population used to derive the T-scores be gender specific, i.e., in men T-scores be calculated based on a male reference population and in women the T-scores be derived from a female reference population.[2] On the other hand, the International Osteoporosis

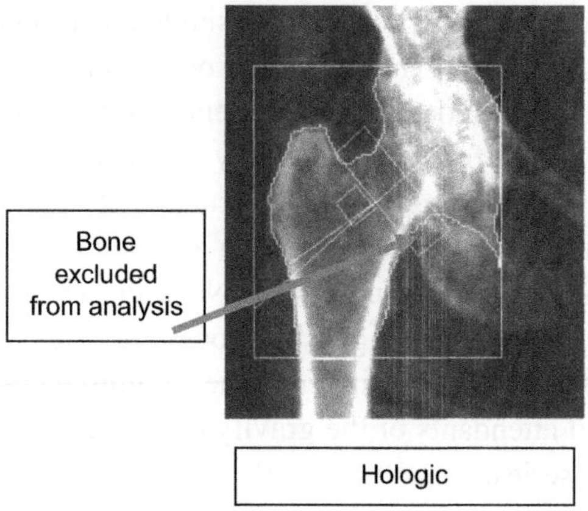

Fig. 6
Software is available to ensure femoral neck box only contains femoral neck and no part of neighboring bones.

Foundation (IOF)[15] recommends using a female Caucasian population for both genders and all races. The International Society for Clinical Densitometry (ISCD)[3] also recommends using a female Caucasian reference population but leaves it to the discretion of individual centers to determine which reference population to use for men.[3]

T-scores are also used in several permutations to estimate fracture risk. This is further discussed in another case in this series. T-scores should not be used to monitor the patient's progress; this is best done by monitoring changes in BMD.

Z-scores represent the number of standard deviations the patient's BMD is compared to an age and gender-matched healthy reference population. Depending on the manufacturers of the bone densitometer, the reference population also may be matched to the subject's ethnic group. *Z*-scores are used in children, adolescents, premenopausal women, and men under the age of 50 years who are then classified as having a "low bone mass for given age" if the *Z*-score is 2 or more standard deviations below that of the reference population or "normal bone mass for given age" if the *Z*-score is less than 2 or more standard deviations below the mean of the reference population. In the absence of fragility fracture(s), the term "osteoporosis" is not recommended in these populations.[2,3]

Some clinicians use Z-scores in postmenopausal women and men over the age of 50 years to determine the extent of workup to identify secondary causes of osteoporosis. A level of −2.0 is sometimes used as a rough guide, but this figure has not been satisfactorily substantiated (Figs. 7–13).

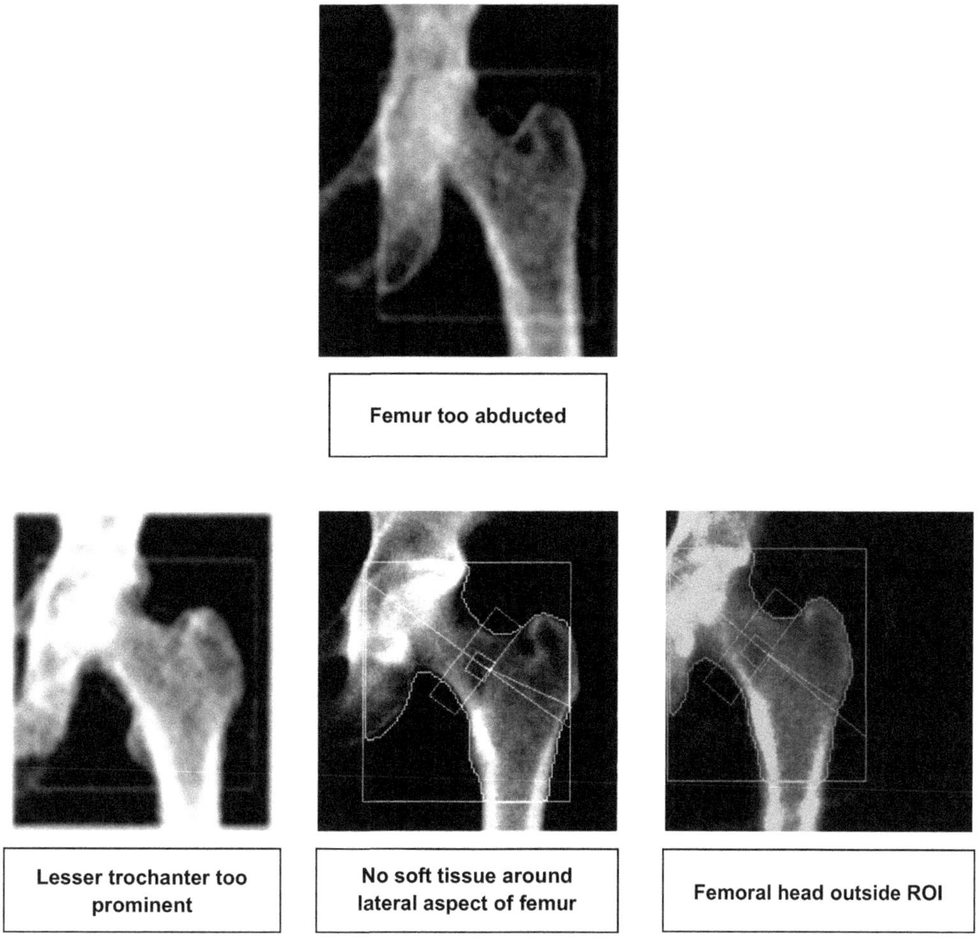

Fig. 7
Some common errors in positioning/analysis of hip scan.

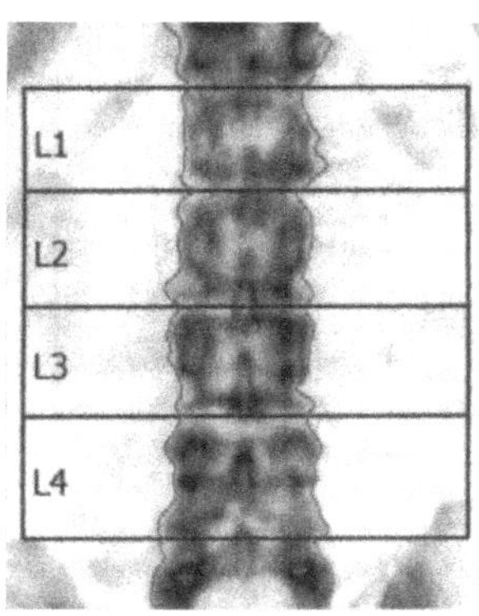

- No artifacts.
- Vertebrae centrally positioned, with equal amount of soft tissue on either side.
- Lower ribs visible.
- Pelvic bones visible.
- Intervertebral discs correctly positioned.
- Half of T12 and of L5 visible.
- Vertebrae correctly identified:
    - L5: appears as block "I" on its side same level as pelvic bone
    - L4: "X" or "H" shaped; L1-3: "U" or "Y" shaped

Fig. 8
Characteristics of a well-positioned DXA scan of the lumbar vertebrae.

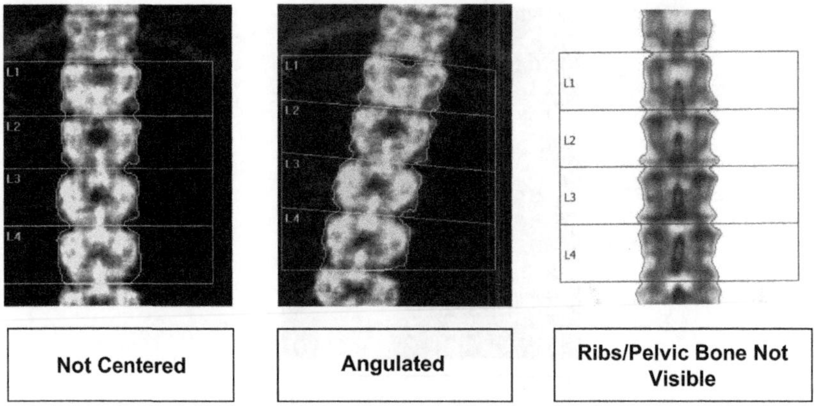

Fig. 9
Some common errors in positioning/analysis of lumbar vertebrae scan: Scan started too low.

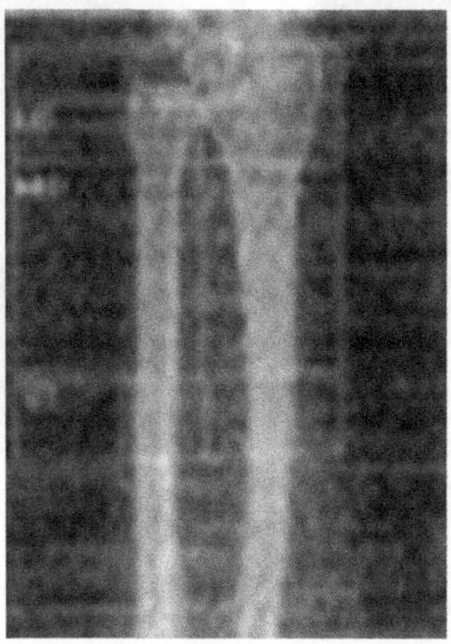

- No Artifacts.
- Radius and ulna parallel, centered, and perpendicular to horizontal line of Region of Interest.
- One row of carpal bone is visible.
- Dense cortical bone in the distal radius is excluded from the ROI

For diagnostic purposes, only the 1/3 (also known as 33%) distal non-dominant radius should be considered.

Fig. 10
Characteristics of a well-positioned DXA scan of the distal radius.

3. ***Match the following T-scores with the diagnostic category:***
   (a) Normal BMD.
   (b) Osteopenia.
   (c) Osteoporosis.
   (d) Severe osteopenia.
   (e) Established osteoporosis.

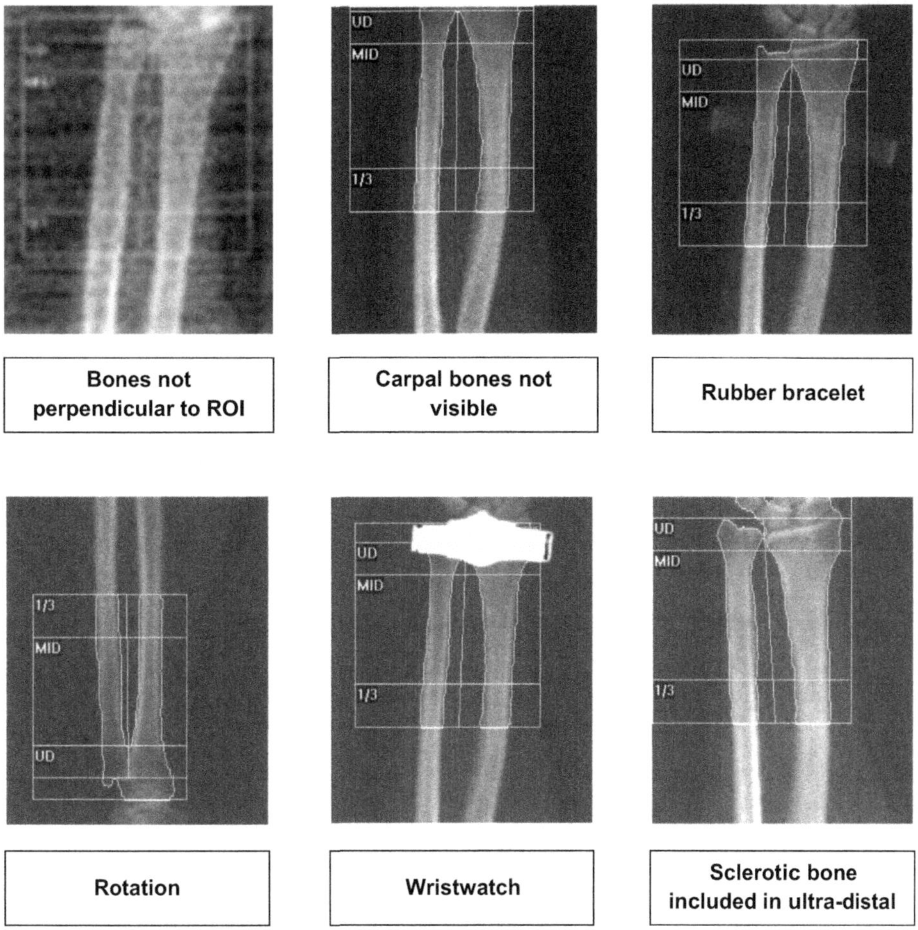

Fig. 11
Some common errors in positioning/analysis of distal forearm scan.

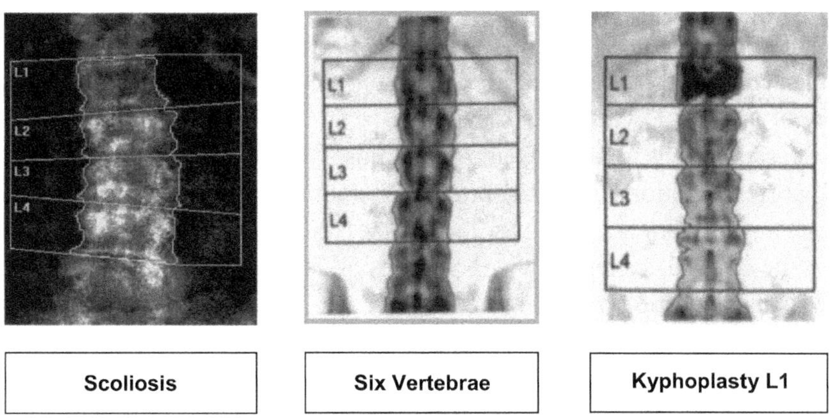

Fig. 12
Select conditions interfering with analysis of lumbar vertebrae scan.

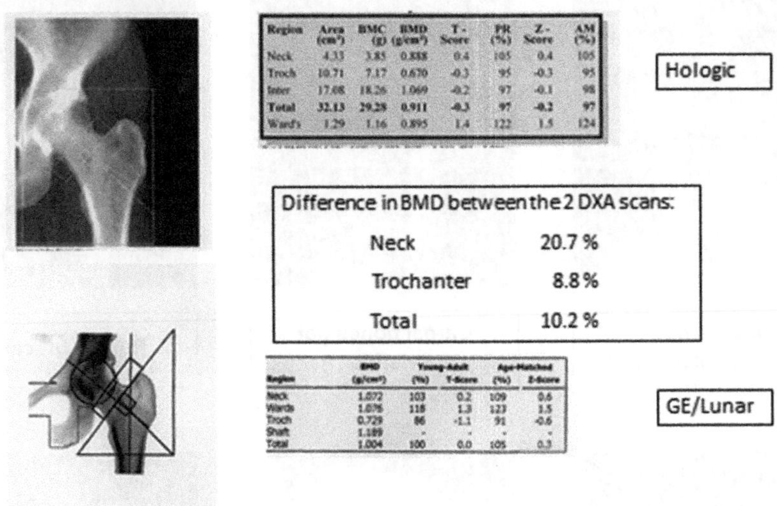

Fig. 13

Different densitometers yield different BMDs. Same patient scanned within minutes on both Lunar and Hologic densitometers.

A. −1.3
B. −3.8
C. −2.4
D. −2.6
E. −0.6

Correct answers: A (b); B (c); C (b); D (c); E (a)

Comment:

According to the WHO guidelines, the patient has a normal BMD if the T-score is −1.0 or higher; osteoporosis if the T-score is −2.5 and lower; and osteopenia if the T-score is less than −1.0, but higher than −2.5 (Fig. 1). There is no "severe osteopenia" category. "Established" osteoporosis refers to the presence of a fragility fracture in addition to a T-score of −2.5 or lower.[1,6]

The T-score levels used for diagnostic purposes are only applicable to those derived by dual energy absorptiometry of the proximal femur (only femoral neck and total hip regions), lumbar vertebrae (at least 2 vertebrae), or distal radius (nondominant one-third or 33% site only). T-scores of other bone sites or derived from other technologies cannot be used for diagnostic purposes.[2,3]

4. ***DI's final densitometric diagnosis is:***
   A. Osteoporosis.
   B. Osteoporosis of the lumbar vertebrae.
   C. Osteopenia of the right femoral neck.
   D. Normal bone density of right total hip.
   E. B, C, and D.

   Correct answer: A

   Comment:

   Only one densitometric diagnosis should be made based on the lowest T-score of the femoral neck, total hip, lumbar vertebrae, or distal one-third radius.[3–6] In DI's case, the lowest T-score is −2.6 in the upper 4 lumbar vertebrae. The final densitometric diagnosis therefore is "osteoporosis."

   When the lumbar vertebrae are considered for the diagnosis of osteoporosis, it should be based on only the AP view (not the lateral view) and at least 2 lumbar vertebrae must be evaluable. The International Society for Clinical Densitometry specifically recommends against basing the diagnosis on the T-score of just one vertebra, sometimes referred as "cherry picking." Ideally the upper 4 lumbar vertebrae should be taken into consideration, but this is not always possible as a number of artifacts may interfere with the accuracy of the measurements.[3–6] Vertebrae that cannot be evaluated should be excluded from the analysis and interpretation. As the printout of most densitometers includes various combinations of the lumbar vertebrae, it should be easy to exclude uninterpretable vertebrae. If this is not possible, the T-score of the remaining evaluable vertebrae should be calculated (Fig. 2), provided there are at least two evaluable vertebrae.

5. ***In dual energy X-ray absorptiometry, the following is/are true concerning the anatomical sites scanned:***
   A. The "total hip" site refers to the area of the femur outlined by the region of interest (ROI) box.
   B. The "total hip" site refers to the area of the femur between the distal part of femoral neck box and the pelvic bone.
   C. The "total hip" site refers to the area of the femur between the proximal part of the femoral neck box and the lower part of the ROI.
   D. "Ward's area" refers to the anatomical area in the femoral neck between the cortical trabeculae.
   E. C and D.

   Correct answer: C

   Comment:

   In dual energy X-ray absorptiometry, the "total hip" area is the area of the femur between the proximal part of the femoral neck box and the lower part of the Region of Interest box

(Fig. 3).[6] It includes neither the hip joint, nor the femoral head, nor the proximal part of the anatomical femoral neck and therefore as such is a misnomer.

"Ward's area" refers to the least mineralized part of the proximal femur. It does not refer to the anatomical Ward's triangle which is the area of the femoral neck outlined by the trabeculae in the lateral cortex and the superior and inferior trabeculae of the femoral neck. As such, therefore, Ward's area also is a misnomer. Given its size and its reproducibility, it is neither used for diagnostic nor monitoring purposes.

Before interpreting the results, it is important to ensure that the patient's position during the scans is satisfactory and that the scans are technically good. Figures at the end of this chapter demonstrate characteristics of good scans of the proximal femur, lumbar vertebrae, and distal radius. If the femoral neck box cannot be placed adequately without including some part of the ischium, software is available to exclude this part of the skeleton from the femoral neck box. Some common errors in positioning and analyzing DXA scans of the proximal femur, lumbar vertebrae, and distal radius are shown in figures at the end of this case study.

The "femoral neck" area is the rectangular area outlined by the femoral neck box. Its exact position differs according to the densitometer used: Hologic densitometers "anchor" the femoral neck box to the greater trochanter, while GE/Lunar densitometers place the femoral neck box at the midpoint of the hip axis. The intertrochanteric area is the area between the greater and lesser trochanter excluding the femoral neck.

In addition to the lumbar vertebrae and distal radius, only the total hip and femoral neck areas should be considered for diagnostic purposes. The total hip and the trochanteric area are also often used for monitoring purposes because of their trabecular bone content which, given its vascularity, responds quicker to medications or disease evolution than cortical bone which is much less vascular.

6. ***In bone densitometry, "Accuracy" refers to:***
   A. The skills of the DXA technologist at positioning patients according to guidelines.
   B. The performance of the densitometer: its ability to accurately calculate BMD.
   C. A quality assurance test that should be done daily before scans are done.
   D. A and C.
   E. B and C.

   Correct answer: E

   Comment:

   The accuracy of a densitometer reflects its ability to correctly measure the mineral content (BMC) and surface area of the bone scanned.[6] The accuracy of each densitometer should be assessed on a phantom every day the densitometer is used, and the results of these accuracy tests should be kept in a logbook. Most densitometers have a built-in mechanism to prevent scans from being done unless the accuracy of the densitometer has been checked that day and that it is within certain specified parameters. This is to ensure that any drift in calibration is detected in a timely manner, thus allowing the manufacturers to take appropriate remedial actions.

7. ***In bone densitometry "Precision and Least Significant Change":***
   A. Are no longer relevant with most modern densitometers.
   B. Are usually done only when results of DXA scans are part of a research program.
   C. Are determined by the make and model of the densitometer used.
   D. A, B, and C.
   E. None of the above.

Correct answer: E

Comment:

Unlike "accuracy" which is largely dependent on the densitometer, "precision" and "Least Significant Change (LSC)" are largely determined by the skills of the DXA technologist at positioning patients to be scanned exactly according to established guidelines.[6] Precision studies are conducted by positioning the patient on the densitometer table, scanning her, then asking her to get off the table, then back on the table, repositioning her, and scanning her again. It can be done by scanning 30 patients twice or 15 patients three times each.[3] It is important to make sure the patient gets off the table in between scans because the main purpose of the precision study is to determine the DXA technologist's ability to reposition the patient in exactly the same position.

The precision of the technologist can be calculated manually according to available formulae[6] or by inputting results of the scans in a spreadsheet available on the ISCD website and following the instructions: www.ISCD.org. If two or more technologists perform DXA scans, the precision of each technologist should be calculated and then the precision of all technologists in the center calculated.[3] This also gives an opportunity to identify technologists whose performance needs improvement. According to ISCD, the minimum acceptable precision is 1.9% (LSC 5.3%) for the lumbar vertebrae, 1.8% (LSC 5.0%) for the total hip, and 2.5% (LSC 6.9%) for the femoral neck.[3] Without knowing the precision and LSC of the center where the scans are done it is not possible to determine whether an observed change is significant or not. For instance, an increase in BMD of say 0.123 is only relevant if the LSC where the DXA scan is done is less than 0.123 but is not significant if the center's precision exceeds this value.

Calculating the center's precision and LSC is therefore neither a "study" nor a "research project," but it is essential for the proper interpretation of serial DXA scans and should be done on a regular basis.[3,6,16] Calculating precision is also recommended whenever there is a change of equipment. Many also suggest repeating the precision and LSC at least at 2-year intervals and whenever there is a change of technologist(s) after giving enough time to adjust to the new environment. Although "precision studies" are not research, informed consent should be obtained from potential subjects, and it is prudent to consult with appropriate Institutional Review Body, Research and Development committee, or other relevant committees.

Many centers identify the first patient on a particular day of the week to have the precision and LSC calculated on a specific bone site if the patient agrees to have a part of her skeleton scanned twice and signs an informed consent form. In this manner precision and LSC are calculated on an ongoing regular basis, and technologists are offered the opportunity to evaluate their skills on an ongoing manner.

There are no phantoms available for precision and LSC calculation, and it is important to ensure that subjects participating in these calculations are similar to the ones scanned in the center.[16] For instance, if most of the patients referred to a center are over the age of say 70 years, it is not appropriate to scan subjects in their thirties to calculate precision and LSC.

8. ***In bone densitometry, cross-calibration:***
   A. Should be done whenever the densitometer is replaced.
   B. Is usually done by the manufacturers.
   C. Is no longer necessary with modern densitometers.
   D. Can be done with available phantom.
   E. A and B.

   Correct answer: A

   Comment:

   Cross-calibration allows for a comparison to be made when patients are scanned on different densitometers. It is done by scanning a series of 30 patients of various age groups and various BMDs once on the "old" densitometer soon to be replaced and on the "new" densitometer.[3] A formula is then developed to "convert" readings of the old densitometer to the new densitometer: www.ISCD.org. Alternatively, the data of both densitometers could be plotted on a graph to convert the BMD as estimated by the old densitometer to readings of the new densitometer.

   There are no phantoms available for cross-calibration.[16] As with precision and LSC calculation, cross-calibration should not be considered "research"[16] but it is prudent to consult with the relevant committee(s) and ensure that informed consent is signed by patients about to be scanned for cross-calibration purposes. If the "old" densitometer is changed without having performed cross-calibration, it is no longer possible to quantify changes in BMD between "old" and "new" densitometers and readings from the new densitometer are then considered as the new baseline.[3] When only hardware, but not the entire system is changed, cross-calibration on 10 patients is sufficient.[3] For more details, the reader is referred to the 2013 ISCD Position Development Conference[3] or the ISCD website.

9. ***The following technologies can be used instead of DXA scans to diagnose osteoporosis:***
   A. Digital X-ray Radiogrammetry (DXR).
   B. Quantitative Ultra-sound (QUS).
   C. Peripheral DXA phalanges (pDXA).
   D. All of the above.
   E. None of the above.

   Correct answer: E

Comment:

None of the three listed techniques can be used to diagnose osteoporosis. Similarly, although a good correlation exists between the results of these techniques and fracture risk, including hip fracture risk, the results cannot be extrapolated to estimate the fracture risk using the FRAX permutation. FRAX is discussed further in other case studies in this series.

None of the previously listed techniques therefore can be used to monitor the patient's response to treatment or disease evolution. Even if readings of DXR, QUS, or pDXA are cross-calibrated with those of DXA scans of the lumbar vertebrae, femoral neck, and total hip, very little is known about the changes induced by medications in the metacarpal bones or calcaneus. Not all bones of the skeleton respond in a similar manner to various therapeutic agents. For instance, when bisphosphonates or teriparatide is administered, the BMD of the distal radius as assessed by DXA sometimes decreases while that of the vertebrae and proximal femur increases. In other words, if only the distal radius were measured, it would not be possible to properly assess the patient's response to treatment with bisphosphonates; in fact, it may be tempting to adjudicate the patient as "nonresponsive" or "getting worse" based on the changes in the distal radius. Without knowing what changes to expect in metacarpal bones or calcaneus, the BMD of these bones, as assessed by DXR, QUS, or pDXA, cannot be used to monitor the patient's response to treatment.

Similarly, relatively little is known about false positive, false negative, specificity, sensitivity, positive predictive and negative predictive power of DXR, QUS, and pDXA compared to conventional DXA. This may result in patients being denied treatment when treatment is indicated, and other patients being treated when no such treatment is indicated. Prescribing unnecessary medication exposes patients to potential adverse events and denying treatment when treatment is indicated may lead to fractures that could have been prevented.

The clinical utility of DXR, QUS, and pDXA is therefore limited, although they are used for some epidemiologic studies, and even their use for screening purposes is questionable because of the potential for false negative results. Neither DXR, nor QUS, nor pDXA at present can replace dual energy X-ray absorptiometry for the management of patients with osteoporosis.

10. ***The following is/are true about Quantitative Computed Tomography (QCT):***
   A. Most CT scanners can be used to perform QCT without any modification being necessary.
   B. The WHO classification based on T-scores can be used with QCT.
   C. QCT data can be incorporated in the FRAX permutation.
   D. A and B.
   E. A and C.

Correct answer: C

Comment:

Quantitative computed tomography (QCT) measures the volumetric bone density, as opposed to dual energy X-ray absorptiometry which measures the areal bone density.[17] As such, therefore, QCT is a more accurate method to measure bone density. Also, unlike DXA, QCT differentiates bone mineral content inside the body of a vertebra as opposed to the extra-vertebral calcifications and can differentiate trabecular from cortical bone.[17] QCT is therefore able to detect small changes in BMD before they become obvious by DXA.

Using a calibration phantom and dedicated analysis software CT scanners can be used for QCT.[17] Unlike DXA scans which cannot be performed in obese patients and those with severe degenerative changes, QCT can be performed in these patients.[17]

QCT data can be incorporated in the FRAX permutation to calculate the 10-year probability of sustaining a hip or major osteoporotic fracture. Radiation exposure is much higher with QCT than with DXA which limits its applicability to monitor patients' progress.[17] Other drawbacks of QCT include the cost of the equipment and the expertise needed.[17] On the other hand, QCTs are increasingly being used as opportunistic tools to detect osteoporosis when patients are having QCTs done for other medical reasons.[18]

Case summary

Analysis of data

Factors predisposing to bone demineralization/osteoporosis

- Female gender.
- Caucasian ethnicity.
- Age: 68 years.
- Status postmenopause, no HRT.
- Sedentary lifestyle.

Factors reducing risk of bone demineralization/osteoporosis

- Negative family history for osteoporosis and fragility fractures.
- No relevant past medical history.
- Good daily calcium intake.
- Well-balanced diet.
- No excessive salt or caffeine intake.
    - No cigarette smoking.
    - No alcohol abuse.

Factors increasing risk of falls/fractures

- Sedentary lifestyle.
- Low BMD/T-scores.
- Age: 68 years.

Factors reducing risk of falls/fractures

- No history of falls.
- No history of fractures.

Diagnosis

- Postmenopausal osteoporosis.

Management recommendations

Treatment(s)

- DI has several treatment options available that are discussed in other cases in this series.

Diagnostic test(s)

- No need, they have been done as part of the annual physical evaluation.

Lifestyle

- DI already is leading a healthy lifestyle. In addition, she may be encouraged to undertake regular physical exercise.
- Follow-up depends on the medication selected and the support the patient needs. This is discussed further in other case studies in this series. Notwithstanding, emphasis should be made on the seriousness of the disease and importance of adhering to the prescribed medication.

Key points

- Osteoporosis is silent until a fracture occurs.
- The diagnosis of osteoporosis can be established by bone densitometry: a T-score of −2.5 or lower in the femoral neck, total hip, lumbar vertebrae, or distal one-third radius of the nondominant forearm.
- The World Health Organization diagnostic categories, based on the T-score:
  - Osteoporosis: T-score −2.5 or lower.
  - Osteopenia: T-score higher than −2.5, but lower than −1.0.
  - Normal bone density: T-score −1.0 or higher.
- The WHO classification can be used only for T-scores of the femoral neck, total hip, lumbar vertebrae (AP view, not lateral), and distal one-third radius of the nondominant forearm. If there are discrepancies between various sites, only one diagnosis should be made based on the lowest T-score of these sites.
- Compressed vertebrae or vertebrae that cannot be reliably interpreted because of artifacts should be excluded from the calculation of the T-score, but at least 2 lumbar vertebrae should be evaluable. If no vertebrae, or only one vertebra can be interpreted, then the lumbar scan should be disregarded and the diagnosis based on the T-score of the femoral neck, total hip, or distal one-third radius.

References

1. Camacho PM, Petak SM, Binkley N, et al. American Association of Clinical Endocrinologists, American College of Endoccrinology Clinical Practice Guidelines for the diagnosis and treatment of postmenopausal osteoporosis – 2020 update. *Endocr Pract.* 2020;26(Suppl 1):1–46. https://doi.org/10.4158/GL-2020-0524SUPPL.
2. Cosman F, de Beur SJ, LeBoff MS, et al. Clinician's guide to prevention and treatment of osteoporosis [published correction appears in Osteoporos Int. 2015 July;26(7):2045–7]. *Osteoporos Int.* 2014;25(10): 2359–2381. https://doi.org/10.1007/s00198-014-2794-2.
3. Schousboe JT, Shepherd JA, Bilezikian JP, Baim S. Executive summary of the 2013 International Society for Clinical Densitometry Position Development Conference on bone densitometry. *J Clin Densitom.* 2013;16(4): 455–466. https://doi.org/10.1016/j.jocd.2013.08.004.
4. Hans D, Downs Jr RW, Duboeuf F, et al. Skeletal sites for osteoporosis diagnosis: the 2005 ISCD official positions. *J Clin Densitom.* 2006;9(1):15–21. https://doi.org/10.1016/j.jocd.2006.05.003.
5. Hamdy RC, Petak SM, Lenchik L, International Society for Clinical Densitometry Position Development Panel and Scientific Advisory Committee. Which central dual X-ray absorptiometry skeletal sites and regions of interest should be used to determine the diagnosis of osteoporosis? *J Clin Densitom.* 2002;5(Suppl):S11–S18. https://doi.org/10.1385/jcd:5:3s:s11.
6. Bonnick SL, Miller PD, Bone Densitometry in Clinical Practice. Application and Interpretation. 2nd ed. Humana Press; 2004.
7. Hamdy R, Kiebzak GM, Seier E, Watts NB. The prevalence of significant left-right differences in hip bone mineral density. *Osteoporos Int.* 2006;17(12):1772–1780. https://doi.org/10.1007/s00198-006-0192-0.
8. Abrahamsen B, van Staa T, Ariely R, Olson M, Cooper C. Excess mortality following hip fracture: a systematic epidemiological review. *Osteoporos Int.* 2009;20(10):1633–1650. https://doi.org/10.1007/s00198-009-0920-3.
9. Office of the Surgeon General (US). Bone Health and Osteoporosis: A Report of the Surgeon General. Rockville (MD): Office of the Surgeon General (US); 2004.
10. Colón-Emeric C, Kuchibhatla M, Pieper C, et al. The contribution of hip fracture to risk of subsequent fractures: data from two longitudinal studies. *Osteoporos Int.* 2003;14(11):879–883. https://doi.org/10.1007/s00198-003-1460-x.
11. Hu J, Zheng W, Zhao D, et al. Health-related quality of life in men with osteoporosis: a systematic review and meta-analysis. *Endocrine.* 2021;74(2):270–280. https://doi.org/10.1007/s12020-021-02792-0.
12. Siris ES, Chen YT, Abbott TA, et al. Bone mineral density thresholds for pharmacological intervention to prevent fractures. *Arch Intern Med.* 2004;164(10):1108–1112. https://doi.org/10.1001/archinte.164.10.1108.
13. Sornay-Rendu E, Munoz F, Garnero P, Duboeuf F, Delmas PD. Identification of osteopenic women at high risk of fracture: the OFELY study. *J Bone Miner Res.* 2005;20(10):1813–1819. https://doi.org/10.1359/JBMR.050609.
14. Siris ES, Adler R, Bilezikian J, et al. The clinical diagnosis of osteoporosis: a position statement from the National Bone Health Alliance Working Group. *Osteoporos Int.* 2014;25(5):1439–1443. https://doi.org/10.1007/s00198-014-2655-z.
15. Kanis JA, Adachi JD, Cooper C, et al. Standardizing the descriptive epidemiology of osteoporosis: recommendations from the epidemiology and quality of life working group of IOF. *Osteoporos Int.* 2013;24 (11):2763–2764. https://doi.org/10.1007/s00198-013-2413-7.
16. Federal Guidance Report No. 14 Radiation Protection Guidance for Diagnostic and Interventional X-Ray Procedures. Interagency working group on medical radiation. Washington, D.C. 20460: U.S. Environmental Protection Agency; 1976.
17. Link TM, Lang TF. Axial QCT: clinical applications and new developments. *J Clin Densitom.* 2014;17 (4):438–448. https://doi.org/10.1016/j.jocd.2014.04.119.
18. Pickhardt PJ, Graffy PM, Perez AA, Lubner MG, Elton DC, Summers RM. Opportunistic screening at abdominal CT: use of automated body composition biomarkers for added cardiometabolic value. *Radiographics.* 2021;41(2):524–542. https://doi.org/10.1148/rg.2021200056.

CHAPTER 6

Osteopenia: Individualizing treatment—Part I☆

Learning objective

- The integration of clinical findings, DXA scan results, FRAX scores, and National Osteoporosis Foundation guidelines to individualize the management strategy for patients with densitometric evidence of osteopenia and/or high falls/fracture risks.

The case study

Reasons for seeking medical help

- AC is concerned about having osteoporosis because of her positive family history: both her mother and grandmother had osteoporosis. Her mother has pronounced kyphosis and her grandmother died a few weeks after sustaining a hip fracture.
- AC had a DXA scan done about 2 weeks prior to her present encounter. It showed evidence of osteopenia: lowest T-score in the upper four lumbar vertebrae: −1.8.

Past medical and surgical history

- No relevant medical or surgical history.
- Menarche at age 12 years, regular menstrual periods.
- Menopause at age 50 years, no hormonal replacement therapy.

Lifestyle

- Exercises regularly three times a week: goes to a fitness center and does a combination of aerobic and resistance exercises. Each session lasts about 60 min. In addition, she often plays tennis: at least 1 h, during weekends.

☆ AC, a 52-year-old Caucasian woman, with osteopenia.

Diagnosis and Treatment of Osteoporosis. https://doi.org/10.1016/B978-0-323-99550-4.00009-5
Copyright © 2024 Elsevier Inc. All rights are reserved, including those for text and data mining, AI training, and similar technologies.

- Drinks daily at least two 8-oz glasses of milk and one glass of orange juice fortified with calcium. She also has a cup of yogurt every day and regularly eats dairy products. She has done so for as long as she can remember.
- Does not smoke cigarettes, never did.
- Consumes alcoholic drinks only in moderation, not exceeding 3 drinks a week.
- Drinks neither caffeinated, nor soda drinks.

Family history

Positive for osteoporosis:

- Mother has pronounced kyphosis.
- Grandmother died after sustaining a hip fracture.

Medication(s)

- Multivitamin tablets, 1 daily.

Clinical examination

- Denies any history of falls, near-falls, or dizzy spells.
- Weight: 130 pounds, height 5′5″, arm span 65″.
- No relevant significant clinical findings.

Laboratory result(s)

About 4weeks prior to her visit, she had a number of laboratory tests done as part of her annual physical examination. All results were within the normal limits, including complete blood count (CBC), comprehensive metabolic panel (CMP), serum 25-hydroxy-vitamin D, and thyroid stimulating hormone (TSH).

DXA and radiological results

Region	BMD	T-score
Left femoral neck	**0.695**	−1.3
Left total hip	**0.712**	−1.2
Lumbar vertebrae	**0.645**	−1.8

FRAX scores (10-year probability of sustaining a fracture):

Hip fracture risk: 0.5%
Other major fractures risk: 6.6%

National Osteoporosis Foundation threshold for initiating pharmacologic treatment: ***Not reached***

Vertebral Fracture Assessment: ***Not done***

Has not experienced repeated falls and/or dizzy spells

Multiple choice questions

1. ***In this patient, risk factors for osteoporosis and low bone mass include:***
   A. Female gender, Caucasian ethnicity.
   B. Age: 52 years.
   C. Status postnatural menopause, no hormonal replacement history.
   D. Positive family history for osteoporosis.
   E. All of the above.
   Correct answer: E
   Comments:
   All of the above are risk factors for low bone mass and osteoporosis.
2. ***In this patient's case, the following is/are correct:***
   A. The densitometric diagnosis is osteopenia.
   B. The main goal of management is to maintain and if possible, increase bone mass.
   C. The fall risk should be thoroughly assessed.
   D. She should be prescribed an antiresorptive medication to increase the bone mass.
   E. A and B.
   Correct answer: E
   Comment:
   AC has densitometric evidence of osteopenia: the lowest T-score is less than −1.0, but higher than −2.5. The densitometric difference between osteopenia and osteoporosis is only the extent of mineralization (bone mineral density—BMD), as determined by DXA scans.

   This patient had only one DXA scan done. At this stage, therefore, it is not possible to determine whether her skeleton is undergoing bone demineralization or has never reached her maximum potential bone mass. Notwithstanding, the BMD, at the time of examination, is below the normal range. The bones are therefore more fragile than those of a normal reference population and the patient's fracture risk is therefore increased, although not sufficiently increased to the extent of needing specific pharmacological therapy for osteoporosis.

The patient's 10-year probability of sustaining a fracture (0.5% and 6.6%, for a hip or major fracture, respectively, as determined by the FRAX scores) is well below the threshold recommended by the National Osteoporosis Foundation to initiate pharmacologic treatment (3% for the risk hip fracture and 20% for other major osteoporotic fractures).

Consequently, if this patient were prescribed medication for osteoporosis, the potential harm, in terms of adverse effects, is higher than the expected benefit associated with a reduction in risk of fractures. The goal of managing this patient therefore is to maintain, and possibly increase the bone mass by nonpharmacological means in order to prevent osteoporosis from developing.

There is no need to pursue the risk of falling as the patient has not sustained any falls and has not experienced any near-falls or dizzy spells. She appears to be physically fit and is leading an essentially healthy lifestyle. Common causes of secondary bone loss have been excluded when she had her annual physical examination. At this stage, therefore, there is no need for any further investigation. However, in about 2years' time, she should be evaluated to reassess the state of her bone health and determine whether there has been any bone loss or gain.

3. ***The following investigations are recommended:***
   A. Serum CTx (carboxyterminal collagen cross-links).
   B. Serum P1NP (Procollagen Type I Intact N-terminal Propeptide).
   C. Bone-specific serum alkaline phosphatase isoenzyme.
   D. All of the above.
   E. None of the above.

   Correct answer: E

   Comment:

   C-Tx is a marker of bone resorption. P1NP and bone-specific alkaline phosphatase are markers of bone formation. There is no need, at this stage, for any of the listed laboratory tests. As AC reached the menopause about 2 years ago, she is probably going through the phase of accelerated bone resorption, and therefore if a medication were needed for her bone mass, it would be an antiresorptive medication. If, on the other hand, AC were much older, for instance in her eighties or nineties, she might respond better to an osteoanabolic agent.

4. ***At this stage the following investigations are recommended:***
   A. Blood chemistry profile.
   B. Serum FSH level.
   C. Serum 25-hydroxy-vitamin D level.
   D. All of the above.
   E. None of the above.

   Correct answer: E

Comment:

This patient has few reversible risk factors that may predispose to osteoporosis and has taken appropriate actions to prevent it: good daily calcium/vitamin D intake, regular physical exercise, and no cigarette smoking. She also had a number of blood tests, and no pathology has been identified. Given the degree of osteopenia, the clinical condition, the fracture risk, and the results of the blood tests there is no indication, at this stage, for any further tests to be done.

A follow-up DXA scan and evaluation of bone status is nevertheless recommended in about 2 years' time to monitor her bone status and determine whether she should start on medication to treat osteopenia.

5. ***The following is/are recommended:***
   A. Increase daily calcium intake or recommend calcium supplements.
   B. Recommend vitamin D supplements.
   C. Increase level of physical activity.
   D. A and B.
   E. None of the above.

Correct answer: E

Comments:

AC is already getting an adequate amount of calcium daily through her diet, estimated to be at least 1200 mg (300 mg per 8 oz. of milk or calcium-fortified orange juice) in addition to the dairy products she regularly consumes. There is therefore no need to recommend further increases in the dietary intake or prescribing calcium supplements as this may lead to hypercalciuria and increase the risk of renal calculi.

Her serum vitamin D level is within the normal range (45 ng/mL). There is therefore no need to recommend vitamin D supplements. As she is getting her daily calcium requirements through food, she is, in all probability, also getting enough vitamin D, as evidenced by the normal serum vitamin D level.

She also is already exercising on a regular basis. As far as her bone health is concerned, there is no need to exercise more.

6. ***The following therapeutic measures may be considered:***
   A. Starting hormonal replacement therapy.
   B. Prescribing an antiresorptive medication such as alendronate 35 mg once a week or risedronate 35 mg once a week or 150 mg once a month, ibandronate 150 mg once a month, or zoledronic acid 5 mg once every 2 years.
   C. Changing estrogen to raloxifene 60 mg once a day.
   D. A, B, or C.
   E. None of the above.

Correct answer: E

Comments:

Although all listed alternatives can be useful in this patient, yet, given the degree of osteopenia, the FRAX scores, and the paucity of risk factors for low bone mass and falls, there is no need for any pharmacologic therapy at this stage. The only recommendation is to continue with her healthy lifestyle and repeat the DXA scan in 2 years' time. The management of her bone health will depend on the change in bone mass over this 2-year period.

Given the adverse effect profile of estrogen and estrogen/progesterone, hormonal replacement therapy is no longer recommended for the management of osteoporosis. It is nevertheless still recommended for the prevention of osteoporosis, provided it is given in the smallest possible dose for the shortest period of time.[1]

7. ***The addition of a bisphosphonate to estrogen:***
   A. Induces greater increases in the bone mineral density.
   B. Interferes with the bioavailability of estrogen.
   C. Increases the potential for adverse effects.
   D. Should be avoided as it may oversuppress the rate of bone turnover.
   E. A and C.

Correct answer: E

Comments:

Bisphosphonates do not interfere with the bioavailability of estrogen. Estrogen, in the USA, is approved for the prevention, but not treatment, of postmenopausal osteoporosis. The Women's Health Initiative study, a large double-blind, placebo-controlled study confirmed benefits derived from Estrogen (ET) and Estrogen/Progesterone (EPT) therapy. For instance, when compared to placebo, EPT reduced hip fractures by 36%, clinical vertebral fractures by 36%, and other osteoporotic fractures by 23. Similarly, ET reduced hip fractures by 39% and clinical vertebral fractures by 38%.[2,3]

These trials also confirmed the potential adverse effects of estrogen and progesterone, including thromboembolic disorders, strokes, dementia, endometrial and breast neoplasia. It is, however, possible that in the Women's Health Initiative study, at least some of these adverse effects were due to the time lag between menopause (i.e., cessation of estrogen production by the ovaries) and initiation of ET and ERT. It has been suggested that if estrogen were administered soon after the onset of the menopause, these adverse effects may have been minimized or prevented.

8. ***A repeat DXA scan is recommended in:***
   A. One year.
   B. Two years.
   C. Five years.
   D. When she becomes 65 years old.
   E. There is no need to repeat the DXA scan.

Correct answer: B

Comment:

One year is too short a period to note any significant change in the BMD as assessed by DXA, especially as the absolute values are so close to the normal range. Five years is too long as her bones may become more demineralized. Two years is a reasonable time. If at that time the BMD has increased, then there will be no need for any pharmacologic agent to be prescribed. If there has been a decrease in bone mass/density, attempts should be made to identify causes of secondary osteoporosis, and if none is identified, specific medication for osteoporosis may be considered. If the bone mass has remained the same, the patient should be encouraged to maintain her lifestyle and another DXA scan will be offered 2 years later.

9. ***The following imaging techniques can be used to follow-up patients treated for osteopenia:***

   A. CT scans.

   B. MRI.

   C. Ultrasound.

   D. Plain X-rays.

   E. None of the above.

   Correct answer: E

   Comments:

   The follow-up imaging of patients treated for osteopenia should be preferably done on the same densitometer, and the precision and accuracy of the DXA scan should be known to ensure that the precision and accuracy of the baseline and follow-up scans are comparable. The least significant change should also be known for the center where scan is done and the technologist performing the scan. These are further discussed in other sections.

10. ***The following may be useful additions to consider:***

   A. Testosterone.

   B. Calcitonin.

   C. Teriparatide (Forteo) or abaloparatide (Tymlos).

   D. All of the above.

   E. None of the above.

   Correct answer: E

   Comment:

   This patient has osteopenia and not osteoporosis. Although the addition of testosterone is also likely to increase the muscle mass, there is a paucity of well-conducted large-scale studies on the effect of adding testosterone to estrogen. Furthermore, testosterone is likely to be associated with a number of adverse effects, including masculinizing effects which most postmenopausal women dislike. The addition of testosterone is therefore not recommended at this stage. Calcitonin has been used for the treatment, not for the prevention of, and for the alleviation of pain postvertebral compression fracture.

Teriparatide and abaloparatide are osteoanabolics approved for the treatment, not prevention of osteoporosis. Furthermore, the cost and the need to administer the medication daily by subcutaneous injections make both medications less likely alternatives for this patient's management.

Case summary

Analysis of data

Factors predisposing to bone demineralization/osteoporosis

- Status postmenopause.
- No hormonal replacement therapy.
- Positive family history of osteoporosis, with history of hip fracture in grandmother and kyphosis in mother.

Factors reducing risk of bone demineralization/osteoporosis

- Physically active lifestyle.
- Regular exercise sessions.
- Good dietary calcium intake.
- Moderate alcohol intake.
- No coffee, no soda drinks.
- No cigarette smoking.

Factors increasing risk of falls/fractures

- None.

Factors reducing risk of falls/fractures

- Physically active lifestyle.
- Regular exercise sessions.
- Moderate alcohol intake.
- Good dietary intake.

Diagnosis

- Osteopenia.
- Ten-year fracture risk does not reach threshold recommended by the NOF to initiate pharmacologic treatment.

Management recommendations

Treatment recommendations

- No pharmacologic recommendation at this stage.
- She is leading a healthy, physically active lifestyle.

Diagnostic test(s)

- None indicated at this stage.

Lifestyle

- None needed. AC is exercising regularly.

DXA and radiologic

- DXA scan in 2 years' time. Sooner if fractures, falls, or near-falls sustained.

Key point

- In patients with densitometric evidence of osteopenia, the FRAX and NOF scores provide guidance as to whether the goal of management should be prevention or treatment.

References

1. Stuenkel CA, Davis SR, Gompel A, et al. Treatment of symptoms of the menopause: an endocrine society clinical practice guideline. *J Clin Endocrinol Metab*. 2015;100(11):3975–4011. https://doi.org/10.1210/jc.2015-2236.
2. Rossouw JE, Anderson GL, Prentice RL, et al. Risks and benefits of estrogen plus progestin in healthy postmenopausal women: principal results from the Women's Health Initiative randomized controlled trial. *JAMA*. 2002;288(3):321–333. https://doi.org/10.1001/jama.288.3.321.
3. Anderson GL, Limacher M, Assaf AR, et al. Effects of conjugated equine estrogen in postmenopausal women with hysterectomy: the Women's Health Initiative randomized controlled trial. *JAMA*. 2004;291(14):1701–1712. https://doi.org/10.1001/jama.291.14.1701.

CHAPTER 7

Osteopenia: Individualizing treatment—Part II☆

Learning objective

- Integrate clinical findings, DXA scan results, FRAX results, and NOF guidelines to develop a management strategy tailored to the individual needs of the particular patient concerned.

The case study

Reason for seeking medical help

- CA, 67 years old, had a DXA scan done 2 weeks ago. She is referred for management of her bone health.

Past medical/surgical history

- Natural menopause at 48 years, started Hormonal Replacement Therapy (HRT) but discontinued it a few months later because of adverse effects.

Lifestyle

- Daily calcium intake, estimated at about 1200 mg.
- Does not smoke cigarettes.
- Consumes alcoholic drinks in moderation, not exceeding three drinks a week.
- Drinks neither coffee nor soda drinks.
- Sedentary lifestyle.

☆ CA is a 67-year-old African American woman who has osteopenia and whose fracture risk exceeds the threshold recommended by the National Osteoporosis Foundation to initiate treatment for osteopenia.

Diagnosis and Treatment of Osteoporosis. https://doi.org/10.1016/B978-0-323-99550-4.00027-7
Copyright © 2024 Elsevier Inc. All rights are reserved, including those for text and data mining, AI training, and similar technologies.

Medication(s)

- Multivitamin tablets once a day.

Family history

- Negative for osteoporosis.

Clinical examination

- Weight: 178 pounds, height 5′4″.
- Mild kyphosis.
- Lying BP 144/89, pulse 78/min; standing blood pressure 140/82, pulse 91/min, regular, no orthostasis.
- Mild osteoarthritic changes affecting both knees. No difficulties standing up. Gait steady.
- No clinical evidence of localizing neurological lesions, no peripheral neuropathy.
- No heart failure, no cervical spondylosis, and no sensitive carotid sinus.
- Timed Get-Up-and-Go test completed in 10.4 s.

Laboratory result(s)

- About 2 weeks prior to visit she had a number of laboratory tests done as part of her annual physical examination. All results were within the normal limits, including complete blood count (CBC), comprehensive metabolic panel (CMP), serum 25-hydroxy-vitamin D level, and serum thyroid stimulating hormone (TSH).

DXA and radiological result(s)

Bone site	BMD	T-scores
Right femoral neck	0.652	−1.7
Right total hip	0.875	−0.6
Left femoral neck	0.621	−2.1
Left total hip	0.852	−0.7
L1–L4	0.645	−1.8

FRAX Scores (10-year probability of fracture):

Hip fracture risk: 4.2%: *EXCEEDED*
Other major fractures risk: 28%: *EXCEEDED*

National Osteoporosis Foundation threshold for initiating treatment: ***REACHED***

Vertebral Fracture Assessment: Not needed/not done

Multiple choice questions

1. ***In CA's case, the following is/are correct:***
   A. The densitometric diagnosis is osteopenia.
   B. The FRAX scores (10-year probability of sustaining a hip or major fracture) exceed the USA-NOF threshold for considering treatment.
   C. Pharmacologic management is recommended.
   D. A and C.
   E. A, B, and C.

   Correct answer: E

   Comment:

   CA has densitometric evidence of osteopenia (the lowest T-score is −2.1 in the lumbar vertebrae, less than −1.0, but higher than −2.5). Her FRAX score, i.e., her probability of sustaining a major osteoporotic or hip fracture in the next 10years (28% and 4.2% for the risk of an osteoporotic major or hip fracture, respectively), exceeds the threshold recommended by the US-National Osteoporosis Foundation to initiate pharmacologic treatment (3% for hip fracture and 20% for other major osteoporotic fractures).[1]

   The goal of managing this patient therefore is to treat the low bone mass as if she had osteoporosis, even though she does not have densitometric evidence of osteoporosis. The risk of sustaining fracture(s) in the next 10years, as per the FRAX algorithm, overrides the densitometric diagnosis.
2. ***The FRAX algorithm:***
   A. Estimates the patient's 5- and 10-year probability of sustaining a hip or major osteoporotic fracture.
   B. Can be applied without including the patient's BMD or T-score.
   C. Can be applied to men aged 40 to 90years.
   D. A, B, and C.
   E. B and C.

   Correct answer: E

   Comment:

   The FRAX algorithm was developed under the auspices of the World Health Organization and first launched in 2008.[2] It estimates the probability of the patient sustaining a hip or major osteoporotic fracture within the next 10years. The permutation can be done with or without the BMD/T-score of the femoral neck. It is available free of charge on the web and has undergone several revisions. FRAX can be applied to men and women between the ages of 40 and 90years.
3. ***The FRAX algorithm:***
   A. Considers the BMD/T-scores of the lumbar vertebrae, total hip, or femoral neck.
   B. Grades risk factors into three categories: mild, moderate, and severe.
   C. Considers the patient's risk of falling.
   D. All of the above.
   E. None of the above.

   Correct answer: E

Comment:

The FRAX algorithm has several limitations including ignoring the BMD of the lumbar vertebrae, one of the first bones to be affected by bone demineralization, and a number of factors that predispose to falls and therefore increase the fracture risk. Furthermore, the answer to all the questions related to risk factors is binary and therefore can only be answered as yes/no. It is therefore not possible to grade these responses; consequently, in the FRAX permutation, there is no difference if the patient is on 2-mg or 40-mg prednisone daily. It also does not consider the patient's daily calcium intake and whether or not she has hypovitaminosis D. Similarly, the risk of falling is not included in the FRAX permutation. Finally, pathologies such as arthritis, muscle weakness, orthostatic hypotension, cardiac arrhythmias, vertebrobasilar insufficiency which also affect the risk of falling and fracturing are not included in the permutation. Falls and fractures are discussed in a different case study.

4. ***In CA's case, the FRAX scores:***
   A. Underestimate the true fracture risk.
   B. Overestimate the true fracture risk
   C. Can be used to monitor her response to therapy.
   D. A and C.
   E. B and C.

   Correct answer: A

   Comments:

   FRAX considers the patient's age, gender, weight, and height in addition to the presence or absence of seven risk factors: a history of fractures, a history of hip fracture in one of the biologic parents, glucocorticoid intake, rheumatoid arthritis, current cigarette smoking, alcohol abuse, and secondary osteoporosis.[2]

   FRAX does not consider factors that increase the risk of falls such as diabetes mellitus, autonomic neuropathy, Parkinson's disease, orthostatic hypotension, arthropathies, and medications, apart from prednisone, that can induce bone demineralization. It therefore underestimates the risk of fractures in these patients. FRAX cannot be used if the patient is receiving pharmacologic therapy for osteoporosis[2] and therefore cannot be used to monitor the patient's response to therapy.

5. ***The Garvan fracture risk calculator (FRC) considers the following:***
   A. Number of falls sustained in the previous 12months.
   B. Number of fragility fractures sustained.
   C. BMD of the lumbar vertebrae or femoral neck.
   D. A and B.
   E. A, B, and C.

   Correct answer: E

   Comment:

   The Garvan FRC estimates the 5- and 10-year probability of sustaining a fracture in women and men aged 60years and older. It considers the BMD of the lumbar vertebrae or femoral neck, the patient's age and weight, and the number of falls sustained during the previous 12 months stratified into 1 and 2 or more than 2 falls. The number of fragility fractures sustained is also stratified into 1, 2, and more than 2.[3]

6. ***The Timed Get-up-and-Go test:***
   A. Is the time taken by the patient to stand up from the sitting position without using the arms of the chair.
   B. Reproducibility and interrater and intrarater variability are very good.
   C. The risk of sustaining a fall is increased if the test is completed in more than 14 s.
   D. A and B.
   E. A, B, and C

   Correct answer: B

   Comment:

   The Timed Get-up-and-Go test is the time taken by the patient to get up from a chair without using arm rests, walk 10 ft, and return to sit on the chair. The patient uses regular footwear and may use a walking aid. The interrater and intrarater variability is very good. Although controversial, it is accepted that the risk of falling, and therefore of fracture, is increased if the test is not completed within 14 s.[4]
7. ***The QFracture score:***
   A. Is based on clinical risk factors.
   B. Includes results of three blood tests: a complete blood picture and comprehensive metabolic profile.
   C. Includes information about alcohol intake.
   D. None of the above.
   E. All of the above.

   Correct answer: A

   Comment:

   The QFracture scale is a 10-year risk algorithm for the patient sustaining a fragility fracture. It is limited to clinical risk factors affecting the fracture risk and is based on data from the UK. One of its main advantages is that it can be calculated entirely based on information available in the patient's clinical records, therefore facilitating retrospective data collection.
8. ***The following is/are true concerning the risk of fractures:***
   A. Most patients who sustain fragility fractures have densitometric evidence of osteoporosis.
   B. Most patients who sustain fragility fractures have densitometric evidence of osteopenia.
   C. The fracture risk of all patients with osteopenia is about the same.
   D. A and C.
   E. B and C.

   Correct answer: B

   Comment:

   The majority of patients who sustain osteoporotic fractures have densitometric evidence of osteopenia and not osteoporosis.[5] Intuitively, the fracture risk of a patient who has a

T-score of −1.1 is much lower than that of a patient who has a T-score of −2.4 and yet, both are in the same densitometric diagnostic category: osteopenia. In these patients it is therefore important to evaluate the patient's fracture risk in order to develop a management strategy tailored to the individual circumstances of the patient. In this respect the FRAX algorithm is quite useful as it adds a different dimension to fracture risk assessment.

9. ***Bone mineral density is:***
   A. The single most important factor affecting fracture risk.
   B. For each standard deviation below that of a normal reference population, fracture rate is about doubled.
   C. In treated patients, medication induced increases in BMD account for most of the fracture risk reduction.
   D. A and B.
   E. A, B, and C.

   Correct answer: D

   Comments:

   It has long been known that the bone mineral density is the single most important factor affecting fracture risk: for each standard deviation below the mean of the reference population, the fracture risk is about doubled.[6] BMD, however, is not the only factor affecting fracture risk, and changes in bone density account for less than half the reduction in fracture risk induced by medications to treat osteoporosis.[7] Several other factors apart from BMD modulate the risk of fractures and are discussed in other case studies.

10. ***The following affect the fracture risk, independently of the BMD:***
   A. Hip axis length.
   B. Femoral neck angle.
   C. Markers of bone resorption.
   D. All of the above.
   E. None of the above.

   Correct answer: D

   Comments:

   The longer the hip axis length is, the more susceptible it is to fracture after being subjected to trauma. Similarly, the less acute the femoral angle is, the more likely it is fracture. These differences may explain the different fracture risks of different ethnic groups.[8,9]

Case summary

Analysis of data

Factors predisposing to bone demineralization/osteoporosis

- Postmenopause, no HRT.

Factors reducing risk of bone demineralization/osteoporosis

- Good daily calcium intake.
- No cigarette smoking.
- No excessive sodium, caffeine, or alcohol intake.

Factors increasing risk of falls/fractures

- None, except for sedentary lifestyle.
- CA has not sustained any falls or near-falls.

Factors reducing risk of falls/fractures

- None.
- CA has not sustained any falls.

Diagnosis

- Postmenopausal osteopenia.
- Fracture risk exceeds threshold established by the National Osteoporosis Foundation to initiate pharmacologic management.

Management recommendations

Treatment(s)

- Antiresorptive medication. At this stage there is no indication for an osteoanabolic medication.

Lifestyle

- Exercises to increase mobility and steadiness.

DXA and radiological

- Repeat DXA scan in 2 years to monitor bone mass and fine-tune management strategy.

Key points

- Patients with osteopenia can have their fracture risk estimated to develop a management strategy tailored to their particular circumstances.
- Several tools are available to estimate the fracture risk.
- If the fall risk cannot be reduced, measures are available to reduce the impact of falling such as hip protectors.

References

1. Cosman F, de Beur SJ, LeBoff MS, et al. Clinician's guide to prevention and treatment of osteoporosis [published correction appears in Osteoporos Int. 2015 Jul;26(7):2045–7]. *Osteoporos Int*. 2014;25(10):2359–2381. https://doi.org/10.1007/s00198-014-2794-2.
2. Kanis JA, Johansson H, Harvey NC, McCloskey EV. A brief history of FRAX. *Arch Osteoporos*. 2018;13(1):118. https://doi.org/10.1007/s11657-018-0510-0.
3. Nguyen ND, Frost SA, Center JR, Eisman JA, Nguyen TV. Development of prognostic nomograms for individualizing 5-year and 10-year fracture risks. *Osteoporos Int*. 2008;19(10):1431–1444. https://doi.org/10.1007/s00198-008-0588—0.
4. Schoene D, Wu SM, Mikolaizak AS, et al. Discriminative ability and predictive validity of the timed up and go test in identifying older people who fall systematic review and meta-analysis. *J Am Geriatr Soc*. 2013;61(2):202–208. https://doi.org/10.1111/jgs.12106.
5. Siris ES, Chen YT, Abbott TA, et al. Bone mineral density thresholds for pharmacological intervention to prevent fractures. *Arch Intern Med*. 2004;164(10):1108–1112. https://doi.org/10.1001/archinte.164.10.1108.
6. Marshall D, Johnell O, Wedel H. Meta-analysis of how well measures of bone mineral density predict occurrence of osteoporotic fractures. *BMJ*. 1996;312(7041):1254–1259. https://doi.org/10.1136/bmj.312.7041.1254.
7. Wasnich RD, Miller PD. Antifracture efficacy of antiresorptive agents are related to changes in bone density. *J Clin Endocrinol Metab*. 2000;85(1):231–236. https://doi.org/10.1210/jcem.85.1.6267.
8. Bonnick SL. Bone Densitometry for Technologists. 2nd ed. Humana Press; 2006.
9. Kanis JA, Harvey NC, Johansson H, Odén A, McCloskey EV, Leslie WD. Overview of fracture prediction tools. *J Clin Densitom*. 2017;20(3):444–450. https://doi.org/10.1016/j.jocd.2017.06.013.

CHAPTER 8

Osteopenia: Individualizing treatment—Part III[☆]

When silent vertebral compression fractures override the densitometric diagnosis

Learning objectives

- The integration of DXA scan results, FRAX algorithm score, NOF guidelines, and patient's clinical condition to develop a management strategy tailored to the individual circumstances of the patient.
- Appreciate that, like osteoporosis, osteopenia is asymptomatic until a fracture is sustained.

The case study

Reason for seeking medical help

- ON is 72-year-old Caucasian woman. She is recovering well from pneumonia and is referred because a plain X-ray of her lungs showed evidence of moderate, wedge vertebral compression fractures of T7, T8, and T9. She denies any trauma to her back and has not experienced any falls, near-falls, or dizzy spells.

Past medical and surgical history

- Natural menopause at age 49 years, has been on hormonal replacement therapy (HRT) since then; still on HRT, good compliance, no adverse effects.
- Menarche at age 12 years, regular menstrual periods until age 49 years.
- Two children aged 59 and 55 years, both in good health.

☆ ON, 72-year-old Caucasian woman with asymptomatic vertebral compression fractures.

Diagnosis and Treatment of Osteoporosis. https://doi.org/10.1016/B978-0-323-99550-4.00032-0
Copyright © 2024 Elsevier Inc. All rights are reserved, including those for text and data mining, AI training, and similar technologies.

Lifestyle

- Physically sedentary lifestyle. Works as a phone operator.
- Good appetite, no weight loss.
- Daily calcium intake about 600mg daily.
- Smokes an average of 10 cigarettes daily. Has tried to stop but was not able.
- Alcohol intake: two to three glasses of wine with dinner, often more during the weekend.
- At least 6 cups of coffee a day and 6 cans of diet Coca-Cola or Pepsi-Cola.
- No recreational drugs.

Medication(s)

- Hormonal replacement therapy: estrogen and progesterone.
- Simvastatin 40mg once a day.
- Multivitamin/mineral tablet supplements.
- Occasional (about once a week) over-the-counter hypnotic.

Family history

- Positive for osteoporosis: mother and maternal grandmother sustained fragility hip fractures.
- Older sister has been diagnosed with osteoporosis and is receiving treatment.

Clinical examination

- Weight 167 pounds, height 5′2″, says she lost about 2″ compared to her height when she was in her thirties. Mild postural kyphosis.
- Alert, cooperative, cognitively intact. Concerned about osteoporosis.
- BP 138/92 sitting; 131/96 standing, no clinical evidence of orthostasis.
- Pulse rate 84/min, regular.
- No difficulties standing up.
- Completes the Timed Up and Go (TUG) test in 8.1 s.
- Clinical examination does not reveal any significant clinical finding.

Laboratory results

About 3weeks before referral she had a number of laboratory tests done. All results were within normal limits, including comprehensive blood count (CBC), comprehensive metabolic panel (CMP), serum vitamin D, parathyroid hormone (PTH), and thyroid stimulating hormone (THS). Serum cholesterol has been marginally elevated for about 2years.

DXA and radiological(s)

- Lowest T-score −1.8 in lumbar vertebrae.
- Vertebral Fracture Assessment: evidence of three vertebral compression fractures: T7, T8, and T9. ON denies any trauma to her back or other parts of her body. She has led a mostly sedentary lifestyle.
- FRAX scores: 2.2% hip and 17% major fracture.

Diagnosis

- Osteoporosis as evidenced by the presence of "silent" vertebral compression fragility fractures.
- The presence of a fragility fracture overrides the densitometric diagnosis of osteopenia and the FRAX derived risks of sustaining a fracture.

> Lowest T-score: −1.8 at L1 to L4
>
> **FRAX Scores (10-year probability of fracture):**
>
> Hip fracture risk: 2.2%
> Other major fractures risk: 17%
>
> **National Osteoporosis Foundation threshold for initiating treatment:** *NOT reached.*
>
> *Evidence of fragility/silent/morphometric vertebral compression fractures, therefore:*
> *Opportunistic diagnosis of osteoporosis.*

Multiple choice questions

1. ***The following is/are true about ON's vertebral compression fractures of T7, T8, and T9:***
   A. They are asymptomatic and part of the normal aging process.
   B. They can be ignored.
   C. Vertebral augmentation procedures should be considered.
   D. A and B.
   E. None of the above.
   Correct answer: E
   Comment:
   Clinically silent vertebral compression fractures are fragility fractures. They are diagnostic of osteoporosis, and therefore cannot be ignored. They should be considered as "warning signs" because once a patient develops a fragility fracture, she/he is likely to sustain further fractures. It is therefore appropriate to investigate these patients for causes of secondary osteoporosis and develop a management strategy tailored to the patient's condition and needs. Often the underlying cause is readily identified, such as

orthostatic hypotension; cardiac arrhythmias; sensitive carotid sinus; low calcium intake; sedentary lifestyle; cigarette smoking; excessive alcohol, coffee, and sodium intake.

It is also important to conduct a full clinical examination to identify a number of conditions that may increase the risk of falls and fractures. In ON's case the vertebral compression fractures are silent, i.e., asymptomatic, and therefore there is no need to consider vertebral augmentation procedures.

2. ***The following is/are true about ON's final diagnosis:***
   A. Osteopenia.
   B. Osteoporosis.
   C. Increased fracture risk.
   D. A and C.
   E. B and C.

   Correct answer: E

   Comments:

   ON has densitometric evidence of osteopenia. However, the presence of the morphometric vertebral compression fractures overrides the densitometric findings as it indicates that her bones are fragile and susceptible to sustaining fractures. This patient therefore needs medication to increase the bone density and reduce the risk of fractures. The National Bone Health Alliance working group recommends that postmenopausal women and men aged 50 years be considered for pharmacological treatment to increase bone mass and therefore reduce the fracture risk. In the USA, the threshold is 3% and 20% for the 10-year risk of sustaining a hip or major fracture, respectively.[1]

3. ***In ON's case, factors increasing the risk of osteoporosis include:***
   A. Age 72 years.
   B. Status postmenopause.
   C. Positive family history for osteoporosis.
   D. Alcohol intake.
   E. A, B, and C.

   Correct answer: E

   Comment:

   Menopause is a risk factor for osteoporosis unless the patient is on hormonal replacement therapy. A positive family history, especially hip fracture, increases the risk of osteoporosis. Alcohol intake exceeding the threshold of two drinks a day for women and three drinks a day for men increases the risk of osteoporosis. Alcohol intake less than that threshold may have a bone mass protective effect. It is, however, not clear whether this benefit is the result of the alcohol intake per se or whether it is due to the patient's lifestyle.

   Patients who consume alcoholic drinks also are at risk of falling: alcoholic drinks may interfere with postural stability and the efficiency of postural reflexes, thus increasing the risk of falls and hence fractures. It also may blunt cognitive functions.

The use of over-the-counter hypnotics is particularly problematic in older patients for a number of reasons, including the often long half-life of these compounds and the potential interactions with other medications or alcohol the patient may be consuming. Excessive caffeine and sodium intake may lead to polyurea and an increased need to get to a toilet frequently and in a relatively short period of time, thus increasing the likelihood of falling and therefore fractures.

4. ***The following laboratory tests are indicated:***
   A. 24-h urinary calcium.
   B. 24-h urinary magnesium.
   C. 24-h urinary sodium.
   D. All of the above.
   E. None of the above.

   Correct answer: E

   Comment:

   At this stage there is no need for any of these laboratory tests.

5. ***The following laboratory tests are recommended:***
   A. Comprehensive metabolic panel.
   B. 25-hydroxy-vitamin D.
   C. 1,25-Di-hydroxy-vitamin D.
   D. All of the above.
   E. None of the above.

   Correct answer: E

   Comments:

   At this stage there is no need for any of these laboratory tests. These tests have been done about 2 weeks prior to her visit.

6. ***In ON's case:***
   A. The FRAX scores reach the threshold recommended by the NOF to initiate pharmacologic treatment.
   B. She should be offered pharmacologic treatment for osteoporosis.
   C. She should be counseled about her dietary intake of calcium or prescribed calcium supplements.
   D. B and C.
   E. All of the above.

   Correct answer: D

   Comment:

   The FRAX scores of 2.2% and 17% (for the probability of sustaining a hip or major fracture, respectively, within 10 years) do not reach the threshold recommended by the National Osteoporosis Foundation (3% or 20% for the 10-year probability of sustaining a hip or major fracture, respectively) to initiate pharmacologic treatment. ON, however, has radiographic evidence of two morphometric vertebral compression fractures that she was not aware of. This is diagnostic of increased bone fragility and overrides the DXA scan results. Pharmacologic management should therefore be considered, as if the patient had densitometric evidence of osteoporosis.[1]

As her serum vitamin D level was within the normal range there is no need to prescribe vitamin D supplements. She should, however, be counseled regarding the dietary calcium intake. Supplements should be prescribed if she cannot increase her dietary calcium intake.

7. ***Pharmacologic management recommendations include:***

A. A Selective Estrogen Receptor Modulator (SERM): raloxifene.
B. An antiresorptive medication: bisphosphonates or denosumab.
C. An osteoanabolic medication: teriparatide or abaloparatide.
D. A and B.
E. None of the above.

Correct answer: D

Comments:

ON needs medication that can increase the bone mass and reduce her fracture risk. Traditionally, pharmacological treatment is initiated with an antiresorptive medication because most patients in the early menopause have an increased rate of bone resorption. Furthermore, the ease of administration, the relative paucity of adverse effects, and the cost of the medication are attractive. These medications will be discussed in other case studies.

8. ***Nonpharmacologic management includes:***

A. Engage in resistive and aerobic exercises.
B. Ensure a well-balanced diet particularly concerning calcium, vitamin D, and protein intake.
C. Limit or avoid alcohol intake.
D. All of the above.
E. None of the above.

Correct answer: D

Comment:

These issues are discussed in another case study.

9. ***ON would benefit from counseling in the following areas:***

A. Adequate dietary calcium and vitamin D intake.
B. Cigarette smoking cessation.
C. Increased physical exercise regularly undertaken.
D. Limit excessive caffeine and soda drinks.
E. All of the above.

Correct answer: E

Comment:

All these issues need to be addressed in an unhurried environment. It is important to get the patient's collaboration to achieve this goal.

10. ***The following follow-up is recommended:***
    A. Repeat DXA scan in 1 year.
    B. Repeat DXA scan in 2 years.
    C. Repeat DXA scan in 5 years.
    D. Repeat the FRAX score in 6 months.
    E. None of the above.

    Correct answer: B

    Comment:

    These issues are discussed in other case studies.

Case summary

Analysis of data

Factors predisposing to bone demineralization/osteoporosis
- Status postmenopause.
- Positive family history for osteoporosis.
- Sedentary lifestyle.
- Cigarette smoking.
- Low daily calcium intake.
- Alcohol intake.

Factors reducing risk of bone demineralization/osteoporosis
- Hormonal replacement therapy since beginning of menopause.
- No excessive caffeine or sodium intake, or limit their intake.

Factors increasing risk of falls/fractures
- Intake of over-the-counter hypnotic tablets.

Factors reducing risk of falls/fractures
- None.

Diagnosis

- Osteoporosis.
- The presence of fragility fractures (T7, T8, and T9) is diagnostic of osteoporosis: "morphometric or opportunistic diagnosis." Pharmacologic treatment is therefore recommended at this stage because the risk of subsequent fractures is increased.

Management recommendations

Treatment(s)

- Antiresorptive medication.

Diagnostic test(s)

- None at this stage.

Lifestyle

- Reduce alcohol intake.

Rehabilitation

- If possible, enroll in a physical exercise program.

DXA and radiological

- DXA scan in 2 years' time, preferably at the same center where the present DXA scan was done to allow for a more accurate comparison of the scans.

Key points

- In order to develop a personalized management plan, the following four issues should be considered:
  1. T-scores.
  2. FRAX (fracture risk assessment) scores.
  3. National Osteoporosis Foundation guidelines.
  4. Vertebral Fracture Assessment.
- The patient's densitometric diagnosis, based on the T-scores, is an important factor considered while developing a treatment plan for patients with low bone mass, but it is not the only factor.
- The FRAX score estimates the patient's probability of sustaining a fracture within the next 10 years and is useful to develop the management strategy. Based on the FRAX probabilities, the National Osteoporosis Foundation has issued guidelines: the threshold to initiate pharmacologic treatment is a 3% and 20% 10-year probability of sustaining a hip and a major fracture, respectively.
- At present, the FRAX algorithm permutation considers only a handful of risk factors and ignores many others. For instance, the patient's cognitive functions and propensity to fall are not considered in the FRAX algorithm, and yet both affect the risk of falls and fractures.
- The clinician's own experience and knowledge about the patient are important to develop a successful management strategy tailored to the individual needs and circumstances of the patient.

Reference

1. Siris ES, Adler R, Bilezikian J, et al. The clinical diagnosis of osteoporosis: a position statement from the National Bone Health Alliance Working Group. *Osteoporos Int.* 2014;25(5):1439–1443. https://doi.org/10.1007/s00198-014-2655-z.

CHAPTER 9

Osteopenia: Individualizing treatment—Part IV☆

Learning objectives

- Individualizing the management strategy for patients with osteopenia and low fracture risk.
- Know when to override the results of the FRAX score and NOF recommendations.
- Appreciate the effect of some medications on fracture risk.
- Recognize the importance of diet, physical exercise, and lifestyle issues when individualizing the management strategy.

The case study

Reason for seeking medical help

Mrs. GH and her family are concerned because she sustained several falls: about two a week for the past few months. These are usually preceded by bouts of dizziness, especially when she tries to stand up from the seated position or when getting out of bed. She is not aware of any palpitations on standing up. She lives on her own but has good social support.

Past medical/surgical history

- Natural menopause at 48 years, no HRT.
- Depression, long standing, on sertraline. No suicidal thoughts.

Personal habits

- Sedentary lifestyle, especially since she started experiencing bouts of dizziness, near-falls, and falls.
- Daily calcium intake about 1200 mg.

☆ H, 66-year-old Asian woman who has osteopenia and sustained repeated falls.

Diagnosis and Treatment of Osteoporosis. https://doi.org/10.1016/B978-0-323-99550-4.00016-2
Copyright © 2024 Elsevier Inc. All rights are reserved, including those for text and data mining, AI training, and similar technologies.

- At least six cups of coffee and three cans of soda a day, used to consume more.
- Smokes about 10 cigarettes a day, used to smoke more. She is planning to stop completely in about 3 months on her birthday.
- About three alcoholic drinks daily, binge drinking about once a month.

Medication(s)

- Sertraline, 15 years.
- Omeprazole, 5 years.
- Furosemide, 2 years.
- Depo-Provera, 4 years.

Family history

- Negative for osteoporosis.
- Married, four children, all healthy.

Clinical examination

- Weight 185 pounds, height 5′5″, historical height 5′8″.
- Mild kyphosis, corrected when asked to stand-up straight.
- No relevant clinical findings.
- Passive movement of the neck does not induce dizzy spells.
- Get-Up-and-Go test completed in 11 s.

Laboratory result(s)

- Complete blood count (CBC), comprehensive blood panel (CMP), 25-hydroxy-vitamin D, and thyroid stimulating hormone (TSH) levels done about 4 weeks ago: within normal limits, except for low serum potassium level: 3.1 mmol/L (normal range 3.6–5.2).

DXA and radiological results

Bone site	T-scores
Right femoral neck	−1.6
Right total hip	−1.3
Left femoral neck	−1.5
Left total hip	−1.2
L1-L4	−2.2

- FRAX scores (with BMD):
  Hip fracture risk: 2.0%
  Major fractures: 11%
- National Osteoporosis Foundation threshold for initiating pharmacologic treatment: NOT REACHED
- Vertebral fracture Assessment: No Vertebral compression fractures

Multiple choice questions

1. ***In Mrs. GH's case:***
   A. The densitometric diagnosis is osteopenia.
   B. The FRAX score does not reach the NOF recommended threshold to initiate pharmacologic treatment for low bone mass.
   C. The FRAX score should be overlooked because of the patient's risk of sustaining repeated falls.
   D. Pharmacologic treatment for low bone mass should be initiated as if the diagnosis were osteoporosis.
   E. All of the above

   Correct answer: E

   Comments:

   Given that the lowest T-score is −2.2 in the upper four lumbar vertebrae, the densitometric diagnosis is "osteopenia." As the FRAX scores are 2.7% and 11% for the 10-year risk of sustaining an osteoporotic hip or major fracture, respectively, they do not reach the threshold recommended by the National Osteoporosis Foundation to initiate pharmacologic treatment for osteopenia.

   As, however, Mrs. GH has sustained a number of falls, her fracture risk is substantially elevated. She therefore should be offered pharmacologic treatment for osteopenia, as if she had osteoporosis. The cause for her repeated falls also should be addressed and she may benefit from hip protectors.
2. ***Depression, Selective Serotonin Reuptake Inhibitors (SSRIs), and bone mass:***
   A. Depression is an independent risk factor for low bone mass.
   B. SSRIs are independent risk factors for low bone mass.
   C. SSRIs interfere with the skeletal serotonergic system.
   D. A and B.
   E. A, B, and C.

   Correct answer: E

   Comment:

   Depression leads to low bone mass through several mechanisms: increased endogenous cortisol production interfering with the hypothalamic-pituitary-adrenal axis resulting in an excessive amount of catecholamines and increased interleukin-6 release; and also by interfering with the release of growth hormone and hypothalamic-pituitary-gonadal axis, resulting in reduced estrogen/testosterone production.[1] SSRIs also interfere with serotonin receptors and transporters in the osteoblasts and osteocytes and are independent risk factors for osteoporosis.[2,3] Other factors include low food intake/inadequate diet, sedentary lifestyle, and lack of exposure to sunlight, which may lead to vitamin D deficiency, which is sometimes associated with proximal myopathy and an increased risk of falling.

3. ***Depo-Provera (medroxyprogesterone acetate—MPA):***
   A. Decreases estrogen production.
   B. Leads to bone demineralization.
   C. The associated BMD loss is totally reversible.
   D. A and B.
   E. A, B, and C.

   Correct answer: D

   Comment:

   By decreasing the serum estrogen levels, MPA induces bone demineralization. The greatest loss is observed during the first 2years of MPA administration. The BMD loss is not totally reversible.[4]

4. ***Proton-pump inhibitors (PPIs) increase the risk of:***
   A. Bone demineralization.
   B. Vertebral fractures.
   C. Fragility fractures.
   D. A and B.
   E. A, B, and C.

   Correct answer: E

   Comment:

   Studies, including at least one prospective study, have shown that PPIs increase the risk of bone demineralization and fragility fractures, including hip fractures. Other studies yielded conflicting results.[5] PPIs decrease calcium absorption, leading to a negative calcium balance, increased parathyroid output, increased bone resorption and bone demineralization, especially if the patient relies on calcium carbonate supplements, which need to be dissolved prior to being absorbed. The dissolution of calcium carbonate requires an acidic medium. The iatrogenic acid suppression also may lead to hypergastrinemia and parathyroid hyperplasia.[5] PPIs also may inhibit osteoclastic proton pumps.[5,6]

5. ***The following is/are true about alcohol consumption:***
   A. Fewer than two units a day do not affect fracture risk.
   B. Two units a day reduce fracture risk.
   C. More than two units a day increase fracture risk.
   D. A and C.
   E. B and C.

   Correct answer: D

Comments:

A study on 5939 men and 11,032 women showed that in both sexes, alcohol consumption exceeding 2 units a day increased the risk of hip fractures (RR 1.68; 95% CI 1.19–2.36), osteoporotic fractures (RR 1.38; 95% CI 1.16–1.65), and any fracture (RR 1.23; 95% CI 1.06–1.43).[7] Alcohol exerts a direct effect on bone cells and modulates factors controlling their activity.[8] Magnesium deficiency may contribute to low bone mass in chronic alcoholism. The "protective" effects of moderate alcohol consumption reported in some observational studies could not be reproduced in controlled studies on experimental animals, suggesting that other factors such as lifestyle changes, including adequate nutritional intake, physically active lifestyle, and avoidance of cigarette smoking, may play a significant role in "protecting" the skeleton.[8]

6. ***Cigarette smoking:***
   A. Increases vertebral fracture risk.
   B. Increases hip fracture risk.
   C. Its negative effect on bone mass is quickly reversed by discontinuing smoking.
   D. A and B.
   E. A, B, and C.

   Correct answer: D

   Comments:

   Cigarette smoking is associated with a smaller bone mass and increased fracture risk. A meta-analysis of 86 studies which included 40,753 subjects showed that cigarette smoking increases vertebral fractures by 13% and 32% in women and men, respectively, and hip fracture risk by 31% and 40% in women and men, respectively. The detrimental effects of cigarette smoking are only partly reversed by smoking cessation.[9]

7. ***Sodium intake and calcium metabolism:***
   A. Excess sodium intake leads to hypercalciuria.
   B. Increasing calcium intake offsets the negative impact of excessive sodium intake.
   C. Potassium reduces the sodium-induced hypercalciuria.
   D. A and B.
   E. A, B, and C.

   Correct answer: E

   Comments:

   Excessive sodium intake induces hypercalciuria through volume expansion and as a result of competition between sodium and calcium ions for the same reabsorption mechanism in renal tubules. In most instances, especially in premenopausal women, hypercalciuria does not lead to a negative calcium balance because of the compensatory increased intestinal calcium absorption.

   Postmenopausal women, however, may not be able to sufficiently increase intestinal calcium absorption and therefore the hypercalciuria may lead to a negative calcium balance resulting in increased parathyroid hormone release and increased bone resorption. This increased bone turnover can be offset by increasing daily calcium intake. Potassium also reduces the sodium-induced hypercalcemia[10]. Processed foods are rich in sodium that is difficult to quantify. Salt substitutes are better than salt because potassium reduces the sodium-induced hypercalciuria.

8. ***The calciuric effect of carbonated beverages is due to their:***
   A. Caffeine content.
   B. Sodium content.
   C. Phosphoric acid content.
   D. A and B.
   E. A, B, and C.

   Correct answer: D

   Comments:

   Caffeine increases the renal calcium loss: each 6oz of caffeine-containing drinks induces a renal calcium loss of 4–6mg,[11] and the nighttime conservation of calcium is insufficient to offset the excess renal calcium loss.[12] Caffeine also has direct deleterious effects on osteoblast function and survival.[13] Intakes of more than 18oz of brewed coffee accelerate bone loss in the lumbar vertebrae in postmenopausal women.[14]

   Sodium, not phosphoric acid, in carbonated drinks also increases urinary calcium excretion.[15] Phosphoric acid binds to calcium in the gastrointestinal track and reduces its bioavailability and absorption. Notwithstanding, it is probably not the carbonated drink, per se, that increases the risk of bone loss but the fact that it replaces the intake of calcium-containing drinks.[15]

9. ***Match the following:***
   (a) Loop diuretics.
   (b) Hydrochlorothiazides.
   (c) Both.
   (d) Neither.
      A. Increase renal calcium excretion.
      B. Decrease renal calcium excretion.
      C. Increase renal potassium loss.
      D. May lead to urinary incontinence.
      E. May induce negative calcium balance and bone demineralization.

   Correct answers: A (a); B (b); C (c); D (c); E (a)

   Comment:

   Loop diuretics increase renal calcium excretion by interfering with its reabsorption at the loop of Henle. Their long-term use may induce a negative calcium balance and bone demineralization. The intake of loop diuretics may lead to hypovolemia which may in turn lead to postural hypotension and bouts of dizziness on standing up or getting out of bed. Thiazide diuretics conserve calcium by increasing calcium absorption at the distal renal tubules thus reducing calcium loss. Loop diuretics and hydrochlorothiazide increase renal potassium loss. All diuretics, particularly loop diuretics, may induce urinary incontinence.

10. ***The following statement(s) is/are true concerning physical exercise:***
    A. In postmenopausal women, walking increases BMD at the lumbar vertebrae and femoral necks.
    B. In postmenopausal women, walking significantly increases the BMD at the lumbar vertebrae but not femoral necks.
    C. In postmenopausal women, walking increases the BMD at the femoral necks but not lumbar vertebrae.
    D. In premenopausal women, high-intensity progressive resistance training increases BMD at the femoral neck and lumbar vertebrae.
    E. In premenopausal women, high-intensity progressive resistance training increases BMD at the femoral necks but not lumbar vertebrae.

    Correct answer: C

    Comment:

    Exercise studies are notoriously difficult to design, conduct, analyze, and interpret given the complexity of the issue and the numerous factors that modulate the response of the skeleton to physical exercise. Notwithstanding, 2 meta-analyses concluded that in postmenopausal women walking increases the BMD at the femoral necks but not lumbar vertebrae,[16] and in premenopausal women high-intensity resistance training increases BMD at the lumbar vertebrae but not femoral necks.[17]

Case summary

Analysis of data

Factors predisposing to bone demineralization/osteoporosis
- Status postmenopause, no HRT.
- Depo-Provera.
- Sedentary lifestyle.
- Excessive caffeine and sodium intake.
- Cigarette smoking.
- Alcohol abuse.
- Depression and antidepressants (SSRI—Sertraline).
- Proton-Pump Inhibitors (Omeprazole).
- Loop diuretics (furosemide).

Factors reducing risk of bone demineralization/osteoporosis
- Negative family history for osteoporosis.
- Good daily calcium intake.
- Normal serum vitamin D level.

Factors increasing risk of falls/fractures
- Several falls and near-falls sustained.

Factors reducing risk of falls/fractures

- Get-Up-and-Go test completed in less than 14 s.

Diagnosis

- Osteopenia.

Management recommendations

- Given the multiple falls/near-falls experienced by Mrs. GH, her risk of sustaining fractures is increased. Repeated falls is a major factor predisposing to fractures, a risk which is not included in the FRAX permutation. Therefore, even though Mrs. GH has only evidence of osteopenia, not osteoporosis, and even though the fracture risk does not reach the threshold recommended by the National Osteoporosis Foundation to initiate treatment, yet pharmacologic treatment is recommended, especially as Mrs. GH has evidence of a low BMD. Other factors increasing the risk of falls should also be incorporated in the management strategy, including the intake of diuretics which may lead to hypovolemia and orthostatic hypotension. Hypokalemia also may lead to dizzy spells.

Treatment(s)

- Pharmacologic management of low bone mass.

Diagnostic tests

- No further tests are recommended at this stage.

Lifestyle

- In addition to pharmacologic management of low bone mass, nonpharmacologic management and lifestyle changes should be emphasized.

DXA and radiologic

- Repeat DXA scan in 2 years to monitor BMD and fine-tune the management strategy.

Key points

- Assessing fracture risk helps develop a management strategy tailored to the individual circumstances of patients with osteopenia.
- Several medications may induce bone demineralization.

References

1. Ilias I, Alesci S, Gold PW, Chrousos GP. Depression and osteoporosis in men: association or causal link? *Hormones*. 2006;5(1):9–16.
2. Bab I, Yirmiya R. Depression, selective serotonin reuptake inhibitors and osteoporosis. *Curr Osteoporos Rep*. 2010;8(4):185–191.
3. Wu Q, Bencaz AF, Hentz JG, et al. Selective serotonin reuptake inhibitor treatment and risk of fractures: a meta-analysis of cohort and case-control studies. *Osteoporos Int*. 2012;23(1):365–375.
4. Wooltorton E. Medroxyprogesterone acetate and bone mineral density loss. *CMAJ*. 2005;172(6):746.
5. Fraser LA, Leslie WD, Targownik LE, et al. The effect of proton pump inhibitors on fracture risk: report from the Canadian multicenter osteoporosis study. *Osteoporos Int*. 2013;24(4):1161–1168.
6. Yang YX. Chronic proton pump inhibitor therapy and calcium metabolism. *Curr Gastroenterol Rep*. 2012;14 (6):473–479.
7. Kanis JA, Johansson H, Johnell O, et al. Alcohol intake as a risk factor for fracture. *Osteoporos Int*. 2005;16 (7):737–742.
8. Sampson HW. Alcohol and other factors affecting osteoporosis risk in women. *Alcohol Res Health*. 2002;26 (4):292–298.
9. Ward KD, Klesges RC. A meta-analysis of the effects of cigarette smoking on bone mineral density. *Calcif Tissue Int*. 2001;68(5):259–270.
10. Heaney RP. Role of dietary sodium in osteoporosis. *J Am Coll Nutr*. 2006;25(Suppl 3):271S–276S.
11. Barger-Lux MJ, Heaney RP. Caffeine and the calcium economy revisited. *Osteoporos Int*. 1995;5(2):97–102.
12. Kynast-Gales SA, Massey LK. Effect of caffeine on circadian excretion of urinary calcium and magnesium. *J Am Coll Nutr*. 1994;13(5):467–472.
13. Tsuang YH, Sun JS, Chen LT, et al. Direct effects of caffeine on osteoblastic cells metabolism: the possible causal effect of caffeine on the formation of osteoporosis. *J Orthoped Surg Res*. 2006;1:7.
14. Rapuri PB, Gallagher JC, Kinyamu HK, Ryschon KL. Caffeine intake increases the rate of bone loss in elderly women and interacts with vitamin D receptor genotypes. *Am J Clin Nutr*. 2001;74(5):694–700.
15. Heaney RP, Rafferty K. Carbonated beverages and urinary calcium excretion. *Am J Clin Nutr*. 2001;74 (3):343–347.
16. Martyn-St James M, Carroll S. Meta-analysis of walking for preservation of bone mineral density in postmenopausal women. *Bone*. 2008;43:521–531.
17. Martyn-St James M, Carroll S. Progressive high-intensity resistance training and bone mineral density changes among premenstrual women: evidence of discordant site-specific skeletal effects. *Sports Med*. 2006;36 (8):683–704.

CHAPTER 10

Screening for osteoporosis☆

Learning objectives

- The importance of screening for osteoporosis.
- Risk factors predisposing to osteoporosis.
- Who, when, and how to screen for osteoporosis.
- Unnecessary laboratory and imaging studies should be avoided.

The case study

Reason for seeking medical help

- SF, a 51-year-old Caucasian woman, is concerned about osteoporosis because the mother of her best friend died about 4 weeks ago after sustaining a fragility hip fracture subsequent to a fall in her carpeted bedroom. SF is asymptomatic and enjoys good health. She is asking whether she should have a DXA scan done.

Past medical and surgical history

- No height loss.
- No history of falls, near-falls, dizzy spells, and no fractures.
- No history of arthritis, no renal calculi, no food allergies, regular bowel functions.
- Menarche at age 12 years, regular menses up to about a year ago.
- Five healthy children aged 25, 23, 21, 19, and 15 years. She breast-fed all, each one for approximately 1 year.

Lifestyle

- She drinks on average one glass (8 oz) of milk and a glass of calcium-fortified orange juice every day. She also has a cup of yogurt (6 oz) daily and regularly eats cheese (at least two slices) and calcium-fortified bread (at least two slices).

☆ SF, 51-year-old postmenopausal Caucasian woman concerned about osteoporosis.

Diagnosis and Treatment of Osteoporosis. https://doi.org/10.1016/B978-0-323-99550-4.00029-0
Copyright © 2024 Elsevier Inc. All rights are reserved, including those for text and data mining, AI training, and similar technologies.

- She drinks only one cup of coffee every morning.
- She avo
- ids salty food.
- She does not consume soda drinks.
- She never smoked cigarettes.
- She drinks a glass of wine four to five times a week with dinner. She does not exceed one small glass.
- She leads an active physical lifestyle. She was in the army for about 25 years and then became a physical education teacher and personal coach. She spends at least an hour, five times a week in a gym doing a combination of aerobic and resistive exercises.

Medication(s)

- Multivitamin tablet once a day.

Family history

- Negative for osteoporosis; both parents are alive, healthy, and lead physically active lifestyles.
- Two older sisters (56 and 54 years) and two younger ones (49 and 47 years) all in good health, on no medication.

Clinical examination

- Weight 107 pounds, height 5′5″, arm span 65″, BMI 18.4. Except during her five pregnancies, SF's weight has always been around 110 pounds. She had been investigated for low body weight about 10 years and again 2 years ago and no pathology was identified. Hyperthyroidism, celiac disease, malabsorption, anorexia nervosa, and the female athlete syndrome have been ruled out.
- No significant clinical finding: no kyphosis, no loss of height, no point tenderness along the vertebral spines, no localized paravertebral muscle spasms, no limitation in the range of movement of the lumbar vertebrae.

Laboratory result(s)

- A complete blood count (CBC), comprehensive metabolic panel (CMP), serum thyroid stimulating hormone (TSH), and 25-hydroxy-vitamin D levels done about 6 weeks ago, as part of her annual medical checkup, were within normal limits.

Multiple choice questions

1. ***In SF's case, the following increase the risk of osteoporosis:***
   A. Female gender.
   B. Caucasian race.
   C. Alcohol consumption.
   D. A and B.
   E. A, B, and C.

   Correct answer: E

   Comments:

   Osteoporosis is the most common metabolic bone disease.[1] It affects both genders and all races, but women more frequently than men, and Caucasians more than Blacks. Fragility fractures are expected to affect about 50% of the female population over the age of 50 years and 25%–30% of the male population.[2]

   Osteoporosis is silent, i.e., asymptomatic, until a fracture is sustained. However, once a fragility fracture is sustained, the risk of further fractures is substantially increased,[3,4] and the long-term outcome often is not good, even after the patient receives excellent orthopedic care. Many patients also enter a downward spiral: pain, limited physical capability, fear of falling, reduced exercise tolerance, withdrawal, unsteadiness, reduced cognitive functions, further gradual withdrawal from physical activities, worsening muscle wasting, sarcopenia, unsteadiness, cognitive impairment, and increased risk of falls and fractures. Once this cycle is entered it is difficult to overcome and reverse.[5]

   An osteoporosis treatment gap has been identified and needs to be addressed: men are less frequently screened for osteoporosis and, compared to women, are less frequently diagnosed and treated.[6,7] Underdiagnosis is a major factor in the development of this treatment gap.[8]

   It is easier, more effective, and cheaper to prevent a fracture than to manage it, rehabilitate the patient, and prevent another fracture from occurring. And yet, many patients with fragility fractures, i.e., the hallmark of osteoporosis, are neither identified nor treated for the osteoporosis.

   Screening is the first step toward identifying patients with, or at risk, of having osteoporosis. To this effect a number of assessment tools have been developed including the Simple Calculated Osteoporosis Risk Estimation (SCORE), Osteoporosis Risk Assessment Instrument (ORAI), Osteoporosis Index of Risk (OSIRIS), DXA-HIP Project, and Osteoporosis Self-Assessment tool.[4,9,10]

   It is sobering to realize that in women over the age of 50years, the projected incidence of osteoporotic fractures exceeds the combined risk of myocardial infarction, strokes, and breast cancer,[11] and yet, osteoporosis remains largely underdiagnosed and undertreated, even after a fragility fracture has occurred. A fragility fracture is defined as a fracture precipitated by trauma that ordinarily would not be expected to result in a fracture.

Sometimes the osteoporotic fracture occurs spontaneously in the absence of trauma or while managing her daily activities and is referred to as "atraumatic fracture."

Women are more susceptible than men to develop osteoporosis, and White women are more at risk of sustaining fractures than African American women. This may be due to several factors including a smaller bone mass, hip axis length, and femoral neck geometry.[12–14] Several other nonmodifiable risk factors affect the risk of fractures, including age, parental history of hip fracture, age of menarche, and menopause.

Seventy to 80% of peak bone mass is genetically determined, and several genes have been associated with osteoporosis and osteoporotic fractures.[15] Twenty to 30% of peak bone mass is determined by nongenetic, potentially reversible factors such as poor nutrition, cigarette smoking, sedentary lifestyles, and lack of physical exercise. Several other risk factors such as older age; parenteral history of fracture, especially hip fractures; age of menarche; and menopause are nonmodifiable. Pregnancy- and lactation-associated osteoporosis has been described. They are nevertheless rare.[16,17]

Alcohol consumption in moderation, i.e., one to two daily serving, is associated with an increased bone density and possibly a reduced fracture risk.[18,19] A cellular mechanism has been advocated for the apparent positive effect of moderate alcohol intake.[20] It is, however, not clear whether these apparent positive effects of moderate alcohol consumption are due to the alcohol intake, per se, or whether they reflect the lifestyle of people who consume alcohol only in moderation, such as leading a more active physical lifestyle and having a better nutritional intake than those who abuse alcohol. Notwithstanding, it is not recommended to encourage nondrinkers to start consuming alcohol to improve their bone health.

In the USA, a standard alcoholic drink is:

12 oz of beer
5 oz of wine
1.5 ounce of spirits

Excessive alcohol consumption, on the other hand, is associated with reduced bone mineral density and increased risk of fractures.[21–24] In addition, excessive alcohol intake interferes with balance, equilibrium, and postural reflexes, thus inducing unsteadiness and increasing the risk of falls and subsequent fractures. Excessive alcohol consumption also has negative effects on gastrointestinal, pancreatic, and hepatic functions which may interfere with the gastrointestinal absorption of calcium, magnesium, and vitamin D metabolism. Excessive alcohol consumption is also often associated with undernutrition and malnutrition. SF consumes alcohol only in moderation, and there is no need to recommend she changes her habits (Table 1).

2. ***SF's low body could be due to:***
   A. The female athlete syndrome.
   B. Anorexia nervosa.

Table 1 Recommended daily calcium and vitamin D intake.[25]

	Calcium		Vitamin D	
Age group	**RDA**[a]	**ULI**[b]	**RDA**[a]	**ULI**[b]
Years	**mg/day**	**mg/day**	**IU/day**	**IU/day**
1–3	700	2500	600	2500
4–8	1000	2500	600	3000
9–18	1300	3000	600	4000
19–50	1000	2500	600	4000
51–70, men	1000	2000	600	4000
51–70, women	1200	2000	600	4000
>70	1200	2000	800	4000

[a]RDA: recommended daily allowance.
[b]ULI: upper level intake.
Adapted from Institute of Medicine (US) Committee to Review Dietary Reference In takes for Vitamin D and Calcium. Ross AC, Taylor CL, Yaktine AL, et al. Dietary Reference Intakes for Calcium and Vitamin D. Washington, DC: National Academic Press; 2011.

C. Malabsorption.
D. Would be significant if she weighed less than she did when she was about 25 years old.
E. B and C.

Correct answer: D

Comments:

As body height, body weight, and body fat are closely intertwined, the Body Mass Index (BMI) is a measure derived from body height and weight and is used in the evaluation of patients with low or elevated body weights. The NIH classifies BMI as follows: underweight: $\leq$18.5, normal weight: 18.5–24.9, overweight: 25–29.9, and obese $\geq$30. SF's BMI is 18.4, marginally below normal.[26] Although all listed conditions are associated with low body weight, it is unlikely that SF has any of these conditions. As she has been menstruating regularly, it is unlikely she has either the female athlete syndrome[27,28] or anorexia nervosa.[29–33] Malabsorption is a possibility. However, in the absence of any other supporting evidence, and given her regular bowel functions, and that she has been previously thoroughly investigated twice for low body weight, malabsorption remains a possibility rather than a probability.[34,35] The normal serum TSH level rules out hyperthyroidism.[36]

A body weight less than 127 pounds, per se, increases the risk of osteoporosis. Similarly, postmenopausal women who weigh less than they did when they were 25 years old have an increased fracture risk (Fig. 1).[14]

Although obese patients are less likely to develop osteoporosis because of the additional weight, obesity may increase the risk of osteoporosis possibly because the

Non-modifiable Risk Factors

- Age[3,11,14,16]
- Gender[11,13,16]
- Ethnicity[1,2]
- Family history of fractures[3,11,13,14]

Modifiable Risk Factors

- Low calcium and vitamin D intake[3,11,13]
- Malnutrition[3,11,13]
- Sedentary lifestyle[60,61]
- Cigarette smoking[37]
- Excessive alcohol[5-10], sodium[30], caffeine [31-34]carbonated drinks[36]
- Quadriceps strength

Intrinsic Factors

- Musculoskeletal disorders
- Neurological disorders
- Cardiovascular disorders
- Respiratory disorders

Extrinsic Factors

- Environmental hazards, including carpet rags, trailing wires
- Inadequate footwear
- Inadequate walking aids

Bone factors

- Bone mineral density[55,56]
- Bone turnover[57,58]
- Hip Axis Length[1]
- Femoral neck angle[2]
- Bone geometry parameters[50]

Inadequate Perception of the Environment

- Inappropriate lighting
- Inadequate glasses
- Glare
- Bifocal glasses

Select Disease States

- Alcohol abuse[5-10]
- Anorexia nervosa[18-22]
- Celiac disease[23-25]
- Cushing's disease[62]
- Depression[63-65]
- Diabetes mellitus[66-67]
- Female athlete syndrome[17]
- Hemiplegia, hemiparesis[68]
- Human immunodeficiency virus[69]
- Hyperparathyroidism[70]
- Hypercalciuria[71,72]
- Hyperthyroidism, including iatrogenic[26]
- Hypogonadism[73,74]
- Hypomagnesemia[75]
- Hypovitaminosis D[76]
- Inflammatory bowel disease[23,24,77]
- Mastocytosis[78]
- Multiple myeloma[79,80]
- Neoplasia[81]
- Obesity[27,28]
- Post bariatric surgery[82,83]
- Post transplant[84]
- Renal impairment[85]
- Rheumatoid arthritis[86]

Select Medications

- Androgen deprivation therapy[89]
- Anti-arrhythmic
- Anticoagulants[90]
- Anticonvulsants[91,92]
- Antiretrovirals[93]
- Aromatase inhibitors[94]
- Cytotoxic/chemotherapy[95]
- Gluco-corticosteroids[96-98]
- Hypnotics
- Hypotensive
- Loop diuretics[99]
- Medroxyprogesterone acetate[100,101]
- Proton pump inhibitors[102-104]
- Psychotropics
- Selective serotonin reuptake inhibitors[105]
- Thiazolidinediones[106]
- Thyroid supplements[102]
- Tricyclic antiepressants[107]

Fig. 1
Factors increasing fracture risk.

increased adipose tissue may be associated with hypovitaminosis D and secondary hyperparathyroidism.[37,38] SF weighs 107 pounds, she is 64″ tall, her BMI is 18.4, just below the normal range.

3. ***Excessive intake of the following increases the risk of bone demineralization and osteoporosis:***
   A. Sodium.
   B. Caffeine.
   C. Phosphoric acid.
   D. A and B
   E. A, B, and C.

   Correct answer: E

   Comments:

All listed food ingredients may induce a negative calcium balance and increase the risk of bone demineralization. Excessive sodium[39] and caffeine intake increases the renal calcium excretion.[40–43] Phosphoric acid, often found in soda and carbonated drinks, binds to calcium in the gastrointestinal track and interferes with the calcium bioavailability.[44] A positive association between caffeine consumption, urinary calcium excretion, and fractures has been documented (Table 2).[45]

A daily protein intake of 0.8 g/kilogram body weight has been shown to minimize postfracture bone demineralization.[46] Cigarette smoking increases the risk of osteoporosis and fractures.[47]

Table 2 Approximate calcium content of select food.[a41]

Calcium content of food, data obtained by surveying labels in food stores	
Milk, 8 oz[b]	300 mg
Milk fortified with calcium, 8 oz	500 mg
Soya milk, 8 oz	500 mg
Chocolate drink with water, 8 oz	300 mg
Chocolate drink with milk, 8 oz	600 mg
Chocolate drink with calcium-fortified milk, 8 oz	800 mg
Orange juice fortified with calcium, 8 oz	300 mg
Yogurt, 6 oz	400 mg
Cheese, 1 slice	100 mg
Cheese, 1 cube, 1″ side	200 mg
Bread, one slice, fortified with calcium	100 mg
Anchovies, 3 oz	125 mg
Sardines, 3 oz	320 mg
Select green vegetables	100 mg

[a]Readers are recommended to check the label of various foods as different brands often contain different amounts of calcium. Food labels usually disclose the % and not mg of calcium. The conversion of % to mg is described in MCQ # 7.
[b]Lactose-free milk, same as milk.

> A well-balanced diet is a sine qua none for the individual to reach and maintain optimum peak bone mass.

4. ***In SF's case, the recommended daily allowance and upper limit intake of calcium are:***
   A. 600 and 2000mg.
   B. 1000 and 2000mg.
   C. 1200 and 2000mg.
   D. 1500 and 2000mg.
   E. There is no upper limit intake: the more calcium one can get, the better it is.

   Correct answer: C

   Comments:

   The Recommended Daily Allowance (RDA) of calcium for women between the ages of 19 and 50years and men between the ages of 19 and 70years is 1000mg.[48] The Upper Level Intake (ULI) or maximum recommended daily intake, especially in the form of tablets, for women 19–50years old is 2500 and for men 19years and older is 2000mg. For women aged 50years and older and men aged 70years and older, the RDA is 1200mg of calcium and the ULI is 2000mg, including calcium obtained from supplements.[48]
   SF's estimated daily calcium intake is at least 1200mg. The calcium content of an eight-ounce glass of milk or calcium-fortified orange juice is about 300mg. A six-ounce cup of yogurt contains about 300mg of calcium. A slice of cheese or a cube of cheese (1in. each side) contains about 100mg. One slice of bread fortified with calcium contains about 100mg of calcium.
5. ***In the USA, on many food packages, the calcium content is expressed as a percentage of the RDA. Converting % to mg:***
   A. In most instances cannot be done given the limited information on the label.
   B. Depends on the type of calcium: carbonate, citrate, gluconate, or lactate.
   C. Is based on an RDA of 1000mg.
   D. Can be done by dropping the % and adding a "0" to the given calcium percentage.
   E. C and D.

   Correct answer: E

   Comments:

   The % RDA is based on a 1000-mg allowance: the RDA for women aged 19–50years and men aged 19–70years.[48] Therefore converting the expressed % to mg can be achieved by dropping the % and replacing it with a "0." For instance, 15% is 150mg and 25% is 250 mg.
6. ***In SF's case, at this stage, the following is/are recommended:***
   A. DXA scan.
   B. qCT lumbar vertebrae.
   C. Ultrasound of the calcaneus.

D. Any of the above.
E. None of the above.

Correct answer: A

Comment:

As SF has few risk factors for osteoporosis, it may be tempting to just reassure her and not to proceed with any further investigation. On the other hand, osteoporosis is a silent disease until a fracture is sustained. But, by that time, it is usually too late, and many patients enter a vicious cycle of further fractures, further handicaps, reduced quality of life, depression, and withdrawal from physical and mental activities. It is, therefore, of paramount importance to prevent fractures, rather than wait until a fracture is sustained and then treat the patient with medication.

Osteoporosis is a silent disease until a fracture occurs

SF is only 51 years old and is at risk of having or developing osteoporosis. She has three major risk factors: first, her ethnicity: Caucasian people tend to have a smaller skeleton than Black people and therefore are more at risk of developing osteoporosis and fracturing a bone. It must nevertheless be emphasized that Black ethnicity, per se, does not offer a protection against osteoporosis. Black people also develop osteoporosis and should be investigated during the asymptomatic phase of osteoporosis, i.e., before a fracture is sustained.

Second, SF is 51 years old and is going through the menopause. This is a critical period in women's lives: they are at risk of losing calcium during the first few years of the menopause, especially if they are not on hormonal replacement therapy. Third, low body weight: even though SF has been investigated twice for low body weight and no underlying pathology has been found, she has a low body weight and is more at risk of sustaining fractures.

On the other hand, SF has a number of factors protecting her from developing osteoporosis and sustaining falls. She also had a normal blood chemistry profile, complete blood picture, serum TSH, and vitamin D levels as assayed prior to seeking medical help for her bone health.

On balance, therefore, it would be appropriate to evaluate SF's bone status. Prevention is better and more effective than treatment and is also much cheaper. Therefore, at this stage, there is a need to further assess/evaluate her bone health, especially as several pharmacological treatments are available: hormonal replacement therapy, raloxifene and bisphosphonates are approved for the prevention of osteoporosis. Undertaking that evaluation also emphasizes to the patient the importance of prevention in the management and prevention of osteoporosis.

7. ***The following is/are true about the FRAX (Fracture Risk Assessment):***
   A. It is a web-based algorithm available, free of charge, but restricted to health care professionals.
   B. It estimates the individual's risk of sustaining fractures of the hip or major fractures in the following 10 years.
   C. It can be calculated with or without including the patient's BMD or T-score of the lumbar vertebrae, femoral neck, or distal one-third radius site.
   D. A, B, and C.
   E. A and B.

   Correct answer: B

   Comments:

   The FRAX tool is an algorithm developed under the auspices of the World Health Organization and unveiled in February 2008.[49,50] It is available on the web, free of charge to all interested parties. The FRAX permutation estimates the risk of sustaining a hip or major fracture within the next 10 years based on the subject's ethnic group, age, gender, weight, height, and seven clinical risk factors: history of fractures, parental history of hip fracture, cigarette smoking, glucocorticoid intake, rheumatoid arthritis, secondary osteoporosis, and excessive alcohol intake.[49,50] It can be calculated with or without BMD/ T-scores of the femoral neck.

   Concern, nevertheless, has been expressed that the FRAX score, calculated without BMD, may fail to identify many women, especially under the age of 65 years, who have osteoporosis and therefore would benefit from a DXA scan.[51] Similarly, in men, by using the FRAX score calculated without BMD, many patients whose fracture risk is increased will not be detected.[52]

8. ***The main strength of the FRAX permutation include:***
   A. It is race and country specific.
   B. It identifies those patients likely to benefit from therapy for osteoporosis.
   C. Its results override the densitometric findings.
   D. B and C.
   E. A, B, and C.

   Correct answer: E

   Comments:

   The FRAX database is gender, race, and country specific. It permutates the patient's risk of sustaining a hip fracture or a major fracture in the following 10years. This estimation is specific for the patient and cannot be extrapolated to other individuals. In order to have maximum impact on the patient or other interested parties, the likelihood of sustaining a fracture is expressed as a percentage. Thresholds also have been established. In the USA, the threshold for recommending the prescription of medication for osteoporosis is 3% for the risk of hip fracture and/or 20% for the risk of major fractures. These thresholds override the densitometric data.[53]

9. ***The following technologies can be used to screen for osteoporosis:***
   A. Digital X-ray Radiogrammetry (DXR).
   B. Quantitative Ultrasound (QUS).
   C. Peripheral DXA phalanges (pDXA).
   D. All of the above.
   E. None of the above.

   Correct answer: D

   Comment:

   Digital X-ray radiogrammetry is a radiological method to assess bone mass of the middle three metacarpal bones of the nondominant hand. It is based on calculating the midpoint width and length of the metacarpal bone and ratio between cortical and trabecular bone.[54–56] Quantitative ultrasound (QUS) studies measure the speed of sound waves (SOS) as transmitted across a bone, typically the calcaneus, and the degree of attenuation (BUA: Broadband ultrasound attenuation). The denser the bone, the quicker is the transmission of sound waves and the less the attenuation.[54,57] Peripheral DXA of the phalanges uses the same technology as DXA but scans the phalanges instead of the lumbar vertebrae, proximal femur, and radius.[54,58]

   The main advantages of these techniques include low cost, portability, convenience, low or no exposure to radiation, short time required to complete the test, and low level of expertise required to perform the scan and interpret the data. DXR also has the added advantage of ready availability as it can be performed with conventional radiology or mammography equipment. QUS and pDXA have gained popularity in health fairs.

   As a good correlation exists between BMD of the calcaneus, DXR, QUS, and pDXA parameters and fracture risk, including hip fracture risk, the results of these tests can be used to estimate fracture risk.[59,60] The main concern with these technologies, however, is the false negative and false positive results. Besides, they can be used neither for diagnostic purposes, nor to monitor the patient's progress.[61]

10. ***Recommendations for screening for osteoporosis include:***
   A. Women aged 65 years and older, even if they have no risk factors for osteoporosis.
   B. Men aged 70 years and older, even if they have no risk factors for osteoporosis.
   C. Adults over the age of 50 years who have risk factors for osteoporosis.
   D. A and B.
   E. A, B, and C.

   Correct answer: E

   Comments:

   Several organizations, including the American College of Endocrinology,[62] National Osteoporosis Foundation (NOF),[63] International Society for Clinical Densitometry (ISCD),[64] American College of Preventive Medicine,[65] and American Association of Clinical Endocrinologists (AACE)[66] recommend screening asymptomatic women aged 65years as well as adults over the age of 50years who have risk factors for osteoporosis or have sustained fractures. NOF[63] and ISCD[64] also recommend screening asymptomatic men aged 70 years and older for osteoporosis even if they have no risk factors for osteoporosis.

The US Preventive Services Task Force[67] recommends screening for osteoporosis in the following groups, regardless of ethnicity:

- Women aged 65 years and older
- Women between the ages of 50 and 65 years if their risk of sustaining a major fracture in the following 10 years (as determined by the FRAX tool, calculated without BMD) is or exceeds the threshold of 9.3% which is the estimated risk of sustaining a major osteoporotic fracture in a hypothetical 65-year-old Caucasian woman who has no additional risk factors for osteoporosis.
- Women 50 years old and older with a BMI less than 21 kg/m^2, daily alcohol use, and parental fracture history.
- Women 55 years old and older with a parental fracture history.
- Women 60 years and older with a BMI less than 21 kg/m^2 and daily alcohol use.
- Women 60 years and older, current cigarette smoker, and daily alcohol intake.

Based on several studies a strategy for universal DXA measurement has been proposed and pharmacological treatment for osteoporosis recommended if the 10-year FRAX score (including BMD measurement and FRAX permutation) is or exceeds 3% for a hip or 20% for major fractures. This cutoff point was selected based on the statistical analysis suggesting that it prevents the greatest number of hip fractures while maintaining acceptable the Numbers Needed to Treat (NNT).[63–68] This threshold is in line with other population studies.

Concern, nevertheless, has been expressed that the FRAX tool alone may not identify many women under the age of 65 years who may benefit from medication for osteoporosis.[51] A number of algorithms have been developed, some are self-administered, to identify those at risk of sustaining fractures.[10]

SF has not lost any height, a relevant finding as loss of height may reflect vertebral compression fractures.[69] There is no evidence of kyphosis, and she has not sustained any fracture which increases the risk of future fractures.[70] Therefore, apart from her low body weight/BMI, SF has very few risk factors for osteoporosis.[71–73] She has an adequate daily calcium intake, leads a physically active lifestyle, exercises regularly, does not consume an excessive amount of sodium or caffeine, does not abuse alcohol, and does not smoke cigarettes. Finally, given her medical history, essentially normal physical examination, and laboratory investigations, it may be tempting to dismiss her and recommend a DXA scan when she is 65 years old.

On the other hand, SF has a low body weight and is going through the menopause which may be associated with bone loss and may further be complicated by a fracture. Once a fracture is sustained, others are likely to follow. A study on 377,561 Medicare beneficiaries revealed that 10% of those who fractured sustained another fracture within a year, 18% within 2 years, and 31% within 5 years.[74]

Osteoporosis is also a silent disease that satisfies all the criteria of a successful, cost-effective, screening program/campaign: First, it is very prevalent: about half the female population over the age of 50 years and a third to one half of the male population over the age of 70 years have osteoporosis and are expected to sustain one or more fragility fracture. In other words, at least half the female population attending an average adult Primary Care, Internal Medicine, or Family Medicine Clinic has osteoporosis. Potential success rate is therefore very high: 50%, i.e., one in two patients attending one of these clinics is likely to have osteoporosis. The odds are still higher in Geriatric Medicine Clinics.

Second, the diagnosis of osteoporosis is very simple, noninvasive, and relatively cheap, with little chance of false positive or false negative results. Third, a number of medications are available that have been shown to significantly reduce the risk of fractures. Finally, the adverse effect profile of many medications for osteoporosis is tolerable.

Conclusion

Taking all these facts into consideration, a screening DXA scan was offered. SF readily accepted the offer. The DXA scan was within normal limits. She was congratulated and a repeat scan was offered in 2 years' time to assess any postmenopausal bone loss. It may be argued that in SF's case the DXA scan was not a "screening" scan but was part of the medical management of her clinical condition: low body weight and postmenopausal status.

Key points

Screening for osteoporosis is indicated in[63–67]:

- Women 65 years of age and older, even if there are no risk factors for osteoporosis.
- Men 70 years of age and older, even if there are no risk factors for osteoporosis.
- Adults between the ages of 50 and 65 if they have risk factors for osteoporosis.
- Adults who have sustained a fracture.
- Adults with a disease predisposing to bone demineralization.
- Adults on medication predisposing to low bone mass.

References

1. LeBoff MS, Greenspan SL, Insogna KL, et al. The Clinician's guide to prevention and treatment of osteoporosis. *Osteoporos Int*. 2022;33:2049–2102.
2. Baim S, Blank R. Approaches to fracture risk assessment and prevention. *Curr Osteoporos Rep*. 2021;19(2):158–165. https://doi.org/10.1007/s11914-021-00659-x.

3. Kanis JA, Johansson H, Harvey NC, et al. The effect on subsequent fracture risk of age, sex, and prior fracture site by recency of prior fracture. *Osteoporos Int.* 2021;32(8):1547–1555. https://doi.org/10.1007/s00198-020-05803-4.
4. Iconaru L, Moreau M, Baleanu F, et al. Risk factors for imminent fractures: a sub study of the FRISBEE cohort. *Osteoporos Int.* 2021;32(6):1093–1101. https://doi.org/10.1007/s00198-020-05772-8.
5. Shorey S, Chan V. Women living with osteoporosis: a meta-synthesis. *Gerontologist.* 2021;61(3):e39–e47. https://doi.org/10.1093/geront/gnz173.
6. Leslie WD, Lix LM, Binkley N. Comparison of screening tools for optimizing fracture prevention in Canada. *Arch Osteoporos.* 2020;15(1):170. Published 2020 October 27 https://doi.org/10.1007/s11657-020-00846-w.
7. Sirufo MM, Ginaldi L, De Martinis M. Bone health in men: still suffer the gender gap. *Osteoporos Int.* 2021;32 (4):791. https://doi.org/10.1007/s00198-021-05843-4.
8. McCloskey E, Rathi J, Heijmans S, et al. The osteoporosis treatment gap in patients at risk of fracture in European primary care: a multi-country cross-sectional observational study. *Osteoporos Int.* 2021;32 (2):251–259. https://doi.org/10.1007/s00198-020-05557-z.
9. Yong EL, Logan S. Menopausal osteoporosis: screening, prevention and treatment. *Singapore Med J.* 2021;62 (4):159–166. https://doi.org/10.11622/smedj.2021036.
10. Erjiang E, Wang T, Yang L, et al. Utility of osteoporosis self-assessment tool as a screening tool for osteoporosis in Irish men and women: results of the DXA-HIP project. *J Clin Densitom.* 2021;24(4):516–526. https://doi.org/10.1016/j.jocd.2021.03.003.
11. Cauley JA, Wampler NS, Barnhart JM, et al. Incidence of fractures compared to cardiovascular disease and breast cancer: the Women's Health Initiative observational study. *Osteoporos Int.* 2008;19(12):1717–1723. https://doi.org/10.1007/s00198-008-0634-y.
12. Cummings SR, Cauley JA, Palermo L, et al. Racial differences in hip Axis lengths might explain racial differences in rates of hip fracture. Study of Osteoporotic Fractures Research Group. *Osteoporos Int.* 1994;4 (4):226–229. https://doi.org/10.1007/BF01623243.
13. Kim KM, Brown JK, Kim KJ, et al. Differences in femoral neck geometry associated with age and ethnicity. *Osteoporos Int.* 2011;22(7):2165–2174. https://doi.org/10.1007/s00198-010-1459-z.
14. Cummings SR, Nevitt MC, Browner WS, et al. Risk factors for hip fracture in white women. Study of Osteoporotic Fractures Research Group. *N Engl J Med.* 1995;332(12):767–773. https://doi.org/10.1056/NEJM199503233321202.
15. Richards JB, Kavvoura FK, Rivadeneira F, et al. Collaborative meta-analysis: associations of 150 candidate genes with osteoporosis and osteoporotic fracture. *Ann Intern Med.* 2009;151(8):528–537. https://doi.org/10.7326/0003-4819-151-8-200910200-00006.
16. Bazgir N, Shafiei E, Hashemi N, Nourmohamadi H. Woman with pregnancy and lactation-associated osteoporosis (PLO). *Case Rep Obstet Gynecol.* 2020;2020:8836583. Published 2020 Nov 12 https://doi.org/10.1155/2020/8836583.
17. Yun KY, Han SE, Kim SC, Joo JK, Lee KS. Pregnancy-related osteoporosis and spinal fractures. *Obstet Gynecol Sci.* 2017;60(1):133–137. https://doi.org/10.5468/ogs.2017.60.1.133.
18. Berg KM, Kunins HV, Jackson JL, et al. Association between alcohol consumption and both osteoporotic fracture and bone density. *Am J Med.* 2008;121(5):406–418. https://doi.org/10.1016/j.amjmed.2007.12.012.
19. Wosje KS, Kalkwarf HJ. Bone density in relation to alcohol intake among men and women in the United States. *Osteoporos Int.* 2007;18(3):391–400. https://doi.org/10.1007/s00198-006-0249-0.
20. Marrone JA, Maddalozzo GF, Branscum AJ, et al. Moderate alcohol intake lowers biochemical markers of bone turnover in postmenopausal women. *Menopause.* 2012;19(9):974–979. https://doi.org/10.1097/GME.0b013e31824ac071.
21. Kanis JA, Johansson H, Johnell O, et al. Alcohol intake as a risk factor for fracture. *Osteoporos Int.* 2005;16 (7):737–742. https://doi.org/10.1007/s00198-004-1734-y.
22. Sampson HW. Alcohol and other factors affecting osteoporosis risk in women. *Alcohol Res Health.* 2002;26 (4):292–298.
23. Maurel DB, Boisseau N, Benhamou CL, Jaffre C. Alcohol and bone: review of dose effects and mechanisms. *Osteoporos Int.* 2012;23(1):1–16. https://doi.org/10.1007/s00198-011-1787-7.

24. Kanis JA, Borgstrom F, De Laet C, et al. Assessment of fracture risk. *Osteoporos Int.* 2005;16(6):581–589. https://doi.org/10.1007/s00198-004-1780-5.
25. Institute of Medicine (US) Committee to Review Dietary Reference Intakes for Vitamin D and Calcium. In: Ross AC, Taylor CL, Yaktine AL, Del Valle HB, eds. *Dietary Reference Intakes for Calcium and Vitamin D.* Washington (DC): National Academies Press (US); 2011.
26. Weir CB, Jan A. BMI classification percentile and cut off points [Updated 2021 June 29]. In: *StatPearls.* Treasure Island (FL): StatPearls Publishing; 2022. [Internet]. Available from: https://www.ncbi.nlm.nih.gov/books/NBK541070/.
27. Nattiv A, Loucks AB, Manore MM, et al. American College of Sports Medicine position stand: the female athlete triad. *Med Sci Sports Exerc.* 2007;39(10):1867–1882. https://doi.org/10.1249/mss.0b013e318149f111.
28. Thein-Nissenbaum J, Hammer E. Treatment strategies for the female athlete triad in the adolescent athlete: current perspectives. Open access. *J Sports Med.* 2017;8:85–95. Published 2017 April 4 https://doi.org/10.2147/OAJSM.S100026.
29. Dalle GR. Eating disorders: progress and challenges. *Eur J Intern Med.* 2011;22(2):153–160. https://doi.org/10.1016/j.ejim.2010.12.010.
30. Warren MP. Endocrine manifestations of eating disorders. *J Clin Endocrinol Metab.* 2011;96(2):333–343. https://doi.org/10.1210/jc.2009-2304.
31. Misra M, Klibanski A. Anorexia nervosa and bone. *J Endocrinol.* 2014;221(3):R163–R176. https://doi.org/10.1530/JOE-14-0039.
32. Grinspoon S, Thomas E, Pitts S, et al. Prevalence and predictive factors for regional osteopenia in women with anorexia nervosa. *Ann Intern Med.* 2000;133(10):790–794. https://doi.org/10.7326/0003-4819-133-10-200011210-00011.
33. Vestergaard P, Emborg C, Støving RK, Hagen C, Mosekilde L, Brixen K. Fractures in patients with anorexia nervosa, bulimia nervosa, and other eating disorders—a Nationwide register study. *Int J Eat Disord.* 2002;32(3):301–308. https://doi.org/10.1002/eat.10101.
34. Stenson WF, Newberry R, Lorenz R, Baldus C, Civitelli R. Increased prevalence of celiac disease and need for routine screening among patients with osteoporosis. *Arch Intern Med.* 2005;165(4):393–399. https://doi.org/10.1001/archinte.165.4.393.
35. Bernstein CN, Leslie WD, Leboff MS. AGA technical review on osteoporosis in gastrointestinal diseases. *Gastroenterology.* 2003;124(3):795–841. https://doi.org/10.1053/gast.2003.50106.
36. Bassett JH, O'Shea PJ, Sriskantharajah S, et al. Thyroid hormone excess rather than thyrotropin deficiency induces osteoporosis in hyperthyroidism. *Mol Endocrinol.* 2007;21(5):1095–1107. https://doi.org/10.1210/me.2007-0033.
37. Compston JE, Watts NB, Chapurlat R, et al. Obesity is not protective against fracture in postmenopausal women: GLOW. *Am J Med.* 2011;124(11):1043–1050. https://doi.org/10.1016/j.amjmed.2011.06.013.
38. Premaor MO, Pilbrow L, Tonkin C, Parker RA, Compston J. Obesity and fractures in postmenopausal women. *J Bone Miner Res.* 2010;25(2):292–297. https://doi.org/10.1359/jbmr.091004.
39. Heaney RP. Role of dietary sodium in osteoporosis. *J Am Coll Nutr.* 2006;25(3 Suppl):271S–276S. https://doi.org/10.1080/07315724.2006.10719577.
40. Tsuang YH, Sun JS, Chen LT, Sun SC, Chen SC. Direct effects of caffeine on osteoblastic cells metabolism: the possible causal effect of caffeine on the formation of osteoporosis. *J Orthop Surg Res.* 2006;1:7. Published 2006 October 7 https://doi.org/10.1186/1749-799X-1-7.
41. Rapuri PB, Gallagher JC, Kinyamu HK, Ryschon KL. Caffeine intake increases the rate of bone loss in elderly women and interacts with vitamin D receptor genotypes. *Am J Clin Nutr.* 2001;74(5):694–700. https://doi.org/10.1093/ajcn/74.5.694.
42. Barger-Lux MJ, Heaney RP. Caffeine and the calcium economy revisited. *Osteoporos Int.* 1995;5(2):97–102. https://doi.org/10.1007/BF01623310.
43. Kynast-Gales SA, Massey LK. Effect of caffeine on circadian excretion of urinary calcium and magnesium. *J Am Coll Nutr.* 1994;13(5):467–472. https://doi.org/10.1080/07315724.1994.10718436.
44. Hallström H, Wolk A, Glynn A, Michaëlsson K. Coffee, tea and caffeine consumption in relation to osteoporotic fracture risk in a cohort of Swedish women. *Osteoporos Int.* 2006;17(7):1055–1064. https://doi.org/10.1007/s00198-006-0109-y.

45. Heaney RP, Rafferty K. Carbonated beverages and urinary calcium excretion. *Am J Clin Nutr*. 2001;74 (3):343–347. https://doi.org/10.1093/ajcn/74.3.343.
46. Rizzoli R, Ammann P, Chevalley T, Bonjour JP. Protein intake and bone disorders in the elderly. *Joint Bone Spine*. 2001;68(5):383–392. https://doi.org/10.1016/s1297-319x(01)00295-0.
47. Ward KD, Klesges RC. A meta-analysis of the effects of cigarette smoking on bone mineral density. *Calcif Tissue Int*. 2001;68(5):259–270. https://doi.org/10.1007/BF02390832.
48. National Institutes of Health. Calcium. https://ods.od.nih.gov/factsheets/Calcium-HealthProfessional/. Accessed 11 May 2022.
49. Kanis JA, Harvey NC, McCloskey E, et al. Algorithm for the management of patients at low, high and very high risk of osteoporotic fractures. *Osteoporos Int*. 2020;31(1):1–12. https://doi.org/10.1007/s00198-019-05176-3.
50. Kanis JA, Johansson H, Oden A, McCloskey EV. Assessment of fracture risk. *Eur J Radiol*. 2009;71 (3):392–397. https://doi.org/10.1016/j.ejrad.2008.04.061.
51. Ghannam S, Blaney H, Gelfond J, Bruder JM. The use of FRAX in identifying women less than 65 years needing bone mineral density testing. *J Clin Densitom*. 2021;24(1):36–43. https://doi.org/10.1016/j.jocd.2020.05.002.
52. Hamdy RC, Seier E, Whalen K, Clark WA, Hicks K, Piggee TB. FRAX calculated without BMD does not correctly identify Caucasian men with densitometric evidence of osteoporosis. *Osteoporos Int*. 2018;29 (4):947–952. https://doi.org/10.1007/s00198-017-4368-6.
53. Kanis JA, Cooper C, Rizzoli R, Reginster JY, Scientific Advisory Board of the European Society for Clinical and Economic Aspects of Osteoporosis (ESCEO) and the Committees of Scientific Advisors and National Societies of the International Osteoporosis Foundation (IOF). European guidance for the diagnosis and management of osteoporosis in postmenopausal women [published correction appears in Osteoporos Int. 2020 January;31(1):209] [published correction appears in Osteoporos Int. 2020 April;31(4):801]. *Osteoporos Int*. 2019;30(1):3–44. https://doi.org/10.1007/s00198-018-4704-5.
54. Bonnick SL. Bone Densitometry in Clinical Practice: Application and Interpretation. 2nd ed. Humana Press; 2004.
55. Dhainaut A, Rohde GE, Syversen U, Johnsen V, Haugeberg G. The ability of hand digital X-ray radiogrammetry to identify middle-aged and elderly women with reduced bone density, as assessed by femoral neck dual-energy X-ray absorptiometry. *J Clin Densitom*. 2010;13(4):418–425. https://doi.org/10.1016/j.jocd.2010.07.005.
56. Wilczek ML, Kälvesten J, Algulin J, Beiki O, Brismar TB. Digital X-ray radiogrammetry of hand or wrist radiographs can predict hip fracture risk—a study In 5,420 women and 2,837 men. *Eur Radiol*. 2013;23 (5):1383–1391. https://doi.org/10.1007/s00330-012-2706-9.
57. Pisani P, Renna MD, Conversano F, et al. Screening and early diagnosis of osteoporosis through X-ray and ultrasound based techniques. *World J Radiol*. 2013;5(11):398–410. https://doi.org/10.4329/wjr.v5.i11.398.
58. Hans DB, Shepherd JA, Schwartz EN, et al. Peripheral dual-energy X-ray absorptiometry in the management of osteoporosis: the 2007 ISCD official positions. *J Clin Densitom*. 2008;11(1):188–206. https://doi.org/10.1016/j.jocd.2007.12.012.
59. Krieg MA, Cornuz J, Ruffieux C, et al. Prediction of hip fracture risk by quantitative ultrasound in more than 7000 Swiss women > or =70 years of age: comparison of three technologically different bone ultrasound devices in the SEMOF study. *J Bone Miner Res*. 2006;21(9):1457–1463. https://doi.org/10.1359/jbmr.060615.
60. Chan MY, Nguyen ND, Center JR, Eisman JA, Nguyen TV. Quantitative ultrasound and fracture risk prediction in non-osteoporotic men and women as defined by WHO criteria. *Osteoporos Int*. 2013;24(3):1015–1022. https://doi.org/10.1007/s00198-012-2001-2.
61. Briot K, Roux C. What is the role of DXA, QUS and bone markers in fracture prediction, treatment allocation and monitoring? *Best Pract Res Clin Rheumatol*. 2005;19(6):951–964. https://doi.org/10.1016/j.berh.2005.06.004.
62. Camacho PM, Petak SM, Binkley N, et al. American Association of Clinical Endocrinologists/American College of Endocrinology Clinical Practice Guidelines for the diagnosis and treatment of postmenopausal Osteoporosis-2020 update. *Endocr Pract*. 2020;26(Suppl. 1):1–46. https://doi.org/10.4158/GL-2020-0524SUPPL.
63. Cosman F, de Beur SJ, LeBoff MS, et al. Clinician's guide to prevention and treatment of osteoporosis [published correction appears in Osteoporos Int. 2015 July;26(7):2045–7]. *Osteoporos Int*. 2014;25 (10):2359–2381. https://doi.org/10.1007/s00198-014-2794-2.

64. Schousboe JT, Shepherd JA, Bilezikian JP, Baim S. Executive summary of the 2013 ISCD position development conference on bone densitometry. *JCD*. 2013;16(4):455–466.
65. Lim LS, Hoeksema LJ, Sherin K, ACPM Prevention Practice Committee. Screening for osteoporosis in the adult U.S. population: ACPM position statement on preventive practice. *Am J Prev Med*. 2009;36(4):366–375. https://doi.org/10.1016/j.amepre.2009.01.013.
66. Watts NB, Bilezikian JP, Camacho PM, et al. American Association of Clinical Endocrinologists Medical Guidelines for clinical practice for the diagnosis and treatment of postmenopausal osteoporosis. *Endocr Pract*. 2010;16(Suppl. 3):1–37. https://doi.org/10.4158/ep.16.s3.1.
67. U.S. Preventive Services Task Force. Screening for osteoporosis: U.S. preventive services task force recommendation statement. *Ann Intern Med*. 2011;154(5):356–364. https://doi.org/10.7326/0003-4819-154-5-201103010-00307.
68. Kwok TCY, Law SW, Leung EMF, et al. Hip fractures are preventable: a proposal for osteoporosis screening and fall prevention in older people. *Hong Kong Med J*. 2020;26(3):227–235. https://doi.org/10.12809/hkmj198337.
69. Bennani L, Allali F, Rostom S, et al. Relationship between historical height loss and vertebral fractures in postmenopausal women. *Clin Rheumatol*. 2009;28(11):1283–1289. https://doi.org/10.1007/s10067-009-1236-6.
70. Chapurlat RD, Bauer DC, Nevitt M, Stone K, Cummings SR. Incidence and risk factors for a second hip fracture in elderly women. The study of osteoporotic fractures. *Osteoporos Int*. 2003;14(2):130–136. https://doi.org/10.1007/s00198-002-1327-6.
71. Siris ES, Brenneman SK, Barrett-Connor E, et al. The effect of age and bone mineral density on the absolute, excess, and relative risk of fracture in postmenopausal women aged 50-99: results from the National Osteoporosis Risk Assessment (NORA). *Osteoporos Int*. 2006;17(4):565–574. https://doi.org/10.1007/s00198-005-0027-4.
72. Schnatz PF, Marakovits KA, O'Sullivan DM. Assessment of postmenopausal women and significant risk factors for osteoporosis. *Obstet Gynecol Surv*. 2010;65(9):591–596. https://doi.org/10.1097/OGX.0b013e3181fc6d30.
73. Kanis JA, Johnell O, De Laet C, et al. A meta-analysis of previous fracture and subsequent fracture risk. *Bone*. 2004;35(2):375–382. https://doi.org/10.1016/j.bone.2004.03.024.
74. Balasubramanian A, Zhang J, Chen L, et al. Risk of subsequent fracture after prior fracture among older women. *Osteoporos Int*. 2019;30(1):79–92. https://doi.org/10.1007/s00198-018-4732-1.

SECTION 2

Pharmacological treatment

CHAPTER 11

Oral bisphosphonates—Initiating and maintaining treatment☆

Learning objectives

- The pharmacology profile of orally administered bisphosphonates.
- Initiating and maintaining pharmacologic treatment with oral bisphosphonates.

The case study

Reason for seeking medical help

- BJ, a retired schoolteacher, is referred for the management of osteoporosis recently diagnosed by bone densitometry performed because her sister fractured her distal right radius and two ribs after tripping on a small rug in her granddaughter's bedroom. BJ also has a strong family history of osteoporosis: her mother, both grandmothers, older sister, and cousin sustained fragility fractures. BJ is, however, asymptomatic and did not sustain any fracture. She also has not experienced any dizzy spells.

Past medical and surgical history

- Natural menopause at age 48 years, no hormonal replacement therapy.
- Menarche at age 13, regular menstrual periods.
- Always enjoyed good health.

Lifestyle

- For the past 14 years she adopted a physically active lifestyle: jogging and gardening daily, weather permitting. Prior to this she led a largely sedentary lifestyle.

☆ BJ, 63-year-old African American woman with osteoporosis.

Diagnosis and Treatment of Osteoporosis. https://doi.org/10.1016/B978-0-323-99550-4.00018-6
Copyright © 2024 Elsevier Inc. All rights are reserved, including those for text and data mining, AI training, and similar technologies.

- Estimated daily dietary calcium intake: average 1000 mg.
- No cigarette smoking.
- No alcohol abuse.
- No excessive sodium or caffeine intake.
- She experienced neither falls nor near-falls.

Medication(s)

- Multivitamin tablets once a day.
- Cholecalciferol tablets 400 units daily.

Family history

- Positive for osteoporosis, as outlined before.
- Two healthy children aged 20 and 16 years.

Clinical examination

- Weight 141 pounds, steady, height 62″, used to be 63″, arm span 62″.
- Mild kyphosis, largely postural.
- No significant clinical findings. BP: 155/81 sitting, 162/82 standing. No evidence of orthostasis, sensitive carotid sinus, vertebrobasilar insufficiency, carotid stenosis, heart failure, arthropathy, and no localizing neurological lesions. Trachea central, no adventitious sounds. Thyroid gland not palpable. No evidence of peripheral vascular insufficiency.
- Get-up-and-Go test completed in 8 s.

Laboratory result(s)

- Comprehensive metabolic panel (CMP): no abnormal finding.
- Serum 25-hydroxy-vitamin D: normal at 42 ng/mL.

DXA and radiological result(s)

- T-scores: right femoral neck −2.7, right total hip −2.3, left femoral neck −2.6, left total hip −2.1, lumbar vertebrae −2.8.
- Vertebral fracture assessment: no evidence of vertebral compression fractures.

Multiple choice questions

1. ***In BJ's case, the following is/are correct:***
   A. The diagnosis is osteoporosis, as per bone densitometry results: lowest T-scores −2.8 at the upper four lumbar vertebrae.

B. Her fracture risk is elevated.
C. As she is essentially asymptomatic, there is no need for any medication for her bones.
D. A and B.
E. A, B, and C.

Correct answer: D

Comment:

The densitometric diagnosis is osteoporosis and is discussed in other chapters. Osteoporosis is essentially an asymptomatic disease until a fracture occurs. The goal of treating asymptomatic patients with osteoporosis, i.e., before a fracture is sustained, is to avoid the increased mortality and morbidity associated with fractures. It must be emphasized that in older people, even under excellent circumstances, fractures, traumatic as well as fragility fractures, are associated with a poor long-term prognosis. Our present armamentarium includes effective medications with a good safely profile and a reasonable cost. Unfortunately, many patients with osteoporosis are still neither diagnosed nor treated for osteoporosis.

2. ***At this stage, in BJ's case, the following medications are recommended as a first choice for her osteoporosis:***
   A. Bisphosphonates, teriparatide, abaloparatide, denosumab, romosozumab, or raloxifene.
   B. Bisphosphonates, teriparatide, abaloparatide, denosumab, or romosozumab.
   C. Bisphosphonates, teriparatide, abaloparatide, or denosumab.
   D. Bisphosphonates or denosumab.
   E. Bisphosphonates.

Correct answer: D

Comments:

BJ's lowest T-score is −2.8 in the upper four lumbar vertebrae. She therefore has densitometric evidence of osteoporosis and is at risk of sustaining fragility fractures, i.e., fractures resulting from trauma that ordinarily would not be expected to result in a fracture: low trauma or low impact fractures. Fragility fractures also can develop spontaneously in the absence of any trauma: atraumatic fractures.

In BJ's case, medications that have been shown to effectively reduce the risk of fractures, especially hip fractures, should be the first choice. The long-term impact of a hip fracture is poor, even if the immediate outcome is excellent: most patients undergoing surgery are able to resume their daily activities, but, in time, the majority sustain more fractures.

A two-year retrospective study on 115,776 patients (72.3% women) showed that hip fractures were the most common second fracture (27.8%). Median time from index to second hip fracture was about 1.5years. In addition, 71.9% of patients with an index hip fracture experienced postsurgery complications. In this group, one-year mortality from any cause after the index hip fracture was 26.2%.[1] Therefore any fracture, especially hip fracture, should be a wake-up call to diagnose and treat osteoporosis. Raloxifene has not been shown to reduce the risk of hip fractures and therefore should not be considered as first-line therapy for BJ. Similarly, ibandronate has been shown to reduce the risk of hip and nonvertebral fractures only in patients with T-scores −3.0 and lower.[2]

Given the patient's age, and time since menopause, it is probable that her skeleton is going through the phase of increased bone resorption and therefore should benefit more from an antiresorptive medication than from an osteoanabolic medication. If there is any doubt, assaying the markers of bone formation and bone resorption should be helpful to confirm the patient's bone status. This information can also be used to motivate the patient to comply with the intake of the orally administered bisphosphonate.

3. ***In BJ's case, the following bisphosphonate should be first choice:***
   A. Alendronate or risedronate.
   B. Ibandronate.
   C. Zoledronic acid.
   D. Any of the above.
   E. A or C.

   Correct answer: E

   Comment:

   The major pivotal trials with fractures as end points have shown that whereas all bisphosphonates reduce the risk of vertebral fractures, not all reduce the risk of hip fracture. Placebo controlled, double-blind, randomized clinical trials have shown that alendronate,[3] risedronate,[4] and zoledronic acid[5] significantly reduce the risk of hip and vertebral fractures. A major clinical trial on ibandronate did not show significant hip fracture risk reductions,[6] although, a subsequent post hoc analysis showed a reduced hip fracture risk in patients with a T-score lower than −3.0.[2]

4. ***Bisphosphonates reduce bone resorption by:***
   A. Selective osteoclast intracellular enzyme inhibition.
   B. Inducing osteoclast apoptosis.
   C. Inhibiting osteoclast activation.
   D. A and B.
   E. A, B, and C.

   Correct answer: E

   Comment:

   Bisphosphonates selectively inhibit the osteoclast intracellular farnesyl pyrophosphate synthase enzyme thus preventing downstream protein prenylation, inhibiting osteoclastic activity, and leading to osteoclast apoptosis.[7]

5. ***Bisphosphonates:***
   A. All have the same basic chemical structure.
   B. Side chains determine their binding affinity and biological half-life.
   C. Side chains determine their enzyme inhibitory activity and antiresorptive potency.

D. B and C.
E. A, B, and C.

Correct answer: E

Comment:

All bisphosphonates have the same basic chemical structure: two phosphonic acid molecules joined to a carbon atom and two side chains. The side chains determine the degree of osteoclastic intracellular enzyme inhibition and affinity of the bisphosphonate to hydroxyapatite crystals. Differences in side chains are responsible for different pharmacologic profiles. Osteoclast enzymatic inhibition is highest with zoledronic acid followed by risedronate, ibandronate, and alendronate. Binding affinity is highest with zoledronic acid followed by alendronate, ibandronate, and risedronate.[8,9]

6. ***Alendronate for the treatment of osteoporosis:***
A. Orally administered, 70 mg, once a week.
B. The tablet should be taken with food to minimize GI adverse effects.
C. At least one hour must elapse between bisphosphonate intake and food intake.
D. All of the above.
E. A and B.

Correct answer: A

Comment:

As only 0.6%–3% of the orally administered bisphosphonate is absorbed through the gastrointestinal tract,[10] any interference with absorption may impact the bioavailability of orally administered bisphosphonates. It is therefore important to ensure the patient takes the medication exactly as directed:

- While fasting and with no other medication, food, or beverage (except water) to prevent food particles or other medications from adhering to the bisphosphonate tablet and interfering with its already low gastrointestinal absorption. As often tap water, bottled water, and especially well water contain impurities or additives, it may be advantageous to take the bisphosphonate with distilled water to ensure least interference and maximal absorption.
- The oral bisphosphonate tablet should be taken with six ounces of water to avoid the tablet adhering to the mucosa in the esophagus and to ensure maximal dispersion and absorption of the bisphosphonate in the stomach.
- After taking the oral bisphosphonate tablet, the patient should refrain from eating or drinking any beverage apart from water for 30 min after taking alendronate or risedronate, or 60 min after ibandronate, to ensure maximal dispersion and absorption of the bisphosphonate. There is therefore no need to fast for longer periods of time.
- Having breakfast, preferably a high fiber breakfast, 30min after taking alendronate or risedronate (60min after ibandronate) ensures that whatever part of the tablet that has not been absorbed in the stomach is coated with the fiber-rich breakfast ingested and

will not irritate the gastrointestinal mucosa. It also is likely to reduce the risk of abdominal pain occurring one to two hours after the ingestion of the bisphosphonate. The maximal absorption of alendronate (and risedronate) occurs within the first half hour following its intake, there is therefore no need to fast for longer than 30 min after swallowing the bisphosphonate tablet. Fasting for more than 30 min may cause the unabsorbed bisphosphonate particles to reach the intestine without being coated by the high fiber breakfast and may irritate the mucosa and induce low abdominal pain.

7. ***In patients with osteoporosis, alendronate:***
   A. Reduces the hip fracture risk.
   B. Reduces the vertebral fracture risk.
   C. Increases the BMD of the lumbar vertebrae and proximal femurs.
   D. All of the above.
   E. B and C.

Correct answer: D

Comment:

The Fracture Intervention Trial showed that over a 3-year period, compared to placebo, alendronate increases BMD at the lumbar vertebrae and proximal femurs and reduces hip fractures by 51%, single morphometric vertebral compression fractures by 47%, multiple vertebral compression fractures by 90%, and nonvertebral fractures by 55%.[2]

The FOSIT (*FOS*amax International *T*rial) study concludes that, when compared to placebo, alendronate administered for 12 months to postmenopausal women (1908 subjects) with a lumbar vertebra T-score of −2.0 or less reduces the risk of nonvertebral fracture by 47%. Similarly, the BMD increased by 4.9%, 2.4%, 3.6%, and 3.0% in the lumbar vertebrae, femoral neck, trochanter, and total hip, respectively.[11]

The administration of oral bisphosphonates for more than 10 years, however, is sometimes paradoxically associated with an increased risk of hip, wrist, and vertebral fractures.[12] This is discussed further in the section on long-term antiresorptive therapy and atypical femoral shaft fractures.

8. ***Risedronate for the treatment of osteoporosis:***
   A. Orally administered, once a week.
   B. Can be taken with a hot drink.
   C. Can be taken after breakfast.
   D. A and B.
   E. All of the above.

Correct answer: E

Comment:

There are, at present, two different formulations of risedronate: the conventional one (Actonel in the USA) and the delayed release formulation (Atelvia in the USA). Conventional risedronate should be taken with the same routine as alendronate. Delayed release risedronate, however, is as effective as conventional risedronate at increasing BMD but can be taken after breakfast.[13]

Risedronate delayed release tablets are formulated in such a way that they can be taken after breakfast without interfering with its pharmacologic activity. This is achieved by the active ingredient being surrounded by a chelating agent and encapsulated in a pH-sensitive envelope that dissolves in an alkaline medium. The tablet therefore cruises unaffected through the stomach. In the alkaline medium of the small intestine, the outer layer is dissolved and releases the chelating agent which binds to cations present in the intestine, thus preventing them from interfering with the bioavailability of risedronate. Pharmacokinetic and pharmacodynamic studies have shown equivalence to the conventional preparation. The delayed release formulation simplifies dosing regimen and improves compliance. Many patients prefer it to the conventional formulation.[13]

9. ***Ibandronate for the treatment of osteoporosis:***
   A. Orally administered, 150mg, once a month.
   B. The tablet must be taken while fasting, in the morning, with no other medication, no food and only water.
   C. A full hour should elapse between the intake of the medication and subsequent food or beverage or medication intake.
   D. All of the above.
   E. None of the above.

   Correct answer: D

   Comment:

   Orally administered ibandronate is available as 150-mg tablets to be taken once a month. Its bioavailability is reduced if the 60-min food/medication/drink (apart from water) abstention period is not observed.[14] Oral ibandronate should be administered with the same caveats outlined before for the oral intake of alendronate. It is also available as an intravenous formulation administered every 3months.

10. ***Adverse effects of orally administered bisphosphonates include:***
    A. Dyspepsia.
    B. Abdominal pain.
    C. Musculoskeletal pain.
    D. All of the above.
    E. A and B.

    Correct answer: D

    Comment:

    All listed adverse effects have been reported after the intake of oral bisphosphonates. Dyspepsia and abdominal pains are due to the irritating property of phosphonic acid molecules on the GI mucosa, hence the need to remain upright and avoid any activity that may increase the risk of gastroesophageal reflux, including jogging and "straightening" a room which involves a certain amount of bending to pick various objects that have been left on the floor.

The abdominal pain, diarrhea, sometimes tenesmus, and occasional fecal incontinence, experienced after the intake of oral bisphosphonates, can be partly relieved by consuming a high fiber meal after the prescribed fast period (30min after the intake of the alendronate and risedronate tablets and 60min after the intake of ibandronate): the fibers bind to the unabsorbed bisphosphonate particles and prevent them from getting in direct contact with, and irritating, the intestinal mucosa.[15] Many patients who cannot tolerate one orally administered bisphosphonate are able to tolerate another one.

Case summary

Analysis of data

Factors predisposing to bone demineralization/osteoporosis

- Postmenopause, no hormonal replacement therapy (HRT).
- Positive family history for osteoporosis, especially hip fracture in a biologic parent.

Factors reducing risk of bone demineralization/osteoporosis

- Physically active lifestyle.
- Good daily dietary calcium intake.
- No cigarette smoking.
- No excessive caffeine, sodium intake.
- No alcohol abuse.

Factors increasing risk of falls/fractures

- None: no factor that may increase the risk of falls, except the patient's age.

Factors reducing risk of falls/fractures

- Physically active lifestyle.
- Normal serum vitamin D level.

Diagnosis

- Postmenopausal osteoporosis.

Management recommendations

Further diagnostic test(s)

- None at this stage. There is no biochemical evidence of impaired renal functions, and the serum vitamin D level is within the normal range.
- Serum bone markers levels can be used to ascertain the baseline rate of bone turnover and monitor the patient's response to treatment.

Treatment(s)

- First-line pharmacologic therapy: antiresorptive, specifically:
  - Orally administered bisphosphonates (alendronate, risedronate, ibandronate).
  - Intravenously administered bisphosphonates such as zoledronic acid once a year or ibandronate every 3 months.
  - Subcutaneously administered denosumab at six-month intervals.
  - Important notice: if there is evidence of renal impairment, bisphosphonates should be avoided as they are excreted by the kidneys. Denosumab is the preferred medication for these patients. However, although denosumab is not nephrotoxic, its administration to patients with impaired renal functions should be monitored.
- Second-line pharmacologic therapy: Osteoanabolic therapy: teriparatide or abaloparatide. However, given the patient's profile, there should be no need for such agents unless there is no response to antiresorptive medication as evidenced by the serum biomarker levels. Even in that case, before switching therapeutic lines, it is important to ascertain the patient is taking the medication exactly as directed and does not have secondary osteoporosis. Both are common causes of poor or nonresponse to antiresorptive therapy.

Follow-up

- Short term: depends on medication prescribed. A follow-up visit, or phone consultation, 4–6 weeks after initiation of treatment may identify noncompliers and emphasize the importance of adopting lifestyle changes, especially to ensure a good daily dietary intake of calcium and vitamin D.
- Two years: repeat DXA scan
- Given the long half-life of bisphosphonates, it is also sometimes recommended that antiresorptives be given initially for a period of 4–6 years and then the medication discontinued for 2–4 years, with DXA scans done at intervals of 2 years and the patient's bone health reevaluated at yearly or every other year intervals.
- These periods of interrupted medication administration are sometimes referred to as "drug holidays." The main objective is to avoid potentially serious long-term adverse effects such as osteonecrosis of the jaw and atypical femoral fracture. Unfortunately, however, in some instances, drug holidays are associated with an increased rate of bone resorption.

Key points

- Bisphosphonates have the same basic chemical formula.
- Different bisphosphonates have different binding affinities to hydroxyapatite crystals in the bone matrix and different degrees of osteoclast inhibitory activity.
- The fracture risk reduction potential is different with different bisphosphonates.
- There are no firm guidelines as to the duration of bisphosphonate therapy.

- Patients on long-term bisphosphonates should be monitored for their potential to develop rare adverse effects, especially osteonecrosis of the jaw and atypical femoral shaft fractures.
- "Drug holidays" are sometimes used to reduce the risk of rare adverse effects.

References

1. Schemistsch E, Adachi JD, Brown JP, et al. Hip fracture predicts subsequent hip fracture: a retrospective observational study to support a call to early hip fracture prevention efforts in post-fracture patients. *Osteoporos Int*. 2022;33:113–122.
2. Chesnut III CH, Skag A, Christiansen C, et al. Effects of oral ibandronate administered daily or intermittently on fracture risk in postmenopausal osteoporosis. *J Bone Miner Res*. 2004;19(8):1241–1249.
3. Black DM, Thompson DE, Bauer DC, et al. Fracture risk reduction with alendronate in women with osteoporosis: the fracture intervention trial. FIT Research Group. *J Clin Endocrinol Metab*. 2000;85 (11):4118–4124.
4. Watts NB, Josse RG, Hamdy RC, et al. Risedronate prevents new vertebral fractures in postmenopausal women at high risk. *J Clin Endocrinol Metab*. 2003;88(2):542–549.
5. Black DM, Reid IR, Boonen S, et al. The effect of 3 versus 6 years of zoledronic acid treatment of osteoporosis: a randomized extension to the HORIZON-pivotal fracture trial (PFT). *J Bone Miner Res*. 2012;27:243–254.
6. Clung MR, Wasnich RD, Recker R, et al. Oral daily ibandronate prevents bone loss in early postmenopausal women without osteoporosis. *J Bone Miner Res*. 2004;19(1):11–18.
7. Kavanagh KL, Guo K, Dunford JE, et al. The molecular mechanism of nitrogen-containing bisphosphonates as antiosteoporosis drugs. *Proc Natl Acad Sci U S A*. 2006;103(20):7829–7834.
8. Rizzoli R. Bisphosphonates for post-menopausal osteoporosis: are they all the same? *QJM*. 2011;104 (4):281–300.
9. Russell RGG. Determinants of structure-function relationships among bisphosphonates. *Bone*. 2007;40(5, Supplement):S21–S25.
10. Chapurlat RD, Delmas PD. Drug insight: bisphosphonates for postmenopausal osteoporosis. *Nat Clin Pract Endocrinol Metab*. 2006;2(4):211–219.
11. Pols HA, Felsenberg D, Hanley DA, et al. Multinational, placebo-controlled, randomized trial of the effects of alendronate on bone density and fracture risk in postmenopausal women with low bone mass: results of the FOSIT study. Fosamax International Trial Study Group. *Osteoporos Int*. 1999;9(5):461–468.
12. Drieling RL, LaCroix AZ, Beresford SAA, et al. Long-term oral bisphosphonate therapy and fractures in older women: the women's health initiative. *J Am Geriatr Soc*. 2017;65(9):1924–1931.
13. McClung MR, Miller PD, Brown JP, et al. Efficacy and safety of a novel delayed-release risedronate 35 mg once-a-week tablet. *Osteoporos Int*. 2012;23(1):267–276.
14. Tankó LB, McClung MR, Schimmer RC, et al. The efficacy of 48-week oral ibandronate treatment in postmenopausal osteoporosis when taken 30 versus 60 minutes before breakfast. *Bone*. 2003;32(4):421–426.
15. Chandran M, Zeng W. Severe oral mucosal ulceration associated with oral bisphosphonate use: the importance of imparting proper instructions on medication administration and intake. *Case Rep Med*. 2021;6620489.

CHAPTER 12

Oral bisphosphonates—Drug holidays and discontinuing therapy

Learning objectives

- Monitor patients on long-term antiresorptive therapy.
- Determine whether to continue or discontinue long-term antiresorptive therapy.
- Determine whether a "Drug holiday" is appropriate in the management of osteoporosis.

The case study

Reasons for seeking medical help

- MR, 62-year-old Caucasian woman, has been diagnosed with osteoporosis about 10 years ago. At that time her T-scores were −3.1 in the lumbar vertebrae, −2.8 in the right femoral neck, and −2.6 in the right total hip. The original DXA scan is not available. Secondary causes of osteoporosis had been ruled out. She was prescribed alendronate. She adheres well with this medication, has incorporated its intake in her daily routine, and is happy to continue taking it. She is essentially asymptomatic.
- Her primary care provider wonders whether the continued administration of a bisphosphonate (for more than 10 years) is appropriate.

Past medical and surgical history

- Natural menopause at age 41 years, no hormonal replacement therapy.
- Menarche at age 13 years.
- No history of fractures.

Lifestyle

- Daily dietary calcium intake estimated to be about 1200 mg.
- Active physical lifestyle, plays tennis at least once a week and jogs about 2 miles twice a week.

Diagnosis and Treatment of Osteoporosis. https://doi.org/10.1016/B978-0-323-99550-4.00033-2
Copyright © 2024 Elsevier Inc. All rights are reserved, including those for text and data mining, AI training, and similar technologies.

- She has not experienced any dizzy spell, falls, or near-falls.
- No excessive sodium, caffeine, or alcohol intake. No cigarette smoking.

Medication(s)

- Alendronate 70 mg once a week.
- Multivitamin tablets once a day.

Family history

- Positive for osteoporosis: mother and both grandmothers sustained fragility hip fractures.

Clinical examination

- Weight 124 pounds, steady, height 62″
- No relevant clinical findings.

Laboratory result(s)

- Comprehensive metabolic panel (CMP): no abnormal findings, eGFR >60 mL/min.
- Serum 25-hydroxy-vitamin D 42 ng/mL.

DXA and radiological result(s)

- T-scores: −2.1 upper 4 lumbar vertebrae, −1.6 right femoral neck, and −1.8 right total hip.
- A comparison of the BMD changes is not possible because the scans were done on different densitometers, in different health care offices, and by different technician. DXA scan illustrations and information about the least significant changes are not available. It transpired that the original scan was done about 10 years ago at a visiting "Health Care Exhibition" that is no longer in business. No other DXA scans during this 10-year period are available.
- Vertebral fracture assessment: no evidence of vertebral compression fractures.
- FRAX scores and 10-year risks of sustaining a hip or major fracture, as per the National Osteoporosis Foundation guidelines: 1.4% and 8% for the risk of a hip or major fracture, respectively. Neither reaches the threshold level recommended by the NOF to initiate pharmacologic treatment: 3% and 20% for the 10-year risk of fractures in the hip or major bones, respectively.

Multiple choice questions

1. ***The following is/are correct:***

   A. There has been a significant improvement in the DXA scans.

B. Continuing alendronate is expected to further improve bone health.
C. Discontinuing alendronate may induce a rebound increased bone resorption phase.
D. None of the above.
E. A and C

Correct answer: C

Comment:

T-scores are used to make a densitometric diagnosis: osteoporosis, osteopenia, or normal bone density. Changes in BMD can be used to determine whether there has been a significant change in the patient's BMD at the various sites examined.

However, as many factors modulate the calculation of the BMD, including make of densitometer, precision, accuracy, least significant change, and possibly, different reference populations used, it is not possible to ensure that the observed "changes" in BMD reflect an actual change and are not due to some artifact and extraneous factor. It is just not possible to compare BMDs if the scans were done on different densitometers, in different centers, and by different technicians, especially as the report sometimes only includes the patient's T-scores, not the BMD, and frequently does not indicate the center's precision, Least Significant Change (LSC), and even reference population. Furthermore, often, especially in older people, increases in lumbar vertebrae BMD are due to degenerative changes and not a genuine increase in BMD.

Changes in BMD, and not T-scores, therefore should be used to monitor the patient's response, or lack of response, to treatment. In this respect, therefore, the validity of available results of the scan done 10 years ago cannot be established because the only parameters reported were the T-scores. There is no mention of the BMD, and the quality of the scan is not addressed. It is therefore possible that the original DXA scan, done about 10 years ago, was of poor quality and unreliable, and therefore cannot be used for clinical purposes. In this case, therefore, it may be more appropriate to disregard altogether the results of the DXA scan done about 10 years ago and to consider the scan done recently as the new baseline.

2. ***At this stage, the most appropriate management strategy includes:***
A. Continue the administration of alendronate.
B. Discontinue alendronate.
C. Prescribe an osteoanabolic medication such as teriparatide or abaloparatide.
D. A and C.
E. B and C.

Correct answer: B

Comment:

Alendronate, like most bisphosphonates, has a very long half-life and therefore can be safely discontinued after it has been administered for a few years. On the other hand, the continued administration of bisphosphonates and other antiresorptive medication increases the risk of rare, but serious adverse effects, such as osteonecrosis of the jaw and atypical femoral shaft fractures. The longer the administration of antiresorptives, the greater the risk. Similarly, discontinuing alendronate therapy decreases the risk of the patient developing osteonecrosis of the jaw and atypical femoral shaft fractures and in many cases, but not all cases, does not lead to a rebound increased bone resorption. The recommendation therefore would be to discontinue alendronate for 2 to 3 years and reevaluate the patient.[1]

3. ***Discontinuing alendronate after 5 years of continuous therapy leads to:***
   A. Declines in BMD, but mean BMD higher than pretreatment BMD.
   B. Declines in BMD, but mean BMD lower than pretreatment BMD.
   C. Increases in markers of bone resorption levels.
   D. Decreases in markers of bone formation levels.
   E. A and C.

   Correct *answer*: E

   Comment:

   A 5-year study was conducted on 1099 postmenopausal women who had completed the 5-year Fracture Intervention Trial (FIT) and were enrolled in the alendronate group. They were then randomly allocated to either alendronate or placebo.[2] Compared to placebo, those on alendronate showed the following mean % changes in BMD[2]:

   - Lumbar vertebrae: +5.26% alendronate versus +1.52% placebo.
   - Total hip: −1.02% alendronate versus −3.38% placebo.
   - Femoral neck: +0.46% alendronate versus −1.48% placebo.
   - Trochanter: −0.08% alendronate versus −3.25% placebo.
   - Total body: +1.01% alendronate versus −0.27% placebo.
   - Forearm: −1.19% alendronate versus −3.21% placebo.

   Similarly, when compared to the baseline BMD values 10 years previously, the BMD increases were significantly higher in those patients who had been on alendronate for 10 years versus those who were on alendronate for only 5 years, followed by 5 years of placebo.

   - Lumbar vertebrae: +14.80% alendronate versus +10.99% placebo.
   - Total hip: +2.41% alendronate versus −0.16% placebo.
   - Femoral neck: +4.75% alendronate versus +2.50% placebo.
   - Trochanter: +5.95% alendronate versus +2.62% placebo.
   - Total body: +3.60% alendronate versus +2.48% placebo.

4. ***In patients who have completed 5 years of alendronate therapy, continuing alendronate* versus *discontinuing alendronate for another 5 years leads to:***
   A. Lower risk of nonvertebral fractures.
   B. Lower risk of clinical vertebral fractures.
   C. Lower risk of hip fractures.
   D. A and B.
   E. A, B, and C.

   Correct answer: B

Comment:

Apart from the decrease in clinical vertebral fractures, there were no differences in the fracture risk among patients who continued with alendronate for 5 years and those who were allocated to the placebo group after completing 5 years of alendronate therapy.[2]

Another retrospective study on postmenopausal women with osteoporosis shows that when bisphosphonates are discontinued after 3 to 5 years of treatment, those who continued to receive the bisphosphonate had a 40% lower risk of sustaining fractures than those who stopped taking bisphosphonates.[3]

5. ***Sequential BMD changes in patients on treatment:***
   A. The greatest increases are seen in the first few years and then tend to become less pronounced.
   B. Larger increases in BMD are associated with greater reductions in fracture risk.
   C. Increases in BMD explain most of the fracture risk reduction.
   D. A and B.
   E. A, B, and C.

   Correct answer: D

   Comment:

   The greatest increases induced by various medications for osteoporosis occur within the first 3 to 4 years and then tend to slow down. Larger increases in BMD, however, are associated with greater reductions in the fracture risk. Other factors, apart from changes in BMD, modulate the fracture risk.[4–6] BMD changes explain less than half of the medication-induced fracture risk reduction. Most medications for osteoporosis affect bone microarchitecture as well as BMD. Changes in bone microarchitecture and strength are not always captured by bone densitometry.

6. ***While considering therapeutic decisions, the following should be noted:***
   A. The rate and direction of change in BMD.
   B. The T-score.
   C. The patient's Z-score.
   D. A and B.
   E. A, B, and C.

   Correct answer: D

   Comment:

   The absolute BMD value, per se, is of little use unless compared to that of previous scans, preferably done on the same densitometer and considering the Least Significant Change (LSC) of the center where the DXA scans are done. The rate and direction of BMD change as well as the T-scores and the serum levels of bone biomarkers are all useful parameters to monitor the patient's response to therapy and determine whether the continued long-term administration of antiresorptives is indicated.[7]

   Changes in the levels of bone biomarkers help determine whether bone resorption and bone formation are increased, decreased, or unchanged. Based on these results, a management strategy individualized for individual patients is developed: patients with a low rate of bone formation are more likely to benefit from an osteoanabolic agent whereas patients with a high rate of bone resorption rate are more likely to benefit from an antiresorptive medication.

In MR's case, unfortunately there are only two points in time: the first scan done about 10years ago, and the second scan done at the time of the visit. As the reliability of the first scan is questionable, it is probably better ignored altogether, especially as there is no information about the patient's adherence with the intake of alendronate.

Bone turnover markers offer a different perspective: if markers of bone formation are suppressed, an osteoanabolic medication is likely to be of benefit. On the other hand, if the markers of bone resorption are elevated, antiresorption medication is recommended. Combining antiresorptive and osteoanabolic medication is not recommended.

If antiresorptives are prescribed, rare long-term complications such as atypical femoral shaft fractures and osteonecrosis of the jaws should be anticipated and avoided while still in the early phase. Patients on long-term antiresorptive therapy should be educated about the early symptoms and signs of atypical femoral shaft fractures and osteonecrosis of the jaw. Both conditions are discussed in separate chapters.

7. ***At this stage the following is recommended:***
   - A. Check gums to ensure she is not likely to have or develop Osteonecrosis of the Jaw (ONJ).
   - B. Perform radiologic studies: plain X-rays or technetium bone scan to ensure she does not have fragility fractures that may lead to atypical femoral shaft fractures.
   - C. Assess the glomerular filtration rate.
   - D. A and B.
   - E. All of the above.

   Correct answer: E

   Comment:

   MR has been on alendronate for about 10years; continuing with this medication or other antiresorptive medication further increases the risk of sustaining rare complications, especially atypical femoral shaft fractures or osteonecrosis of the jaw. It is therefore appropriate to assess these patients for both adverse effects and discontinue the bisphosphonate. Discontinuing the bisphosphonate is associated with a reduced risk of rare adverse effects.

8. ***Alternatively, alendronate may be discontinued and replaced by:***
   - A. Raloxifene.
   - B. Denosumab.
   - C. Zoledronic acid.
   - D. A, B, or C.
   - E. None of the above.

   Correct answer: E

Comment:

At this stage, there is no need for either continuing with alendronate or switching to another antiresorptive or osteoanabolic medication.

9. ***"Drug holidays"***
   A. Should be considered in many patients on antiosteoporosis treatment for more than 5 years.
   B. Reduce the risk of adverse events, especially rare adverse effects such as osteonecrosis of the jaw and atypical femoral shaft fracture.
   C. Promote patient adherence with medication.
   D. A and B.
   E. A, B, and C.

   Correct answer: E

   Comment:

   The concept of "Drug holidays" is gaining popularity especially as adherence to the "drug" often entails changes in lifestyle and the "drug" is prescribed for an essentially asymptomatic condition.[6,8,9] Also, patients may be more motivated if they knew the medication is prescribed for a finite period of time.

   Bisphosphonate drug holidays are based on the fact that bisphosphonates are incorporated and kept in the bone matrix until they are released during bone resorption. As such, therefore, their biological half-life could extend for a number of years and their antiresorptive activity and fracture risk reduction continue for a long time: one or more years after the administration of the bisphosphonate has stopped. Discontinuing the medication reduces the risk of rare adverse effects, such as osteonecrosis of the jaw and atypical femoral shaft fractures.

10. ***A "bisphosphonate drug holiday" should be considered in patients:***
    A. Treated with bisphosphonates for 3–5 years.
    B. No longer at high fracture risk.
    C. The patient is keen to discontinue the medication.
    D. A and C.
    E. A, B, and C.

    Correct answer: E

    Comment:

    There is ample evidence that the risk/benefit ratio of bisphosphonates is in favor of benefit in the first 3–5 years of their administration.[8,9] After this period, the balance may move slightly in the opposite direction. Three to 5 years is therefore a good landmark to reevaluate the patient's osteoporosis and determine whether on balance, continuing the medication is likely to offset potential adverse effects. Factors that need to be considered include the changes in BMD, the T-scores, biomarkers, and the patient's attitude toward taking the medication: patients who dislike taking the medication are more likely to adhere to it if they knew the intake was for a finite period.

The underlying principle of drug holidays does not apply to nonbisphosphonate therapy for osteoporosis, even other antiresorptives such as denosumab, because their biological effects are often quickly reversed once the medication is stopped.

Case summary

Analysis of data

Factors predisposing to bone demineralization/osteoporosis

- Age: 62 years old.
- Early natural menopause: at age 41 years. No hormonal replacement therapy.

Case summary

Factors protecting against bone demineralization/osteoporosis

- Alendronate therapy, prescribed about 10 years ago. MR is taking the medication as directed, has not experienced adverse effects, and, if recommended is happy to continue taking that medication.
- Good daily calcium intake from food.
- Active physical lifestyle.
- No excessive sodium, caffeine, and alcohol intake.
- No evidence of hypovitaminosis D.
- No cigarette smoking.

Factors increasing risk of falls/fractures

- Positive family history of fragility fractures: patient's mother and both grandmothers sustained fragility fractures.

Factors reducing risk of falls/fractures

- Physically active lifestyle.
- Good adherence to alendronate tablets.

Diagnosis

Osteopenia as per densitometric evidence: T-scores between −2.5 and −1.0.

Results of the DXA scan done about 10 years ago will be rejected.

Management recommendations

Treatment(s)

- Stop alendronate therapy: she has been taking it for about 10 years.
- After the initial assays of bone markers, reevaluate BMD, bone turnover, and vitamin D status.

Diagnostic test(s)

- No diagnostic tests are recommended at this stage. However, in order to evaluate future changes in bone turnover, bone markers such as C-Tx, P1NP, and bone-specific alkaline phosphatase will establish a baseline against which future assessments will be made. For similar reasons a baseline serum vitamin D level is also recommended.

Lifestyle

- Maintain a physical active lifestyle.
- Ensure a well-balanced diet with good calcium and vitamin D intake.

Key points

- Continuing antiresorptive therapy for more than 5 years increases the risk of rare complications such as osteonecrosis of the jaw and atypical femoral shaft fractures.
- "Drug holidays" should be considered after 5 years of completed antiresorptive medication. Caution, however, should be exercised with denosumab as its cessation may lead to a rebound increase in bone resorption and risk of fragility fractures, especially multiple vertebral fractures.

References

1. Cosman F, Cauley JA, Eastell R, et al. Reassessment of fracture risk in women after 3 years of treatment with zoledronic acid: when is it reasonable to discontinue treatment. *J Clin Endocrinol Metab*. 2014;99:4546–4554.
2. Black DM, Schwartz AV, Ensrud KE, et al. Effects of continuing or stopping alendronate after 5 years of treatment. The fracture intervention trial long-term extension. *JAMA*. 2006;296:2927–2938.
3. Mignot MA, Taisne N, Legroux I, et al. Bisophosphonate drug holidays in postmenopausal osteoporosis: effect on clinical fracture risk. *Osteoporos Int*. 2017;28(12):3431–3438.
4. Hochberg MC, Greenspan S, Wasnich RD, et al. Changes in bone density and turnover explain the reductions in incidence of nonvertebral fractures that occur during treatment with anti-resorptive agents. *J Clin Endocrinol Metab*. 2002;87(4):1586–1592.
5. Wasnich RD, Miller PD. Antifracture efficacy of anti-resorptive agents are related to changes in bone density. *J Clin Endocrinol Metab*. 2000;85(1):231–236.
6. Cummings SR, Karpf DB, Harris F, et al. Improvement in spine bone density and reduction in risk of vertebral fractures during treatment with anti-resorptive drugs. *Am J Med*. 2002;112(4):281–289.
7. Lewiecki EM, Watts NB. Assessing response to osteoporosis therapy. *Osteoporos Int*. 2008;19(10):1363–1368.
8. Chang LL, Eastell R, Miller PD. Continuation of bisphosphonate therapy for osteoporosis beyond 5 years. *N Engl J Med*. 2022;386(15):1467–1469.
9. Bonick SL. Going on a drug holiday? *J Clin Densitom*. 2011;14(4):377–383.

CHAPTER 13

Oral bisphosphonates—Long term: 13 years

Learning objectives

- Evaluation of patients on long-term antiresorptive therapy.
- When and how to discontinue long-term bisphosphonate therapy.

The case study

Reasons for seeking medical help

- VP is a 74-year-old Caucasian woman, diagnosed with osteoporosis about 12 years ago after sustaining a fragility vertebral fracture while watching, at home, a movie with her daughter. The diagnosis of osteoporosis was confirmed by DXA scan: lowest T-score −3.0 and −2.9 for the left total hip and femoral neck, respectively. At that time, secondary causes of osteoporosis had been ruled out. She was prescribed alendronate, but could not tolerate the gastrointestinal adverse effects.
- She was switched to risedronate, tolerated it, and adhered well to this medication, but is now experiencing heart burn and abdominal discomfort after taking the medication. She would prefer not to continue taking that medication for her osteoporosis especially as she is essentially asymptomatic except for the abdominal pain and discomfort after taking risedronate.
- About 11 years ago, shortly after starting risedronate therapy, she was detailed as a missionary teacher to teach geography at schools in Africa where bone densitometry was not readily available. She nevertheless was able to get risedronate shipped and has been taking it regularly. She is now back in the USA and is on no other medication. She has no plans to return to Africa.

Past medical and surgical history

- Natural menopause at 45 years, no HRT.
- Menarche at age 12 years, regular menstrual periods.

Diagnosis and Treatment of Osteoporosis. https://doi.org/10.1016/B978-0-323-99550-4.00030-7
Copyright © 2024 Elsevier Inc. All rights are reserved, including those for text and data mining, AI training, and similar technologies.

Lifestyle

- Active physical lifestyle. She spends about an hour, three times a week, exercising in a gymnasium.
- Daily dietary calcium intake: about 1300 mg.
- No excessive sodium, caffeine, alcohol, and no cigarette smoking.

Medications

- Risedronate 35 mg once a week. VP is taking the medication exactly as directed.
- Multivitamin tablets once a day.

Family history

- Positive for osteoporosis: mother sustained bilateral fragility hip fractures.

Clinical examination

- Weight 142 pounds, steady, height 64″
- Get-Up-and-Go Test: completed in 9 s.
- No relevant clinical findings. No clinical evidence suggestive of atypical femoral shaft fracture or osteonecrosis of the jaw.

Laboratory results

- Comprehensive metabolic profile: no abnormal findings, eGFR >60 mL/min.
- Serum 25-hydroxy-vitamin D 46 ng/mL.

DXA and radiologic results

VP had only three DXA scans done: baseline, about 5 years later, and the last one a few weeks ago. Given that VP had her DXA scans done on different densitometers, by different densitometrists, in different centers, and also different countries, it is not possible to adequately evaluate the results and compare those of the present scan with the previous scans. Notwithstanding, the VFA shows evidence of T7 vertebral compression fracture. VP does not recall being subjected to any significant trauma on her back. The vertebral compression fracture is therefore a fragility fracture, and the final diagnosis is "established osteoporosis," i.e., densitometric evidence of osteoporosis and the presence of a fragility fracture.

Multiple choice questions

1. ***The following laboratory tests are recommended:***
   A. Serum CTX (Serum cross-linked C-telopeptide of type I collagen).
   B. Serum P1NP (Procollagen Type I Intact N-terminal propeptide).
   C. Serum vitamin D.
   D. Comprehensive metabolic profile.
   E. A and B.
   Correct answer: E
   Comment:
   The comprehensive metabolic profile and serum vitamin D levels have been assayed about 3 weeks prior to this encounter and are within the normal range. There is no need to repeat these analyses. The serum CTX level is 54 pg/mL, well below the normal range of 100–1000 pg/mL. It is suggestive of a reduced rate of bone resorption in line with the intake of risedronate, an antiresorptive medication that VP has been taking for the past 10 years. Similarly, the serum P1NP is suggestive of a reduced rate of bone formation in line with the drug-induced low rate of bone turnover.
   The serum vitamin D level is within normal limits. Parameters of renal functions are of particular interest as they will guide the choice of medication. Having this data available before seeing the patient helps determine the various options available without any delay.
2. ***The data about VP suggest that:***
   A. She has not been adhering to the medication.
   B. She has secondary osteoporosis.
   C. She never had osteoporosis.
   D. A and C.
   E. None of the above.
   Correct answer: E
   Comment:
   VP has been adhering to risedronate therapy as evidenced by the low serum CTX level. Osteoporosis is the diagnosis as evidenced by the fragility vertebral compression fracture she sustained some time ago. It is not possible to be more specific as to the occurrence of the vertebral compression fracture as it is "silent," i.e., asymptomatic and occurs without the patient knowing that a vertebra is being crushed. This is not the case in patients sustaining clinical or symptomatic fractures that are usually associated with severe, often very severe, pain.
   The presence of a fragility fracture is diagnostic of osteoporosis and overrides the densitometric diagnosis. There is no indication that she has secondary osteoporosis. A DXA scan is nevertheless indicated as it can be used as a baseline against which the

patient progress can be noted. Her T-scores are −3.0 in the upper four lumbar vertebrae, −2.9 and −2.8 in the left and right femoral neck, and −2.5 and −2.6 in the total right and left hip, respectively. The T-score of the nondominant distal 1/3 radius is −2.6.

3. ***In VP case, at this stage, the following is recommended:***
   A. Discontinue risedronate.
   B. Prescribe delayed release risedronate formulation.
   C. Prescribe teriparatide.
   D. All of the above.
   E. None of the above.

   Correct answer: A

   Comment:

   Given that her fasting serum CTX level is below the normal range indicating that her bone turnover rate is probably oversuppressed, the antiresorptive medication (risedronate) should be discontinued. An osteoanabolic agent such as teriparatide or abaloparatide may be considered to stimulate bone formation. Given the degree of osteoporosis, however, she also could be a good candidate for romosozumab which has a dual effect: stimulating bone formation and inhibiting bone resorption.

4. ***Before comparing the present densitometric findings to previous ones, the following should be ascertained:***
   A. The least significant change of the center is known.
   B. The same densitometer has been used for all the scans.
   C. If there has been a change of densitometers, cross-calibration studies have been conducted.
   D. A and C.
   E. A, B, and C.

   Correct answer: E

   Comment:

   As deviations from optimum patient positioning on the densitometer may give rise to different results, precision studies are conducted to determine the technologist's skills at repositioning patients in exactly the same position. Precision studies are done by scanning a patient, then asking her to get off the densitometer table, then repositioning her and scanning her again. This is repeated either twice in 30 patients or three times in 15 patients. This has been discussed in the chapter on bone densitometry. The data are then entered in a formula (available on the ISCD website) and the precision of the technologist performing the scans is calculated. From the precision study, the Least Significant Change (LSC) is calculated to determine the smallest change in BMD, for that particular technologist, using that particular densitometer, that is statistically significant, usually with a 95% level of confidence. LSC may be expressed as a percentage or an absolute value and should be known before interpreting any change in BMD. ISCD recommends that LSC be calculated separately for each technologist.

Precision studies and LSC calculation are not considered research but are quality assurance programs. It is nevertheless advisable to get clearance from the local Institutional Review Body where the scans are done. ISCD also recommends that changes not exceeding LSC be reported as "nonsignificant."

5. ***Cross-calibration studies:***
   A. Should be done when densitometers are changed.
   B. Are not needed because formulae are available to convert results.
   C. Are done by the manufacturers before delivering the new densitometer.
   D. Can be done on the office staff or by using specially designed phantoms.
   E. A and D.

   Correct answer: A

   Comment:

   Cross-calibration studies should be done before changing densitometers and are necessary because results from different densitometers often cannot be compared as different manufacturers use different methods to produce the two waves of energy for densitometry, use different algorithms to separate soft from bone tissue, and sometimes use different anatomical sites, but use the same terminology. For instance, the "femoral neck" site is the area of the femoral neck adjacent to the greater trochanter for Hologic densitometers, whereas for GE/Lunar densitometers it is the area at the midpoint of the hip axis. These two areas may be anatomically distinct and therefore cannot be directly compared, hence the need for cross-calibration studies.

   During cross-calibration studies a number of patients are scanned on both densitometers (the one about to be changed and the new model) and the results are plotted on a chart which can then be used to "convert" results obtained on one densitometer to the other. It is not recommended to use office staff to conduct cross-calibration studies as in most instances they do not represent patients being scanned. At the time of writing this manuscript, no phantoms are available for cross-calibration studies. Although formulae are available to convert data sets and are used for epidemiological studies, they are not sufficiently sensitive and specific to be used for clinical purposes.

6. ***Match the following:***
   (a) Least significant change.
   (b) Cross-calibration study.
   (c) Accuracy study.
   (d) Precision study.
      A. Performed when the densitometer is about to be changed.
      B. Phantoms can be used.
      C. Reflects the technologist's skills at positioning the patient on the densitometer table.
      D. Needs to be known when evaluating changes in BMD
      E. Reflects the sensitivity of the densitometer.

Correct answers: A (b); B (c); C (d); D (a); E (c)

Comment:

Sequential changes in BMD cannot be evaluated unless the LSC for the particular center where the scans are done is known. This is discussed further in the section on bone densitometry. Results of scans obtained from different densitometers cannot be compared unless cross-calibration studies have been done. It is therefore essential for these studies to be conducted prior to changing the densitometer. Although phantoms are available to check the accuracy and therefore sensitivity of the densitometer to accurately measure the bone mineral content and surface area of the bone scanned, no such phantoms are available to cross-calibrate densitometers.

7. ***VP should be offered a "drug holiday" because:***
   A. She has been on risedronate for about 12 years.
   B. Her lowest T-score is −3.0 in the upper four lumbar vertebrae.
   C. Her CTX is low.
   D. A and C.
   E. None of the above.

   Correct answer: D

   Comment:

   VP should not be offered a "drug holiday" because she has "established osteoporosis" as evidenced by her densitometric data and also the fragility fractures she sustained. Her fracture risk is therefore high/very high and she should be prescribed medication to reduce the risk of fractures by increasing bone mass, i.e. osteoanabolic medications such as teriparatide or abaloparatide.

   Risedronate should be stopped because of the risk of developing serious adverse effects such as osteonecrosis of the jaw (ONG) or atypical femoral fractures (AFF). For similar reasons other antiresorptive agents should not be prescribed as they may increase the risk of ONJ and AFF. Given that she has significant osteoporosis (T-score of −3.0 in the upper four lumbar vertebrae) and that the bone turnover is low as evidenced by the low serum bone marker levels, she no longer needs antiresorptive medication and may respond to an osteoanabolic medication that will stimulate bone growth. Romosozumab is unique as it is the only medication presently available that has a dual effect: increasing bone formation and reducing bone resorption.

8. ***In VP's case, follow-up should include:***
   A. Repeat DXA scan 1 year.
   B. Repeat DXA scan 2 years.
   C. Repeat CTX in 1 to 6 months.
   D. A and C.
   E. B and C.

   Correct answer: E

Comment:

A repeat DXA scan in 2 years is recommended. Changes in BMD are not likely to be significant in DXA scans done earlier than 2years. Assaying bone biomarkers will confirm that the rates of bone formation and bone resorption have changed after discontinuing risedronate and prescribing an osteoanabolic medication or romosozumab.

9. ***The following is/are recommended:***
   A. Clinical examination of both upper femurs.
   B. Plain X-ray of both upper femurs.
   C. Technetium bone scan.
   D. A and B.
   E. A, B, and C.

Correct answer: D

Comment:

An atypical femoral shaft fracture is one of the most serious adverse effects of long-term antiresorptive therapy. It usually first presents with tenderness along the upper shaft of the femur, and the patient may experience some pain when she stands on the affected leg. As the condition progresses the patient experiences pain aggravated by standing, walking, and especially running or jogging. An initial partial or incomplete fissure fracture can then be seen in the X-ray; eventually, the fissure fracture extends and becomes a full fracture.

Radiological features are characteristic: initially there appears to be a swelling of the bone and then a fissure fracture appears, cutting transversally across the shaft of the femur. Sometimes both sides are affected, albeit to different degrees. A technetium bone scan reveals an increased uptake on the site(s) of the fracture. Surgery is recommended while the fracture is still localized to one side of the femoral shaft. Atypical femoral shaft fractures are discussed in a separate chapter.

10. ***The following also is recommended:***
   A. A full examination of the mouth, especially gums.
   B. Ascertain the integrity of upper and lower gums.
   C. Identify localized pain/tenderness in both gums.
   D. None of the above.
   E. All of the above.

Correct answer: E

Comment:

Osteonecrosis of the Jaw (ONJ) is a major adverse effect of long-term antiresorptive therapy for osteoporosis. Although it may occur spontaneously, it usually complicates tooth extraction. The initial presentation is an exposed area after a tooth extraction: similar to a "dry socket" which does not heal. Discomfort and pain are the initial presentations. At this stage the clinical examination reveals the presence of an exposed/ulcerated area that eventually becomes infected. Sinuses and fistulae eventually develop. ONJ and AFF are discussed in other case studies.

Case summary

Analysis of data

Factors predisposing to bone demineralization/osteoporosis
- Status post natural menopause, no hormonal replacement therapy.
- The presence of a fragility vertebral fracture (T7).
- Positive family history: mother sustained bilateral fragility hip fractures.

Factors protecting against bone demineralization/osteoporosis
- Good daily calcium intake.
- Good well-balanced diet.
- Physically active lifestyle.
- No excessive sodium, no excessive caffeine, and no cigarette smoking.
- She has been taking risedronate, an orally administered bisphosphonate for approximately 12 years.

Factors increasing risk of falls/fractures
- None

Factors reducing risk of falls/fractures
- Physically active lifestyle.
- Good well-balanced diet.
- Completed the Get-Up-and-Go test in 9 s.
- Serum vitamin D level within normal range.

Diagnosis

- The complete diagnosis is: established osteoporosis as manifested by:
  1. Fragility fracture of T7.
  2. Densitometric evidence of osteoporosis: lowest T-score of −3.0 in the upper four lumbar vertebrae.
  3. Status post long-term bisphosphonate therapy, i.e. increased risk of osteonecrosis of the jaw (ONF) and Atypical Femoral Fractures (AFF). These are discussed at the end of this section.

Management recommendations

Treatment recommendation(s)

- Discontinue risedronate.
- Panoramic X-ray of the jaws, because of possible ONJ.
- Prescribe an osteoanabolic medication or romosozumab.
- Review and reassess bone health in 2 years' time.

Lifestyle changes

- None, maintain level of physical activity.

Key points

- Patients with osteoporosis who are prescribed antiresorptive medication should be followed up regularly to ensure compliance and avoid rare adverse effects such as atypical femoral shaft fractures and osteonecrosis of the jaw.
- A DXA scan, assays of biomarkers of bone resorption and bone formation, and a panoramic X-ray of the jaws to comprehensively assess the patient's bone health and formulate a management strategy tailored to the individual needs of the patient.

CHAPTER 14

Oral bisphosphonates—Lack of response☆

Learning objectives

- Evaluation of patients on long-term bisphosphonate therapy for drug resistance.
- Recognize lifestyle habits that can interfere with bisphosphonate efficacy.

The case study

Reasons for seeking medical help

Mrs. BF, a 54-year-old Asian woman, comes for a follow-up visit. She had been diagnosed with postmenopausal osteoporosis about 2 years ago: Her lowest T-score was −2.7 in the left total hip. The DXA scan done at that time also showed that she had sustained multiple fragility vertebral compression fractures. Clinical examination and laboratory investigations (CBC, blood chemistry profile, and serum vitamin D level) did not reveal a secondary cause for her osteoporosis. Alendronate 70mg once a week was prescribed. Mrs. BF maintains that she takes the medication as directed and has not experienced any adverse effect.

Past medical and surgical history

- Postmenopausal osteoporosis diagnosed about 2 years ago. On alendronate therapy.
- Reached a natural menopause at the age of 51 years. She preferred not to take hormonal replacement therapy because she was afraid of breast cancer.
- Three children; all breast-fed. She could not remember whether or not she was taking calcium supplements on a regular basis during pregnancy and lactation.

Personal habits, lifestyle, and daily routine

- She dislikes milk and dairy products. The average daily calcium intake is about 500 mg.
- No cigarette smoking.
- No alcohol intake.
- Sedentary lifestyle.

☆ BF, 54-year-old Asian woman not responding to oral bisphosphonates.

Diagnosis and Treatment of Osteoporosis. https://doi.org/10.1016/B978-0-323-99550-4.00013-7
Copyright © 2024 Elsevier Inc. All rights are reserved, including those for text and data mining, AI training, and similar technologies.

Medications

- Alendronate 70mg once a week started about 2 years ago. Mrs. BF maintains that she takes that medication exactly as directed by her physician.
- Over-the-counter calcium supplements amounting to 1200 mg daily.
- Ibuprofen for back pain, 400mg as required. On average she takes about six tablets a week.

Family history

- Negative for osteoporosis.

Clinical examination

- Weight 140 pounds, height 5′2″, arm span 65″.
- No relevant significant clinical findings except for evidence of osteoarthritic changes in her hands and knees. She admits that she had these signs for a number of years.

DXA scan results

	Baseline		Baseline		2 years later	2 years later
Site	BMD	T-scores	BMD	T-scores	% BMD change	LSC %
Right total hip	0.721	−2.5	0.689	−2.9	−4.5	3.1
Left total hip	0.688	−2.7	0.657	−2.9	−5.1	3.2
Lumbar vertebrae	0.991	−1.1	0.975	−1.3	−1.6	3.0
Left distal radius	0.447	−2.3	0.446	−2.3	−0.2	3.0

Note: There is evidence of moderate vertebral wedge compression fractures of L2 and L3.

Multiple choice questions

1. ***In Mrs. BF the observed changes in BMD:***
   A. Are significant in both hips only.
   B. Are not significant in the lumbar vertebrae and the distal radius.
   C. Are not significant in the distal radius.
   D. A and B.
   E. A, B, and C.
   Correct answer: E
   Comments:
   When comparing the changes in DXA scans over a period of time, it is the percentage change in BMD that matters, not the changes in T-scores. If the change exceeds the Least Significant Change of the Center (LSC) in the center where the DXA scan is done then that change is significant.

   Although the changes did not alter the diagnostic classification of the patient they are significant as they indicate that the bisphosphonate administered has not been able to increase the BMD or even maintain it at its original level.

This patient's osteoporosis appears to be resistant to alendronate. True resistance to alendronate, however, is very rare. The three most common causes of apparent "resistance" to alendronate or other orally administered bisphosphonates are first the patient not taking the medication as directed, second the patient not getting enough calcium and/or vitamin D and is therefore not able to build up bone. Third, the patient has secondary osteoporosis.

2. ***In Mrs. BF's case the following inquiries should be made:***
   A. Exactly how is she taking alendronate?
   B. What type of liquid is she using to take alendronate?
   C. Is she taking any other medications with alendronate?
   D. A and B.
   E. A, B, and C.

   Correct answer: E

   Comments:

   Alendronate, like other orally administered bisphosphonates, has to be taken on its own, with no other medication. It should be taken with plain water. It may be even better if it were taken with distilled water which contains nothing but water as opposed to tap water, well water, and bottled water which may contain a number of additives or contaminants. Minerals and other additives or contaminants may interfere with the bioavailability of orally administered bisphosphonates. Even filtered water may contain some contaminants. Well water is usually rich in minerals which may interfere with the bioavailability of alendronate and other orally administered bisphosphonates.

   It is important to ascertain that the patient is taking the medication exactly as directed. Often patients, not realizing the importance of taking the medication exactly as directed, may take it with coffee, orange juice, or some beverage other than plain water. Similarly, they may take it with mineral water or well water that may be rich in minerals. All these beverages may interfere with the absorption of bisphosphonates and reduce their bioavailability. Even if the patient states that she is taking the medication as prescribed, it behooves the clinician to ascertain that this indeed is how she should be taking it.

3. ***In Mrs. BF case the following inquiries should also be made:***
   A. How long does she wait before taking any other medication(s)?
   B. How long does she wait before eating after taking the alendronate tablet?
   C. When does she take her calcium supplements?
   D. A and B.
   E. A, B, and C.

   Correct answer: E

   Comments:

   All these questions are relevant. If another medication is taken within 30min of ingesting the orally administered bisphosphonate, it may interfere with its bioavailability and hence efficacy. Similarly, if the patient ate within half an hour of taking the medication, food may interfere with the bioavailability of the bisphosphonate.

Mrs. BF stated that in order to remember taking her medications (alendronate, calcium, vitamin D, and mineral supplements), she takes them all at the same time. She thought it would be a good idea to take all her medications "for bone health" at the same time, even if one tablet, the bisphosphonate, is taken only once a week. It is therefore probable that the concomitant intake of calcium and other supplements interfered with the bioavailability of the bisphosphonate, reduced its absorption, and therefore effectiveness at reducing the rate of bone resorption which translated into a further loss of bone mass as evidenced by the BMD changes over the past 2 years. Finally, to be significant, the change in BMD should exceed the least significant changes of the center where the DXA scan is done.

4. ***At this stage the following investigations are recommended:***
   A. Blood chemistry profile.
   B. Serum estradiol level.
   C. Serum FSH level.
   D. Serum protein electrophoresis.
   E. None of the above.

   Correct answer: A

   Comments:

   The blood chemistry profile is indicated to assess renal functions to ensure her kidney functions have not deteriorated. This is an important finding affecting the treatment strategy as bisphosphonates are not recommended in patients with impaired renal functions. Assaying the serum vitamin D level will help ensuring she is not developing vitamin D deficiency. This also could be suspected if the serum alkaline phosphatase level has increased since the previous analysis, even though it may remain within the normal range.

   Apart from these assessments, renal functions, and vitamin D status, at this stage, there is no need for any other blood test to be done. Mrs. BF has been fully investigated as far as her bone status is concerned about 2 years ago. The most probable reason for her nonresponse to alendronate is that she was taking it with dietary supplements which most probably interfered with its bioavailability and efficacy to increase bone density.

   If vitamin D deficiency is suspected, the serum vitamin D metabolites could be assayed. The 25-hydroxy-cholecalciferol (or 25-hydroxy-vitamin D) represents the cumulative vitamin D obtained through diet and exposure to ultraviolet sunrays. In vitamin D deficiency, the level of 25-OH vitamin D is reduced. 1,25-di-hydroxy-cholecalciferol does not reflect the patient's vitamin D status but rather the ability of the kidneys to hydroxylate 25-OH vitamin D at the 1-position, under the influence of circulating parathyroid hormone, to produce 1,25-di-hydroxy-vitamin D, the most active vitamin D metabolite. In vitamin D deficiency as the calcium levels tend to drop, the parathyroid hormone production is increased. This in turn increases the rate of hydroxylation of 25(OH) vitamin D to 1,25-di-hydroxy-vitamin D. The levels of the latter often remain within the normal range.

5. ***Following the oral ingestion of bisphosphonates:***
   A. Most of the bisphosphonate is readily absorbed from the stomach.
   B. Most of the absorption takes place within the first 30 min following the ingestion.
   C. Less than 50% of the orally administered dose is absorbed.
   D. A and B.
   E. B and C.

   Correct answer: E

   Comments:

   Most of the absorption of alendronate and risedronate takes place within the first 30 min after their ingestion. This period is 60 min for ibandronate. As a very small amount of the orally administered bisphosphonate is absorbed, any interference with its absorption may significantly reduce the amount absorbed, and hence efficacy of the bisphosphonate.

6. ***The following statement(s) is/are true:***
   A. Patients taking oral bisphosphonates should be encouraged to have breakfast 30 min after taking alendronate or risedronate and 60 min after taking ibandronate.
   B. The longer the patient can refrain from eating after taking the bisphosphonate the better will the results be.
   C. The bisphosphonate should be taken with at least 6 oz of water, but the larger the quantity of water the better it will be.
   D. A and C.
   E. A, B, and C.

   Correct answer: A

   Comments:

   It may be beneficial for the patient to have some food, preferably high-fiber food, after the period of abstinence, i.e. 30 min for alendronate and risedronate and 60 min after ibandronate. Eating food after the 30-min period has elapsed will allow the ingested food to coat the bisphosphonate particles that have not been absorbed and prevent them from irritating the gastrointestinal mucosa. High-fiber food is preferred to low-fiber food as the fiber is not digested and therefore will be evacuated while still coating the bisphosphonate particles, thus preventing them from irritating the gastrointestinal mucosa and avoiding the pain and heartburn the patient may experience.

   Waiting for longer periods before eating will allow some of the unabsorbed bisphosphonate particles (i.e., most of the ingested tablet) to get in contact with the gastrointestinal mucosa and irritate it, thus causing abdominal discomfort and pain.

   Six to eight ounces of water is the optimum amount to administer the bisphosphonate. Smaller amounts may not be sufficient to disperse the contents of the ingested tablet sufficiently to maximize its absorption. More than 8oz is likely to distend the stomach and gastroesophageal area particularly in older patients and induce nausea.

7. ***The most likely cause for Mrs. BF's apparent resistance to alendronate is:***
   A. She is not taking alendronate as directed.

B. She stopped taking alendronate.
C. She's not getting enough calcium.
D. She has secondary osteoporosis.
E. Any of the above

Correct answer: E

Comments:

Poor compliance is one of the main reasons for nonresponse to orally administered bisphosphonates. It is therefore important for the patient to fully understand how to take that medication and why it is so important to meticulously follow these directions. It may be appropriate to contact the patient 4–6 weeks after prescribing the orally administered bisphosphonate to ensure that the medication is taken exactly as directed and the patient has not experienced any adverse effect.

Follow-up:

Mrs. BF was told that, most probably, the reason for her nonresponse to the oral bisphosphonates is that she was not complying with the intake of this medication. The importance of taking that medication exactly as directed was further emphasized during her clinic visit. She appeared to understand the implications. Other treatment options were offered but she preferred to continue with oral alendronate once a week. A follow-up phone call to Mrs. BF about 6 weeks after the original encounter revealed that she is now taking the medication as directed and has not experienced any adverse effect. She stated she will make sure to take alendronate regularly and as directed.

8. ***If the orally administered bisphosphonate is continued the following follow-up regimen is recommended to ascertain that the medication is taken as directed:***

A. Compare baseline fasting C-telopeptide to that done 1 to 3 months later.
B. Repeat DXA scan in 6 months' time.
C. Repeat DXA scan in 2 years' time.
D. A and B.
E. A and C.

Correct answer: E

Comments:

Assaying the fasting C-telopeptide blood level at baseline and 2–3 months after the weekly self-administration of the oral bisphosphonate has resumed will indicate whether the patient is complying with the intake of that medication and whether it has been successful at reducing the rate of bone resorption.

If 2–3 months after reinitiating alendronate therapy there has been no significant reduction of the fasting serum C-telopeptide blood level, then either the patient is still not complying with the intake of alendronate or it is not absorbed in the gastrointestinal tract. In either instance there needs to be a change in the management strategy.

Follow-up:

The baseline fasting serum C-telopeptide level was 658pg/mL, 8weeks later it was 342 pg/mL, indicating that the rate of bone resorption has been significantly reduced. The patient was appraised of the results, encouraged to continue taking the bisphosphonate as directed, and to ensure an adequate daily calcium and vitamin D intake. She can now be reassured that, as long as she takes alendronate as directed, she should respond well and not experience gastrointestinal adverse effects. Her BMD is likely to increase and the risk of further fractures decreased.

A repeat DXA scan done 2 years later showed increases of 5.6%, 6.1%, and 7.3% in the right and left total hip scan and lumbar vertebrae, respectively. These increases are significant as they all, and each one, exceed the least significant change.

9. ***If it is felt the patient will not comply with the intake of the orally administered bisphosphonate, the following is/are treatments options:***
   A. Zoledronic acid iv infusion once a year.
   B. Denosumab 60mg sc at 6-month intervals.
   C. Teriparatide 20mcg sc daily.
   D. A or B.
   E. Any of the above.

   Correct answer: D

   Comments:

   Given that the patient is only 54years old, and reached menopause when she was 51years old, her rate of bone resorption is likely to be increased. She therefore would benefit most from an antiresorptive medication than from an osteoanabolic one. Therefore, although all three medications are effective at managing osteoporosis, in this patient's case, antiresorptive medications should be the first ones to prescribe. The ease of their administration also increases the likelihood of good compliance.

10. ***The time that should be allowed to elapse between the ingestion of the bisphosphonate and eating or taking any other medication is:***
    A. 30min with alendronate.
    B. 30min with risedronate.
    C. 60min with ibandronate.
    D. 30min with all orally administered bisphosphonates.
    E. A, B, and C.

    Correct answer: E

    Comments:

    In order to maximize the absorption of bisphosphonates it is recommended that they be taken while the patient is fasting and that 30min (for alendronate and risedronate) and 60min (for ibandronate) elapse between the ingestion of the bisphosphonate and the consumption of food and drinks apart from plain water.

Key points

- True resistance to bisphosphonates is rare.
- To be significant, the change in BMD must exceed the least significant change.
- Oral bisphosphonates should be taken exactly as directed in order to maximize the potential benefits and minimize the potential adverse effects.
- Taking bisphosphonates at the same time as dietary supplements or any other medication may interfere with their efficacy.

CHAPTER 15

Zoledronic acid—Annual infusions☆

Learning objectives
- Osteoporosis is silent until a fracture is sustained.
- Osteoporosis is underdiagnosed and undertreated.
- The pharmacologic profile of zoledronic acid: efficacy and adverse effects.

The case study

Reason for seeking medical help

- AJ is a 72-year-old man. Two weeks ago, while spending the weekend with his son and grandchildren, he sustained a fragility femoral neck fracture after tripping, in the carpeted bedroom, over an electric cord he had not noticed. He underwent a total hip replacement and recovered well. He is independent with most of his daily activities. He lives with his wife in a ground floor condominium and has good social support. He is referred for the management of osteoporosis. Secondary causes of osteoporosis have been ruled out.

Past medical and surgical history

- No relevant past medical history—no history of repeated falls, and no dizzy spells.
- He had been diagnosed with osteoporosis about 2years ago when he sustained a hip fracture while working in his garage: he tried to reach for a tool on a high shelf, lost his equilibrium, and fell. He responded well to surgery and was prescribed alendronate, but could not tolerate it. He was then switched to risedronate but could not tolerate it also because of the upper gastrointestinal adverse events he experienced. His primary care provider changed risedronate to ibandronate. AJ, however, continued to experience the same upper gastrointestinal adverse events and stopped taking the medication without notifying his primary care provider.
- Always enjoyed good health.

☆ AJ, 72-year-old Caucasian man, 2 weeks postfragility hip fracture.

Diagnosis and Treatment of Osteoporosis. https://doi.org/10.1016/B978-0-323-99550-4.00011-3
Copyright © 2024 Elsevier Inc. All rights are reserved, including those for text and data mining, AI training, and similar technologies.

Lifestyle

- Physically independent and mentally good up to time of fracture.
- Sedentary lifestyle but travels frequently: at least once a month to visit family and friends.
- Daily dietary calcium intake estimated to be about 1000 mg.
- No cigarette smoking, no alcohol abuse.
- Low salt and caffeine intake.
- One cocktail every day before dinner, two on weekends.

Medication

- Multivitamin tablets, once a day.

Family history

- Mother sustained fragility hip fracture.

Clinical examination

- Weight 161 pounds, steady, height 5′7″.
- No pain but appears anxious.
- Able to ambulate independently, but hesitant and unsteady.
- No evidence of neurologic deficit, no localized weakness, no tremors, cerebellar functions intact.
- Moderate osteoarthritic changes in knees and hands.

Laboratory result(s)

- Comprehensive metabolic panel (CMP): normal, eGFR>60 mL/min.
- Serum 25-hydroxy-vitamin D level: 52 ng/mL.

DXA and radiological result(s)

- Lumbar vertebrae: −2.8.
- Hips: neither hip could be scanned because of the fractures sustained.
- Left distal radius: −2.5.
- Vertebral fracture assessment: no vertebral fractures noted.

Multiple choice questions

1. ***The following is/are true concerning fragility hip fractures in men:***
   A. Are diagnostic of osteoporosis and are associated with a worse prognosis than fragility hip fractures in women.
   B. Up to one-third of the patients die within a year of the fracture.
   C. Less than 10% of men and 25% of women who sustain an osteoporotic fracture are treated for osteoporosis.
   D. A and B.
   E. A, B, and C.

   Correct answer: E

   Comments:

   Fragility fractures, i.e., fractures occurring in the absence of trauma (atraumatic fractures) or as a result of trauma that ordinarily would not be expected to give rise to a fracture (low trauma or low impact fractures), are diagnostic of osteoporosis.

   It is estimated that one in four men over the age of 50 years is expected to sustain an osteoporotic fracture,[1] and approximately half of the female population over the age of 50 years is expected to sustain a fragility fracture. Hip fractures are life-changing events. The mortality and morbidity associated with hip fractures are worse in men than in women: about one-third die within 1 year of the fracture.[2] Osteoporosis, particularly in men, remains underdiagnosed and undertreated: less than 10% of men who have sustained a hip fracture are treated for osteoporosis.[3] Several guidelines have been published to help identify and treat these patients.[4,5]

   Osteoporosis, nevertheless, still remains an asymptomatic, silent disease and often patients who have sustained a fragility fracture deny having a diagnosis of "Osteoporosis": "I just fractured my hip.... It's only a fracture; I do not have osteoporosis" are frequent comments made by patients and often reinforced by the lack of urgency from the patient's health care providers. As already mentioned, a fragility fracture is diagnostic of osteoporosis on par with, for instance, ketoacidosis being diagnostic of diabetes mellitus. No health care provider would manage a patient's ketoacidosis and ignore the underlying diagnosis of diabetes mellitus. The same should apply to fragility fractures, which are often the first manifestation of the underlying problem: osteoporosis, hence the remark that "osteoporosis is a silent disease" albeit until a fragility fracture occurs. Osteoporosis in men is discussed in another case study in this series.

2. ***Factors affecting outcome after sustaining a fragility hip fracture include:***
   A. Prefracture level of cognitive functioning.
   B. Prefracture level of physical independence.
   C. Comorbidities prior to the fracture.
   D. A, B, and C.
   E. B and C.

Correct answer: D

Comment:

The level of cognitive functioning prior to sustaining the fracture is the single most important prognostic factor for resuming prefracture function.[6] The level of physical independence and prefracture comorbidities also affect the prognosis. The longer the period of physical inactivity after sustaining a fracture, the more likely are the skeletal muscles to waste, and atrophy, leading to instability, weakness, increased risk of further falls and fractures. Physical rehabilitation should start as soon as possible after surgical fracture repair. Patients' motivation for return to their own environment should be kept high.

3. ***When administered within 90 days after a hip fracture, compared to placebo, over a 2-year period, annual Zoledronic acid (ZA) intravenous infusions reduced:***
   A. Clinical fractures by 35%.
   B. Vertebral fractures by 46%.
   C. Overall mortality by 28%.
   D. A and C.
   E. A, B, and C.

Correct answer: E

Comment:

These are the results of the "**H**ealth **O**utcomes and **R**educed **I**ncidence with **Z**oledronic acid **On**ce yearly—Pivotal **F**racture **T**rial: **HORIZON—PFT**." It is an international, randomized, double-blind, placebo controlled, clinical trial on men and women who sustained a hip fracture and underwent surgical repair in the 90days prior to enrollment in the study.[7] A subsequent analysis demonstrated the positive effects of ZA when administered as early as 2 weeks after the fracture occurred.

4. ***The likelihood of the patient being diagnosed and treated for osteoporosis after sustaining a fragility fracture is:***
   A. 60%.
   B. 50%.
   C. 45%.
   D. 33%.
   E. 25%.

Correct answer: E

Comment:

It is difficult to rationalize how it is possible that only one of every four patients who sustain an osteoporotic fragility fracture is diagnosed and treated for osteoporosis, even though it is well established that fragility fractures, per se, are diagnostic of osteoporosis. Furthermore, once an osteoporotic fracture has occurred, the risk of sustaining further fractures is substantially increased and the morbidity and mortality after sustaining an osteoporotic fracture are also significantly increased. The irony is that we now have effective, relatively safe, and cheap medications that can reduce the risk of vertebral, nonvertebral, and even hip fractures.

5. ***Following a fragility osteoporotic fracture, the risk of sustaining, within 18 months, a subsequent hip fracture is approximately:***
   A. 72.5%.
   B. 64%.
   C. 56%.
   D. 43%.
   E. 28%.

   Correct answer: E

   Comment:

   A large retrospective cohort study which included 115,776 patients, 65 years of age and older, who sustained a hip fracture, revealed that a subsequent second hip fracture occurred in 27.8% of the patients who sustained a hip fracture. The median time to a second hip fracture was approximately 18months postindex event. The one-year mortality rate from any cause after the index hip fracture was 26.2%.[8] There is a need to recognize that at present a number of medications are commercially available to significantly reduce the risk of further fractures, including hip fractures. The judicious use of these medications should ensure maximal benefit and minimal adverse effects.

6. ***Zoledronic acid (ZA) is effective for the:***
   A. Treatment and prevention of postmenopausal osteoporosis.
   B. Treatment and prevention of glucocorticoid-induced osteoporosis.
   C. Treatment of men with osteoporosis.
   D. A, B, and C.
   E. A and B.

   Correct answer: D

   Comments:

   ZA is useful for the management of the previously mentioned conditions.[9] At the end of 3 years, compared to placebo, ZA infusions reduced hip fractures by 41%, morphometric vertebral fractures by 70%, and clinical vertebral fractures by 77% in postmenopausal women with osteoporosis.[10,11] It is also effective in postmenopausal women with osteopenia[12] and men with osteoporosis and osteopenia.[3,13–17] ZA is also useful for the prevention and treatment of osteoporosis in patients on glucocorticoids,[18] patients on aromatase inhibitors[19] those with metastatic bone disease,[20] those with HIV-induced bone loss,[21] and to prevent poststroke bone demineralization.[22]

7. ***Zoledronic acid (ZA):***
   A. ZA is an intravenously administered bisphosphonate.
   B. Overcomes issues related to adherence with oral bisphosphonates.
   C. Should not be administered if the creatinine clearance is 35 mL/min or less.
   D. Should not be administered to patients with hypocalcemia.
   E. All of the above.

   Correct answer: E

   Comments:

   ZA is a bisphosphonate administered once a year by intravenous infusion. It overcomes many issues related to adherence (compliance and persistence) to oral bisphosphonate therapy.

   AJ is a good candidate for ZA: he could tolerate neither alendronate, nor risedronate, nor ibandronate, and his travel schedule is such that adherence to oral bisphosphonates is likely to be low. Denosumab is another alternative, discussed in another case study.

   As ZA is excreted by the kidneys, its administration is not recommended to patients with a creatinine clearance of 35 mL/min or less and caution should be exercised when administered with potentially nephrotoxic medications, including, and especially, nonsteroidal antiinflammatory medications as they can be obtained over the counter, without a medical prescription. Transient elevations in serum creatinine levels were observed in 1.3% of patients receiving ZA infusion as opposed to 0.4% of those receiving placebo infusions. However, within 30 days of the infusion the serum creatinine levels returned to the preinfusion levels.[23]

   Hypocalcemia may occur in patients who rely on the mobilization of calcium from the skeleton to the circulatory compartment to maintain the serum calcium level within a narrow range. By suddenly inhibiting bone resorption, ZA may reduce calcium flow from bones to circulation, thus inducing hypocalcemia or aggravating an existing one. ZA should not be administered to patients with hypocalcemia.

8. ***The Acute Phase Reaction (APR) following ZA iv infusion:***
   A. Affects about 18% of bisphosphonate naïve patients, but only about 9% of patients previously exposed to bisphosphonates.
   B. Presents as fatigue, headaches, generalized aches and pains, myalgia, bone/joint pains, and low-grade fever.
   C. Is significantly reduced if the patient takes acetaminophen 1000mg or a nonsteroidal antiinflammatory drug before the infusion.
   D. Is an allergic reaction.
   E. A, B, and C.

   Correct answer: E

   Comments:

   The APR is probably the result of a large bisphosphonate dose administered over a short period of time (15–30 min). It is also seen, albeit to a much lesser extent, when oral monthly doses of bisphosphonates are taken for the first time. Patients with the APR experience a variety of symptoms, including generalized aches or pains, low-grade fever, malaise, and fatigue occurring 1 or 2 days after the infusion and lasting 3–5 days. Occasionally it may last longer.

The APR is seen more frequently in bisphosphonate naïve patients than in those who had been on oral bisphosphonates and is less frequent and less severe after the second and subsequent infusions. It is not an allergic reaction. The incidence and severity are reduced by the intake of acetaminophen before the infusion.[24] Although nonsteroidal antiinflammatory medications also reduce its severity, they should be used cautiously given their potential nephrotoxicity.[25]

9. ***The musculoskeletal pain experienced after the administration of ZA:***
   A. Is usually localized to the lower back, hips, upper legs, and occasionally ribs.
   B. Is part of the acute phase reaction.
   C. Usually occurs within hours of the ZA administration.
   D. Is usually relieved spontaneously within a few days of the ZA administration.
   E. A, C, and D.

   Correct answer: A

   Comment:

   Patients may develop moderate to severe pain in the lower back, hips, upper thighs, and occasionally ribs after the intravenous or oral administration of bisphosphonates. Unlike the APR which occurs within a few days of ZA administration, musculoskeletal pains occur any time. The underlying mechanism of musculoskeletal pain postadministration of bisphosphonates is poorly understood. It can be related to hypovitaminosis D and compensatory secondary hyperparathyroidism associated with an increased bone turnover rate and bone vascularity resulting in a higher concentration of bisphosphonate in the bone microenvironment leading to increased production of proinflammatory cytokines and triggering a localized inflammatory response.[25,26] There is also some evidence to suggest that patients who develop an APR have a better BMD response than those who do not experience it.[27]

10. ***Adverse effect(s) reported after ZA administration include:***
    A. Arrhythmias.
    B. Atrial fibrillation.
    C. Myocardial infarction.
    D. A and B.
    E. All of the above.

    Correct answer: E

    Comment:

    Atrial fibrillation occurred in 6.9% of the patients on ZA as opposed to 5.3% of the patients on placebo. The onset of arrhythmias typically was more than 30days after ZA iv infusion, casting doubt on a cause-and-effect relationship.[27]

Very rarely, diffuse, severe, unilateral ocular and orbital inflammation including corneal endotheliitis, anterior uveitis, and scleritis has been reported within 12h of the zoledronic acid intravenous infusion. Topical steroids, and high-dose systemic corticosteroids as well as referral to expert opinion, may be recommended.[28,29]

Case summary

Analysis of data

Factors predisposing to bone demineralization/osteoporosis in AJ's case

- Diagnosed with osteoporosis about 2 years ago, postfragility fracture; no treatment.
- Sedentary lifestyle.
- Positive family history for osteoporosis, especially mother sustaining fragility hip fracture.

Factors reducing risk of bone demineralization/osteoporosis in AJ's case

- Good daily calcium intake.
- No cigarette smoking.
- No alcohol abuse.
- Low salt and caffeine intake.

Factors increasing risk of falls/fractures

- Two fragility hip fractures.
- Falls sustained.
- Hazardous home environment: trailing electric cords.
- Positive family history: mother sustained fragility hip fracture.

Factors reducing risk of falls/fractures

- Physically independent up to time of fracture.

Diagnosis

Established osteoporosis, i.e., densitometric evidence of osteoporosis and fragility hip fracture.

Management recommendations

Pharmacological treatment

- Zoledronic acid is the drug of choice for this patient who sustained a fragility fracture about 2 weeks prior to referral. He could tolerate neither risedronate, nor alendronate, nor ibandronate administered orally. Given his lifestyle, especially the frequent travel, he is likely to fully adhere with neither the intake of orally administered bisphosphonates nor daily subcutaneous injections of teriparatide or abaloparatide. Zoledronic acid infusions are not associated with any GI adverse effects. Compliance is usually good especially if the patient is motivated. Another alternative medication for AJ is denosumab. This is discussed in another case study in this series.

Diagnostic tests and follow-up

- No further testing required: secondary causes of osteoporosis have been ruled out; eGFR > 60 mL/min, and serum 25-hydroxy-vitamin D and calcium levels are within normal limits: 52 ng/mL and 9.2 mg/mL, respectively.
- One year: assay serum vitamin D, calcium, and creatinine, prior to second ZA infusion.
- Two years: DXA scan and assay serum vitamin D, calcium, and creatinine prior to third ZA infusion.

Lifestyle

- Encourage he continues with his physically and mentally active lifestyle.
- Ensure adequate daily calcium and vitamin D intake preferably from food, but failing this from supplements.

Rehabilitation

- Rehabilitation until physically independent.
- Prevent postfall syndrome.

References

1. Diab DL, Watts NB. Updates on osteoporosis in men. *Endocrinol Metab Clin North Am.* 2021;50:239–249.
2. Brauer C, Coca-Perraillon M, Cutler D, Rosen A. Incidence, and mortality of hip fractures in the United States. *JAMA.* 2009;302:1573–1579.
3. Szulc P, Kaufman JM, Orwoll ES. Osteoporosis in men. *J Osteoporosis.* 2012;675984.
4. Qaseem A, Snow V, Shekell P, et al. Screening for osteoporosis in men: a clinical practice guideline from the American College of Physicians. *Ann Intern Med.* 2008;148:680–684.
5. Watts N, Adler R, Bilezikian J, et al. Osteoporosis in men—an endocrine Society clinical practice guideline. *J Clin Endocrinol Metab.* 2012;97:1802–1822.
6. Samuelsson B, Hedstrom MI, Ponzer S, et al. Gender differences and cognitive aspects on functional outcome after hip fracture – a 2-years' follow-up of 2,134 patients. *Age Ageing.* 2009;38(6):686–692.
7. Lyles KW, Colon-Emeric CS, Magaziner JS, et al. Zoledronic acid and clinical fractures and mortality after hip fracture. *N Engl J Med.* 2007;357:1799–1809.
8. Schemitsch E, Adachi JD, Brown JP, et al. Hip fracture predicts subsequent hip fracture: a retrospective observational study to support a call to early hip fracture prevention efforts in post-fracture patients. *Osteoporos Int.* 2022;33:113–122.
9. Eriksen EF, Lyles KW, Colon-Emeric CS, et al. Antifracture efficacy and reduction of mortality in relation to timing of the first dose of zoledronic acid after hip fracture. *J Bone Miner Res.* 2009;24(7):1308–1313.
10. Black DM, Delmas PD, Eastell R, et al. Once-yearly zoledronic acid for treatment of postmenopausal osteoporosis. *N Engl J Med.* 2007;356(18):1809–1822.
11. Black DM, Reid IR, Boonen S, et al. The effect of 3 versus 6 years of zoledronic acid treatment of osteoporosis: a randomized extension to HORIZON-PFT. *J Bone Miner Res.* 2012;27:243–254.
12. McClung M, Miller P, Recknor C, et al. Zoledronic acid for the prevention of bone loss in postmenopausal women with low bone mass: a randomized controlled trial. *Obstet Gynecol.* 2009;114(5):999–1007.
13. Boonen S, Reginster J-Y, Kaufman J-M, et al. Fracture risk and zoledronic acid therapy in men with osteoporosis. *N Engl J Med.* 2012;367:1714–1723.
14. Boonen S, Orwoll E, Magaziner J, et al. Once-yearly zoledronic acid in older men compared with women with recent hip fracture. *J Am Geriatr Soc.* 2011;59(11):2084–2090.

15. Ruza I, Mirfakhraee S, Orwoll E, Gruntmanis U. Clinical experience with intravenous zoledronic acid in the treatment of male osteoporosis: evidence and opinions. *Ther Adv Musculoskelet Dis*. 2013;5(4):182–198.
16. Spiegel R, Nawroth PP, Kasperk C. The effect of zoledronic acid on the fracture risk in men with osteoporosis. *J Endocrinol Invest*. 2014;37(3):229–232. https://doi.org/10.1007/s40618-013-0038-5.
17. Sim IW, Ebeling PR. Treatment of osteoporosis in men with bisphosphonates: rationale and latest evidence. *Ther Adv Musculoskelet Dis*. 2013;5(5):259–267.
18. Reid DM, Devogelaer JP, Saag K, et al. Zoledronic acid and risedronate in the prevention and treatment of glucocorticoid induced osteoporosis (HORIZON): a multicenter, double-blind, double-dummy, ramdomised controlled trial. *Lancet*. 2009;373(9671):1253–1263.
19. Hines SL, Sloan JA, Atherton PJ, et al. Zoledronic acid for treatment of osteopenia and osteoporosis in women with primary breast cancer undergoing adjuvant aromatase inhibitor therapy. *Breast*. 2010;19(2):92–96.
20. Polascik TJ, Mouraviev V. Zoledronic acid in the management of metastatic bone disease. *Therapeut Clin Risk Mange*. 2008;4:261–268.
21. Poole KE, Loveridge N, Rose CM, et al. A single infusion of zoledronate prevents bone loss after stroke. *Stroke*. 2007;38(5):1519–1525.
22. Huang J, Meixner L, Fernandez S, et al. A double-blind, randomized controlled trial of zoledronate therapy for HIV-associated osteopenia and osteoporosis. *AIDS*. 2009;23(1):51–57.
23. Boonen S, Sellmeyer DE, Lippuner K, et al. Renal safety of annual zoledronic acid infusions in osteoporotic postmenopausal women. *Kidney Int*. 2008;74:641–648.
24. Wysowski DK, Chang JT. Alendronate and risedronate: reports of severe bone, joint and muscle pain. *Arch Intern Med*. 2005;165:346–347.
25. Crotti C, Watts NB, De Santis M, et al. Acute phase reactions after zoledronic acid infusion: protective role of 25 hydroxyvitamin D and previous oral bisphosphonate therapy. *Endocr Pract*. 2019;24(5):405–410.
26. Black DM, Reid IR, Napoli N, et al. The interaction of acute-phase reaction and efficacy for osteoporosis after zoledronic acid: HORIZON pivotal fracture trial. *J Bone Miner Res*. 2021;1–8.
27. Pazianas M, Compston J, Huang CL. Atrial fibrillation, and bisphosphonate therapy. *J Bone Miner Res*. 2010;25 (1):2–10.
28. Procianoy F, Procianoy E. Orbital inflammatory disease secondary to a single-dose administration of zoledronic acid for treatment of postmenopausal osteoporosis. *Osteoporos Int*. 2010;21:1057–1058.
29. Umunakwe OC, Herren D, Kim SJ, Kohanim S. Diffuse ocular, and orbital inflammation after zoledronate infusions – case report and review of the literature. *Digit J Ophthalmol*. 2017;23(4):109–112.

CHAPTER 16

Receptor activator of nuclear factor kappa-B ligand (RANK-L) inhibitor—Denosumab☆

Learning objectives

- Appreciate the mode of action of denosumab, its efficacy, and adverse effects.
- Develop a management strategy to follow up patients on denosumab.

The case study

Reason for seeking medical help

NB is a 58-year-old Caucasian woman diagnosed with osteoporosis about 3 months ago. She was prescribed alendronate but could not tolerate the upper gastrointestinal adverse effects she experienced, did not appreciate the "prolonged" routine involved in taking oral bisphosphonates, and did not wish to continue with these tablets, other oral bisphosphonates, or any medication for osteoporosis. She emphasizes that she is essentially asymptomatic; has not sustained any fractures, falls, or near-falls; and does not experience dizzy spells. She believes she therefore does not need any medication with adverse effects to treat a disease that is largely asymptomatic! It took quite some time to convince her of the natural history of osteoporosis and the importance of treating the disease before a fracture occurs.

Past medical and surgical history

- Osteoporosis, diagnosed about 3 months ago by bone densitometry. DXA scan results: T-scores left femoral neck −2.6, left total hip −2.2, L1–L4: −2.8.
- No evidence of fractures.
- Natural menopause at age 51 years, no HRT.

☆ NB, 58-year-old Caucasian woman with osteoporosis, could not tolerate oral bisphosphonates.

Diagnosis and Treatment of Osteoporosis. https://doi.org/10.1016/B978-0-323-99550-4.00004-6
Copyright © 2024 Elsevier Inc. All rights are reserved, including those for text and data mining, AI training, and similar technologies.

Lifestyle

- Daily dietary calcium intake about 1200 mg.
- No excessive caffeine, sodium, or alcohol intake.
- No cigarette smoking.
- Active physical lifestyle: jogs about 2 miles every weekday and cycles about 5 miles during most weekends.

Medication

- No medication.

Family history

- Older sister: fragility hip fracture, about 6 months ago.

Clinical examination

- Weight 151 pounds, height 62″.
- Get-Up-and-Go test completed in 7 s.
- No relevant clinical findings. No fractures, no orthostatic hypotension, no arrhythmias, no clinical evidence of sensitive carotid sinus, no arthropathies, no cervical spondylosis, and no localizing neurological lesions.

Laboratory results

- CBC, CMP, TSH within normal limits.
- Serum vitamin D: 42 ng/mL.

Multiple choice questions

1. ***After reviewing treatment options, NB chose denosumab. The following is/are true about denosumab:***
   A. Antiresorptive agent.
   B. Human antibody with high specificity.
   C. Excreted by the kidneys.
   D. A and B.
   E. A, B, and C.
   Correct answer: D
   Comment:
   Denosumab is a highly specific, fully human, monoclonal antibody that specifically binds to Receptor Activator Nuclear Factor-Kappa-beta Ligand (RANK-L), thus preventing the

activation of RANK which in turn prevents the recruitment of preosteoclasts to form osteoclasts, maturation of osteoclasts, and their subsequent activation.[1] Denosumab is neither metabolized nor excreted by the kidneys. It therefore can be administered to patients with mild to moderately impaired renal functions. It is nevertheless important to monitor the serum calcium level to prevent hypocalcemia.[2] Denosumab is well tolerated. When given a choice, more patients (92%) prefer denosumab to alendronate.[3]

2. ***In postmenopausal women with osteoporosis, compared to placebo, over a 3-year period, denosumab reduced the risk of:***
   A. Hip fractures by 40%.
   B. Vertebral fractures by 68%.
   C. Nonvertebral fractures by 20%.
   D. A and B.
   E. A, B, and C.

   Correct answer: E

   Comment:

   These are the results of the pivotal phase 3 study, a 3-year randomized double-blind, placebo-controlled study, which included 7868 postmenopausal women between the ages of 60 and 90years and with a T-score of −2.5 or lower at lumbar vertebrae or total hip. Exclusion criteria included women who had a T-score of −4.0 or lower, one severe or more than two moderate vertebral compression fractures, and those with a serum vitamin D level lower than 12ng/mL. Neutralizing antibodies did not develop in any of the subjects.[4]

3. ***In postmenopausal women with osteoporosis, compared to placebo, over a 3-year period, denosumab induced the following changes:***
   A. Lumbar vertebrae BMD increased by 9.2%.
   B. CTX decreased by 72%.
   C. P1NP decreased by 76%.
   D. A and B.
   E. A, B, and C.

   Correct answer: E

   Comment:

   In this study, at the end of the 3-year period, compared to placebo, patients on denosumab had an average 9.2% increase in lumbar vertebrae BMD (95% CI 8.2–10.1) and 6.0% total hip (95% CI 5.2–6.7). Serum CTX (C-telopeptide of type I collagen), a marker of bone resorption, decreased by 86%, 72%, and 72% at month 1, 6, and 36, respectively, and serum intact procollagen type I N-terminal propeptide (P1NP), a marker of bone formation, decreased by 18%, 50%, and 76% at month 1, 6, and 36, respectively.[4]

   The BMD increases were further enhanced in the Extension study: compared to baseline, patients who had been for 5years on denosumab had mean increases of 13.7% at the lumbar vertebrae, 7.0% total hip, 6.1% femoral neck, and 2.3% at 1/3 radius (all $P < 0.001$).[5] Patients who had been on denosumab for 10years had a 21.7% increase in BMD of the lumbar vertebrae and 9.2% in the total hip.[6]

4. ***In the initial 3 years of the FREEDOM trial, the main adverse effects of denosumab included:***
   A. Increased risk of cellulitis/skin infections.
   B. Systemic infections.
   C. Cutaneous/mucosal lichenoid drug eruptions.
   D. A and C.
   E. A, B, and C.

   Correct answer: E

   Comment:

   In this study, eczema, cellulitis, and serious infections occurred more frequently in patients on denosumab than those on placebo. These trends, however, were not maintained in the extension study.[4–6]

5. ***Possible long-term adverse effects include:***
   A. Osteonecrosis of the jaw.
   B. Atypical femoral shaft fracture.
   C. Increased risk of bone loss and fractures after stopping denosumab.
   D. All of the above.
   E. A and B.

   Correct answer: D

   Comment:

   Like most other antiresorptive medications, the risk of osteonecrosis of the jaw and atypical femoral shaft fractures is increased in patients on long-term denosumab therapy. The fracture risk is also increased in patients who discontinue denosumab and are not prescribed another antiresorptive medication.[7,8]

   The increased risk of vertebral fractures has been observed in patients who discontinue denosumab injections and may occur as early as missing just one single dose by about a month, i.e., 7 months from the previous subcutaneous dose.[9]

6. ***Contraindications to the administration of denosumab include:***
   A. Patients 80 years of age and older.
   B. Hypercalcemia.
   C. Creatinine clearance less than 35 mL/min.
   D. Hyperparathyroidism.
   E. None of the above.

   Correct answer: E

   Comment:

   Old age is not a contraindication to the administration of denosumab. A retrospective study on 60 female patients, mean age 83.9± years, treated with denosumab every 6 months for 12 months showed significant increases in the BMD of the lumbar vertebrae:

3.02±2.74% ($P = .000$), femoral neck 3.10±6.90% ($P = .005$), and total hip 2.89±5.80 ($P = .002$). Similarly, the serum bone marker levels of the C-terminal telopeptide type I collagen and osteocalcin declined significantly after 12 months of treatment: −34.8 ± 45.9% ($P = .002$) and −35.5 ± 38.9% ($P = .004$), respectively.[10]

By reducing the rate of bone resorption and therefore the mobilization of calcium from bones to circulation, denosumab may induce or worsen an existing hypocalcemia. It is therefore contraindicated in patients who have hypocalcemia. Checking the serum calcium level prior to the administration of denosumab is recommended.

As denosumab is not excreted by the kidneys, it can be safely administered to patients with impaired renal functions. Care should nevertheless be exercised as these patients' calcium homeostasis is precarious. Denosumab is not contraindicated in patients with hyperparathyroidism.

In patients with normal serum calcium and vitamin D levels, normal renal functions, and administered 1-g calcium carbonate and 800 IU cholecalciferol daily, the administration of denosumab was followed by significant increases in serum parathyroid hormone level at 1-month, returning to baseline at 6 months: baseline serum PTH: 34.8 ± 2.8; 1 month: 62.4 ± 13.3 and 6 months 40.7 ± 4.0 pg/mL.

7. ***Discontinuation of denosumab therapy is associated with:***
   A. Increased fracture risk.
   B. Decreases in BMD.
   C. Increases in markers of bone turnover.
   D. B and C.
   E. A, B, and C.

Correct answer: E

Comment:

Discontinuation of denosumab is associated with increases in bone turnover, decreases in BMD, and an increased vertebral fracture risk, especially multiple vertebral compression fractures, often more than the pretreatment fracture risk.[11]

"Drug holidays" when denosumab is discontinued are therefore not recommended in patients who have been on denosumab unless some other antiresorptive medication is prescribed when the administration of donepezil is stopped.

The increased fracture risk after discontinuing denosumab can be as early as 7 months after the last injection, i.e., postponing the intake of denosumab by as short a period as 1 month can be sufficient to trigger an increased rate of bone resorption and an increased risk of fractures sustaining fractures. Most fractures nevertheless occur between 9 and 19 months of discontinuance of denosumab. This "rebound phenomenon" may lead to multiple vertebral compression fractures.[11] It can be, at least partly, avoided if the cessation of denosumab is followed by the administration of a bisphosphonate.[7,12–15] Unfortunately, in some instances, the denosumab rebound-associated vertebral fractures continue despite reinstitution of denosumab.[12]

8. ***When denosumab is combined with teriparatide, over a 12-month period, compared to either medication on its own, changes in the following parameters are significant:***
   A. Increases in BMD.
   B. Decreases in fracture risk.
   C. Decreases in markers of bone resorption.
   D. A and C.
   E. A, B, and C.

   Correct answer: D

   Comment:

   At the end of a 12-month period, the combination of denosumab and teriparatide induced larger increases in the BMD and more pronounced changes in bone turnover markers than either medication alone. The mean increases in BMD at the lumbar vertebrae were 6.2%, 5.5%, and 9.1% for the teriparatide, denosumab, and combination group, respectively. Changes in femoral neck BMD were 0.8%, 2.1%, and 4.2% and in the total hip were 0.7%, 2.5%, and 4.9%, respectively. Markers of bone resorption (CTX) were decreased more in the denosumab and combination group than in the teriparatide group. Markers of bone formation (osteocalcin and P1NP) increased more with teriparatide than either denosumab alone or denosumab combined with teriparatide. Fracture risk reduction was not assessed given the short duration of the study: 12 months.[16]

9. ***Match the following:***
   (a) Denosumab.
   (b) Bisphosphonates.
   (c) Both.
   (d) Neither.
      A. Embedded in bone matrix.
      B. Stimulate osteoblast receptors.
      C. Cleared by reticuloendothelial system.
      D. Recycling occurs after medication is discontinued.
      E. Inhibit osteoclast intracellular enzymes.

   Correct answers: A (b); B (d); C (a); D (b); E (b)

   Comment:

   The antiresorptive effect of bisphosphonates and denosumab is mediated differently.[17] Bisphosphonates become embedded in the bone matrix calcified hydroxyapatite crystals until released by the acidic environment created by the osteoclasts during bone resorption. Once engulfed by osteoclasts they inhibit intracellular enzymes, interfere with bone-resorbing activity, and induce apoptosis. Denosumab prevents the activation, differentiation, maturation, and activation of osteoclasts by binding with RANK-L which stimulates RANK surface receptors.

   Denosumab is cleared by the reticuloendothelial system and is not excreted by the kidneys. It therefore can be administered safely to patients with impaired renal functions.

Bisphosphonates are cleared through renal excretion. Neither bisphosphonates nor denosumab is metabolized by the liver. "Recycling" occurs as bisphosphonates are released from the bone matrix to the circulation. No recycling occurs with denosumab.

10. ***In patients on hormonal ablation therapy, denosumab:***
    A. In men with prostate cancer, increases BMD, reduces bone turnover and fracture risk.
    B. In women with breast cancer, increases BMD, reduces bone turnover and fracture risk.
    C. In men and women, adverse effects were similar to placebo.
    D. A and B.
    E. A, B, and C.

    Correct answer: E

    Comment:

    In men with prostate cancer on hormonal ablation therapy, over a 3-year period, compared to placebo, denosumab reduced the risk of new vertebral fractures at 12 months: 0.3% denosumab, 1.9% placebo; 24 months: 1.0% versus 3.3%; and 36 months: 1.5% versus 3.9%. Denosumab also induced increases in BMD and decreases in bone turnover markers.[14] Similarly, in women with nonmetastatic breast cancer on aromatase inhibitors, over a 2-year period, compared to placebo, denosumab reduced the risk of nonvertebral fractures, increased BMD, and decreased bone turnover.[15,16]

Case summary

Analysis of data

Factors predisposing to bone demineralization/osteoporosis

- Status postmenopause, no HRT.
- Caucasian race.
- Positive family history for osteoporosis and fragility fractures: older sister sustained fragility hip fracture.

Factors protecting against bone demineralization/osteoporosis

- Good daily dietary calcium intake.
- Active physical lifestyle.
- No alcohol abuse, no cigarette smoking, no excess sodium or caffeine.

Factors increasing risk of falls/fractures

- None.

Factors reducing risk of falls/fractures

- Active physical lifestyle.

Diagnosis

Osteoporosis, as diagnosed by bone densitometry: a T-score of −2.5 or lower in one of the hips, lumbar vertebrae, or distal one-third radius. No fractures.

Management recommendations

Further tests

- None at this stage.

Medications

- Denosumab 60 mg sc at 6-month intervals.

Lifestyle

- Maintain present healthy lifestyle.

Follow-up

- 6, 12, and 18 months visits, before the administration of denosumab, to ensure the serum calcium level is within the normal range and renal functions are normal prior to next denosumab sc injection.
- 2 years: DXA scan, serum calcium level, and serum vitamin D level prior to fourth denosumab injection.

Key points

- Denosumab is useful in the management of osteoporosis in postmenopausal women and men.
- Denosumab reduces vertebral and nonvertebral fracture risk.
- Denosumab is well tolerated.
- Discontinuation of denosumab is sometimes associated with a rebound increase in bone turnover rate, a decreased BMD, and an increased fracture risk, especially multiple vertebral compression fractures. This "rebound phenomenon" can be minimized by the timely administration of other antiresorptive or osteoanabolic medication.

References

1. Delmas PD. Clinical potential of RANKL inhibition for the management of postmenopausal osteoporosis and other metabolic bone diseases. *J Clin Densitom.* 2008;93:2149–2157.
2. Nitta K, Yajima A, Tsuchiya K. Management of osteoporosis in chronic renal disease. *Intern Med.* 2017;56 (24):3271–3276.

3. Kendler DL, Macarios D, Lillestol MJ, et al. Influence of patient perceptions and preferences for osteoporosis medication on adherence behavior in the denosumab adherence preference satisfaction study. *Menopause*. 2014;21(1):25–32. https://doi.org/10.1097/GME.0b013e31828f5e5d.
4. Cummings SR, San Martin J, McClung MR, et al. Denosumab for prevention of fractures in postmenopausal women with osteoporosis. *N Engl J Med*. 2009;361:756–765.
5. Papapoulos S, Chapurlat R, Libanati C, et al. Five years of denosumab exposure in women with postmenopausal osteoporosis: results from the first ten years of the FREEDOM extension. *J Bone Miner Res*. 2012;27 (3):694–701.
6. Bone HG, Wagman RB, Brandi ML, et al. 10 years of denosumab treatment in postmenopausal women with osteoporosis: results from the phase 3 randomised FREEDOM trial and open-label extension. *Lancet Diabetes Endocrinol*. 2017;5(7):513–523.
7. Anastasilakis AD, Makras P, Yavropoulou MP, Tabacco G, Naciu AM, Palermo A. Denosumab discontinuation and the rebound phenomenon: a narrative review. *J Clin Med*. 2021;10:152–180.
8. Bauer DC, Abrahamsen B. Bisphosphonate drug holiday in primary care: when and what to do next? *Curr Osteoporos Rep*. 2021;19:182–188.
9. Brown JP, Roux C, Torring O, et al. Discontinuation of denosumab and associated fracture incidence. *J Bone Mine Res*. 2013;28(4):746–752.
10. Everts-Graber J, Reichenbach S, Gahl B, Ziswiler HR, Studer U, Lehmann T. Risk factors for vertebral fractures and bone loss after denosumab discontinuation: a real-world observational study. *Bone*. 2021;115830.
11. Jeong C, Ha J. The effect of densosumab on bone mass in super-elderly patients. *J Bone Metab*. 2020;27 (2):119–124.
12. Tsai JN, Uihlein AV, Lee H, et al. Teriparatide and denosumab, alone, or combined, in women with postmenopausal osteoporosis: the DATA study randomized trial. *Lancet*. 2013;382(9886):50–56.
13. Hanley DA, Adachi JD, Bell A, Brown V. Denosumab: mechanisms of action and clinical outcomes. *Int J Clin Pract*. 2012;66(12):1139–1146.
14. Smith MR, Egerdie B, Hernandez TN, et al. Denosumab in men receiving androgen-deprivation therapy for prostate cancer. *N Engl J Med*. 2009;361:745–755.
15. Scaturro D, de Sire A, Terrana P, et al. Early denosumab for the prevention of osteoporotic fractures in breast cancer women undergoing aromatase inhibitors: a case control retrospective study. *J Back Musculoskelet Rehabil*. 2021;1:1–6.
16. Ellis CK, Bone HG, Chlebowski R, et al. Randomized trial of denosumab in patients receiving adjuvant aromatase inhibitors for nonmetastatic breast cancer. *J Clin Oncol*. 2008;26:4875–4882.
17. Zeytinoglu M, Naaman SC, Dickens LT. Denosumab discontinuation in patients treated for low Bone density and osteoporosis. *Endocrinol Metab Clin North Am*. 2021;50:205–222.

CHAPTER 17

Sclerostin inhibitor (SERM): Raloxifene☆

Learning objectives

- Raloxifene: Therapeutic profile: efficacy and adverse effects.
- Estrogen/progesterone: uses, limitations, adverse effects.

The case study

Reason for seeking medical help

Mrs. KA, 65-year-old woman is concerned about osteoporosis because her mother recently sustained a fragility hip fracture.

Past medical/surgical history

- Natural menopause at 51 years, no HRT.
- Menarche at 13 years, regular menstrual periods.
- No relevant past medical history.
- Asymptomatic, always enjoyed good health.

Personal habits

- Sedentary lifestyle.
- Daily dietary calcium intake about 1200 mg.
- No excessive sodium, caffeine, alcohol, or carbonated drinks.
- No cigarette smoking.

Medication

- Multivitamin one tablet daily.
- Cholecalciferol 1000 units daily.

☆ KA, 65-year-old Caucasian woman with osteoporosis.

Diagnosis and Treatment of Osteoporosis. https://doi.org/10.1016/B978-0-323-99550-4.00005-8
Copyright © 2024 Elsevier Inc. All rights are reserved, including those for text and data mining, AI training, and similar technologies.

Family history

- Mother sustained fragility hip fracture.

Clinical examination

- Weight 165 pounds, steady; height 65″.
- No significant clinical findings.
- Get-Up-and-Go test completed in 8.3 s.

Laboratory investigations

- Comprehensive metabolic profile, TSH, serum vitamin D levels within normal limits.

DXA scan results

- Left total hip −2.1, left femoral neck −1.9, L1–L4 −2.5.

Multiple choice questions

1. ***In postmenopausal women hormonal replacement therapy (HRT):***
   A. Increases lumbar vertebrae and proximal femur BMD.
   B. Reduces risk of vertebral and hip fractures.
   C. Is associated with significant adverse events.
   D. A and B.
   E. A, B, and C.
   Correct answer: E
   Comment:
   The Women's Health Initiative (WHI) study documents that in postmenopausal women HRT reduces fracture risk, including hip fractures, but is associated with a number of adverse events, including coronary artery disease events, thromboembolism, breast cancer, strokes, urinary incontinence, and dementia.[1,2] HRT is now no longer recommended for the treatment of osteoporosis unless alternate therapies are not appropriate. It may be used for the prevention of osteoporosis if given in the smallest effective dose and for a short period of time.[3] The "smallest effective dose" is determined by vasomotor symptom relief.[3]
   There is also epidemiological evidence that reduced estrogen production by the ovaries is associated with an increased fracture risk. A population study on 80,955 postmenopausal women (mean age 68.8 years) documented that as HRT use decreased from 85% in July 2002 to 18% in December 2008 the age-adjusted hip fracture risk

increased from 3.9 to 5.67 per 1000 women. The increased risk was observed as early as 2 years after cessation of hormonal therapy, steadily increased thereafter and was inversely correlated to T-scores.[4]

2. ***The WHI enrolled postmenopausal women:***
   A. 1–5 years postmenopause.
   B. T-score −2.5 or lower in the vertebrae.
   C. T-score −2.0 to −2.5 and a moderate vertebral compression fracture.
   D. No estrogen intake for at least 3 months.
   E. All of the above.

   Correct answer: D

   Comment:

   The WHI study was a randomized, double-blind, placebo-controlled study on postmenopausal women, 50–79 years old, comparing placebo to estrogen (0.625 mg) in hysterectomized women or estrogen (0.625 mg) and progesterone (2.5 mg) in nonhysterectomized women. The study was devised in such a manner that it be terminated should the potential harm outweigh the potential benefit(s) of estrogen and estrogen/progesterone. The primary endpoint was coronary heart disease events, and neither fractures nor BMD changes. Secondary endpoints, however, included fractures, strokes, thromboembolism, cancer, and all-causes mortality. Enrollment was not based on T-scores. A wash out period of 3 months was required for participants who had been on HRT.

   The estrogen/progesterone study (16,608 participants) was prematurely terminated because the adverse events (increased risk of breast cancer, coronary artery disease events, strokes, and pulmonary emboli) outweighed beneficial effects (reduced fractures and colon cancer).[5] The estrogen only study (10,739 participants) also was subsequently prematurely terminated because of increased incidence of strokes in the estrogen group.[2]

3. ***Hormonal Replacement Therapy (HRT) and risk of coronary artery disease (CAD) events:***
   A. Estrogen increases the risk of coronary artery disease in all age groups.
   B. The risk is increased regardless of presence or absence of CAD.
   C. The risk is increased regardless of estrogen dose.
   D. All of the above.
   E. None of the above.

   Correct answer: E

   Comment:

   A secondary analysis of WHI data showed that adverse cardiovascular events occurred primarily in women 70 years and older and less frequently in those 60 years or younger or within 10 years of the menopause.[6] Other studies document that HRT reduces the risk of cardiovascular events if initiated within 10years of menopause and in women who have no preexisting atherosclerosis.[7,8] The patient's age and underlying CAD therefore may modulate CAD adverse events.[9] Lower doses of estrogen such as 0.3mg daily have been shown to prevent bone loss at the lumbar vertebrae and hips in early postmenopausal women.[10]

4. ***Match the following:***
   (a) Raloxifene.
   (b) Estrogen.
   (c) Both.
   (d) Neither.
      A. Reduced risk of hip fractures.
      B. Reduced risk of colon cancer.
      C. Increased hot flashes.
      D. Increased risk of breast cancer.
      E. Increased thromboemboli.

   Correct answers: A (b); B (b); C (a); D (b); E (c)

   Comment:

   Estrogen with or without progesterone reduces the risk of fractures, including hip fractures, but increases the risk of breast cancer.[1,2] Raloxifene reduces the risk of vertebral, but not hip fractures.[11] Other potentially serious adverse events include deep vein thrombosis, thromboembolism, and strokes. Leg cramps, flu-like symptoms, arthralgias, peripheral edema, and excessive sweating also have been reported.

5. ***Estrogen increases the risk of:***
   A. Dementia.
   B. Strokes.
   C. Urinary incontinence.
   D. A and B.
   E. A, B, and C.

   Correct answers: E

   Comments:

   Estrogen, in doses of 0.625mg daily, increases the risk of gall bladder disease, dementia, strokes, and urinary incontinence in postmenopausal women.[1,2]

6. ***Raloxifene:***
   A. Is a selective estrogen receptor modulator (SERM).
   B. Reduces vertebral and nonvertebral fractures.
   C. Reduces the risk of breast cancer.
   D. A and C.
   E. A, B, and D.

   Correct answer: D

Comment:

Raloxifene is a SERM with estrogen receptor agonistic activity on bone tissue: decreasing bone resorption and turnover, increasing BMD and reducing vertebral, but not nonvertebral fractures.[11] Raloxifene has an estrogen receptor antagonist activity on breast and uterine tissue, thus reducing the risk of breast cancer (ER positive) and uterine cancer.[12,13]

7. ***Raloxifene is contraindicated in patients with a history of:***
   A. Venous thrombosis.
   B. Retinal vein thrombosis.
   C. Pulmonary embolism.
   D. A and C.
   E. A, B, and C.

   Correct answer: E

   Comment:

   Raloxifene increases the risk of venous thromboembolism and therefore should not be administered to patients with a history of venous thrombosis or susceptible to venous thrombosis, including patients with the antiphospholipid antibody syndrome.[11,12,14,15] Similarly, it is prudent to discontinue the use of raloxifene at least 72 h prior to an anticipated prolonged period of immobilization, including transoceanic flights.

8. ***Raloxifene is not recommended in patients who:***
   A. Smoke cigarettes.
   B. Have transient ischemic attacks.
   C. Have hypertension and/or atrial fibrillation.
   D. B and C.
   E. A, B, and C.

   Correct answer: E

   Comment:

   Compared to placebo, patients on raloxifene have a higher incidence of fatal strokes (2.2 versus 1.5 per 1000 person years), but no increase in the overall risk of strokes or coronary events.[9,16,17]

9. ***Raloxifene can be used for the:***
   A. Prevention of osteoporosis.
   B. Primary prevention of coronary heart disease.
   C. Secondary prevention of coronary artery disease.
   D. A and B.
   E. A, B, and C.

   Correct answer: A

   Comment:

   Raloxifene can be used for the prevention of osteoporosis but neither for the primary nor secondary prevention of coronary artery disease. Raloxifene should not be administered to premenopausal women.

10. ***After considering various medications, Mrs. KA decided to go on raloxifene. Appropriate reasons for prescribing it include:***
    A. Ease of administration.
    B. Good patient adherence.
    C. Mrs. KA's fracture risk.
    D. A and C.
    E. A, B, and C.

    Correct answer: E

    Comments:

    Raloxifene is easily administered: it can be taken any time of the day, with or without food. Given Mrs. KA's T-scores, her risk of sustaining a hip fracture is only marginally increased compared to the risk of vertebral fractures. Raloxifene is therefore a reasonable choice as it reduces the risk of vertebral fractures.

Case summary

Analysis of data

Factors predisposing to bone demineralization/osteoporosis
- Status postmenopause, no HRT.
- Positive family history of osteoporosis.
- Sedentary lifestyle.

Factors reducing risk of bone demineralization/osteoporosis
- Good daily calcium intake.
- No excessive sodium or caffeine intake.
- No cigarette smoking.

Factors increasing risk of falls/fractures
- Mother sustained fragility hip fracture.
- Get-Up-and-Go test completed in less than 10 s.

Factors reducing risk of falls/fractures
- None.

Diagnosis

- Postmenopausal osteoporosis, as determined by bone densitometry.

Management recommendations

Treatment recommendation(s)

- Antiresorptive medication.

Diagnostic test(s)

- None at this stage.

Lifestyle

- Enroll in exercise program

DXA scans

- At 2 years to monitor bone mass.

Key points

- Raloxifene reduces the risk of vertebral, but not nonvertebral fractures in postmenopausal women with osteoporosis.
- Estrogen is not recommended for the treatment of osteoporosis, unless other therapies are not appropriate.
- Estrogen can be used for the prevention of osteoporosis if given in the smallest dose for a short period of time.
- Raloxifene reduces risk of estrogen receptor positive breast cancer.
- Main adverse effects of raloxifene include hot flushes, deep venous thromboses, and leg cramps.

References

1. Cauley JA, Robbins J, Chen Z, et al. Effects of estrogen plus progestin on risk of fracture and bone mineral density: the women's health initiative randomized trial. *JAMA*. 2003;290:1729–1738.
2. Anderson GL, Limacher M, Assaf AR, et al. Effects of conjugated equine estrogen in postmenopausal women with hysterectomy: the women's health initiative randomized controlled trial. *JAMA*. 2004;291:1701–1712.
3. North American Menopause Society. Estrogen and progesterone use in postmenopausal women 2010 position statement of the North American Menopause Society. *Menopause*. 2010;17:242–255.
4. Karim R, Dell RM, Greene DF, et al. Hip fracture in postmenopausal women after cessation of hormone therapy: results from a prospective study in a large health management organization. *Menopause*. 2011;18:1172–1177.
5. Rossouw JE, Anderson GL, Prentice RL, et al. Risks and benefits of estrogen plus progestin in healthy postmenopausal women: principal results from the women's health initiative randomized controlled trial. *JAMA*. 2002;288(3):321–333.
6. Manson JE, Hsia J, Johnson KC, et al. Estrogen plus progestin and the risk of coronary heart disease. *N Engl J Med*. 2003;349:523–534.
7. Grodstein F, Manson JE, Colditz GA, et al. A prospective, observational study of postmenopausal hormone therapy and primary prevention of cardiovascular disease. *Ann Intern Med*. 2000;133:933–941.
8. Salpeter SR, Walsh JM, Greyber E, Salpeter EE. Coronary heart disease events associated with hormone therapy in younger and older women. *J Gen Intern Med*. 2006;21:363–366.
9. Gallagher JC, Levine JP. Preventing osteoporosis in symptomatic postmenopausal women. *Menopause*. 2011;18(1):109–118.

10. Lindsay R, Gallagher JC, Kleerkoper M, Pickar JH. Effect of lower doses of conjugated equine estrogens with and without medroxyprogesterone acetate on bone in early postmenopausal women. *JAMA*. 2002;287:2668–2676.
11. Delmas PD, Ensrud KE, Adachi JD, et al. Efficacy of raloxifene on vertebral fracture risk reduction in postmenopausal women with osteoporosis: four-year results from a randomized clinical trial. *J Clin Endocrinol Metab*. 2002;87:3606–3617.
12. Recker RR, Mitlak BH, Ni X, Krege JH. Long-term raloxifene for postmenopausal osteoporosis. *Curr Med Res Opin*. 2011;27:1755–1761.
13. Vogel VG, Constantino JP, Wickerham DL, et al. Effects of tamoxifen vs raloxifene on the risk of developing invasive breast cancer and other disease outcomes. *JAMA*. 2006;295:2727–2741.
14. Burshell AL, Song J, Dowsett SA, et al. Relationship between bone mass, invasive breast cancer incidence and raloxifene therapy in postmenopausal women with low bone mass or osteoporosis. *Curr Med Res Opin*. 2008;24:807–813.
15. Raloxifene Package Insert, 2018.
16. Collins P, Mosca L, Geiger MJ, et al. Effects of the selective estrogen receptor modulator raloxifene on coronary outcomes in the raloxifene use for the heart trial. *Circulation*. 2009;119:922–930.
17. D'Amelio P, Isai GC. The use of raloxifene in osteoporosis treatment. *Expert Opin Pharmacother*. 2013;14 (7):949–956.

CHAPTER 18

Sclerostin inhibitor (SERM): Romosozumab☆

Learning objectives

- Understand bone turnover, its various components, and how they can be manipulated.
- Recognize the role of sclerostin and romosozumab in bone turnover.
- Identify patients who are suitable candidates for romosozumab.

The case study

Reasons for seeking medical help

- RE is a 74-year-old Caucasian woman who, about 2 weeks ago, sustained a fragility fracture of her left hip after tripping on a toy her great grandchild had left on the carpet. The fracture was surgically reduced and healed well. She is now physically independent.
- About 15 years ago she sustained a Colles' fracture of the right radius and was diagnosed with osteoporosis. The fragility fracture of the right radius healed well. She was prescribed alendronate but could not tolerate it. It was then changed to risedronate, but she also could not tolerate it. She is on no medication for osteoporosis.
- Given her impaired renal functions: creatinine clearance 20mL/min, she was not considered for either orally administered bisphosphonates or zoledronic acid intravenous infusions. RE preferred not to be prescribed medication that has to be self-administered daily such as teriparatide or abaloparatide. She also was concerned that because of her osteoarthritic changes she may not be able to self-administer subcutaneous injections.
- She seems amenable to denosumab, 6-monthly subcutaneous injections administered by a health care provider but is concerned that as she travels extensively visiting children, grandchildren, and great-grandchildren and is very often away from home, she may not be able to ensure regular 6-monthly subcutaneous injections.

☆ RE, 74-year-old Caucasian woman with impaired renal functions.

Diagnosis and Treatment of Osteoporosis. https://doi.org/10.1016/B978-0-323-99550-4.00015-0
Copyright © 2024 Elsevier Inc. All rights are reserved, including those for text and data mining, AI training, and similar technologies.

Past medical and surgical history

Apart from one vertebral fragility fracture of T7, and a Colley sustained, RE has been enjoying good health. Her two fractures healed well. She is physically independent and mentally good. She lives on her own in a retirement community and travels extensively.

Lifestyle

- Physically active lifestyle. When not traveling she enjoys going for walks, playing golf, and swimming at least three times a week.
- Body weight: steady at about 120 pounds
- She enjoys three cups of hot tea a day. No alcoholic drinks, no cigarette smoking, no excessive salt intake.
- Good nutritional intake, daily calcium intake estimated to be about 1500 mg; oral vitamin D intake about 800 units.

Medications

- She is not taking any medication, except for the occasional analgesic.

Family history

- All family members are in good health.

Clinical examination

- Osteoarthritic changes affecting hands and knees, but not interfering with her daily activities.
- Clinical examination essentially within normal limits. She just had her annual physical examination. No significant signs detected. BP 152/82 sitting, 154/85 standing, no orthostasis. No arrhythmias, no clinical evidence of sensitive carotid sinus, carotid stenosis, and no vertebrobasilar insufficiency. No clinical evidence of cervical spondylosis. Heart sounds clearly audible, no added sounds, no ectopic beats, no JVD, no clinical signs of heart failure. No edema of the lower limbs. Chest clear. Examination of the chest and abdomen does not reveal any significant signs.
- Timed Get-Up-and-Go test, completed within 8.2 s

Laboratory results

- CBC, CMP, GFR, and TSH, all essentially within normal range.

DXA and radiologic results

- T-scores:
  Left total hip: −2.7.
  Left femoral neck: −2.5.
  Right total hip: −2.5.
  Left femoral neck: −2.4.
  Distal 1/3 left radius: −2.6.
- Vertebral fracture assessment: evidence of moderate vertebral compression fracture at T7.

Multiple choice questions

1. ***Romosozumab:***
   A. Is a monoclonal antibody against sclerostin.
   B. Suppresses bone resorption.
   C. Stimulates bone formation.
   D. A and B.
   E. A, B, and C.
   Correct answer: E
   Comment:
   Bone is a dynamic tissue which constantly undergoes remodeling to accommodate for the mechanical demands of the body: a solid, mechanical stress-sustaining skeleton, and the metabolic needs of the body: a readily accessible, well-stocked calcium and mineral reservoir. Osteoblasts are the bone-forming cells and osteoclasts are the bone-resorbing cells. These two mechanisms of bone formation and bone resorption are responsible for changes in bone mass, density, and mechanical strength throughout life and are referred to as bone turnover.

   The bone remodeling cycle is initiated by osteocytes in response to changes of the body's need for calcium or by the physical mechanical stress on individualized foci in the skeleton. The phase of increased bone resorption by the activated osteoclasts is dynamic and ready to change according to skeletal activities and demands for calcium and other minerals. This period is followed by a reversible phase when the osteoclasts, having met the demands imposed on them, withdraw from the cavities they have created while resorbing bone tissue and make room for the osteoblasts to refill the resorbed areas. The osteoblasts then either become osteocytes, buried in the skeleton, ready to become active again, or become bone-lining cells, also ready to respond to appropriate stimuli. The main goal is to maintain a healthy skeleton and a well-stocked calcium and mineral reservoir.

   Sclerostin inhibits the differentiation of precursor cells into mature bone-forming osteoblasts and decreases bone formation.[1] Conversely, inhibiting sclerostin binding to osteoblasts allows an increase of osteoblastic activity and bone mass.

Sclerostin was originally discovered in patients with sclerosteosis and van Buchem disease, two rare inherited diseases characterized by an increased bone mass, deformities, characteristic facial features, and nerve compression due to the expanding skeleton.

Romosozumab is a humanized monoclonal antibody developed to inhibit the effects of sclerostin and increase the bone mass. It is used in the management of osteoporosis.[2–5] The elimination half-life of romosozumab is estimated to be 12.6 days after the administration of three doses. Whereas the inhibited rate of bone resorption is maintained throughout the course of therapy, the increased rate of bone formation returns to the original pretreatment levels after the 9th month of regular monthly administration. After cessation of therapy markers of bone formation, bone resorption and BMD gradually return to baseline levels.[2]

2. ***Romosozumab is administered:***
   A. Daily
   B. Once a week
   C. Once a month
   D. Once every 3 months
   E. Once every year

   Correct answer: C

   Comment:

   Romosozumab is administered subcutaneously, once a month, for 12 months. It is recommended that on completion of the 12-month period, the patient be prescribed an antiresorptive medication.[2]

3. ***A comparison of the effects of denosumab and romosozumab shows that after a 12-month period:***
   A. The increase in BMD of the lumbar vertebrae is about the same in both groups.
   B. Patients on denosumab have significant increases in the serum P1NP.
   C. Significantly more patients who sustained fragility fractures were in the denosumab group.
   D. All of the above.
   E. None of the above.

   Correct answer: E

   Comment:

   A retrospective, observational cohort study was conducted on women with postmenopausal osteoporosis to compare the efficacy of denosumab to that of romosozumab. In this study one of the two medications was administered to 69 matched patients. At the end of a 6-month period, patients in the romosozumab group had mean increases in the lumbar vertebrae, total hip, and femoral neck BMD of 7.4%, 3.4%, and 3.0%, respectively. Those on denosumab had increases of 6.0%, 2.4%, and 2.0% in the lumbar vertebrae, total hip, and femoral neck, respectively. Similarly, in patients on romosozumab the increases at the end of the 12-month period were 12.5%, 6.0%, and 5.5% for the lumbar vertebrae, total hip, and femoral neck, respectively. Patients on denosumab had a decrease in the P1NP of 63.1% at 6months and 68.2% at 12months in the serum P1NP level, an index of bone formation. Patients on romosozumab had decreases of P1NP of 5.9% and 5.6% at 6 and 12 months, respectively.[6] These results have been replicated in other similar studies and suggest that the magnitude of changes in BMD and bone markers is more pronounced in previously untreated patients.[7,8]

4. ***The use of oral antiresorptive medications is limited by:***
   A. Frequency of adverse effects.
   B. Poor adherence rates.
   C. Severity of adverse effects.
   D. A and B.
   E. A, B, and C.

   Correct answer: D

   Comment:

   The intake of oral bisphosphonates is cumbersome: the tablet has to be taken in the morning, while the patient is fasting and has to be taken with 6 oz of water and then the patient has to fast for about half an hour. Other issues related to the intake of oral bisphosphonate are discussed in another case study. Adherence to the intake of oral bisphosphonates is problematic.

5. ***The anabolic response to the administration of romosozumab as determined by changes of P1NP, a marker of bone formation, is approximately:***
   A. A 5% increase.
   B. A 50% increase.
   C. A 150% increase.
   D. 1-month duration.
   E. Lasts about 1 week.

   Correct answer: C

   Comment:

   The increase in bone formation induced by romosozumab, as measured by changes in P1NP, a marker of bone formation, is quite robust: reaching approximately 150% of baseline value. It is, however, short lived and normalizes back to baseline in about 9 months. A second course of romosozumab after one year of no treatment (i.e., romosozumab then placebo, then romosozumab again) induced further increases in the BMD of the lumbar vertebrae (12.4%) and total hip (5.5%). If, however, the second course of romosozumab is administered after completion of the first course, followed by a course of denosumab (i.e., romosozumab, denosumab, then romosozumab), then the increases of BMD are smaller: 2.3% in the lumbar vertebrae and unchanged in the total hip.[9]

6. ***Inclusion criteria for the "Fracture Study in Postmenopausal Women" (FRAME study) include:***
   A. Postmenopausal women between the ages of 55 and 90 years.
   B. Lumbar vertebrae T-score ≤2.0.
   C. Serum vitamin D level <20 ng/mL.
   D. None of the above.
   E. All of the above.

   Correct answer: A

   Comments:

   The FRAME study included postmenopausal women between the ages of 55 and 90 years, who had osteoporosis as evidenced by a T-score of −2.5 or lower at the total hip or femoral neck. Patients who had sustained a hip fracture or had evidence of a severe or more than two moderate vertebral compression fractures were excluded from the study.
7. ***After 12 months, compared to placebo, the following is/are true about the results of the FRAME study (Fracture Study in Postmenopausal Women):***
   A. BMD of the lumbar vertebrae increased by 13.3%.
   B. BMD of the total hip increased by 6.9%.
   C. BMD of the femoral neck increased by 5.9%.
   D. B and C.
   E. A, B, and C.

   Correct answer: E

   Comment:

   The first part of the FRAME study included 7180 postmenopausal women aged 55–90 years, with a T-score of ≤2.5 at the total hip or femoral neck, randomly allocated to romosozumab (3589 patients) or placebo (3591 patients). The first part of the study lasted 12months. At the end of this period, all participants were prescribed denosumab 60 mg every 6 months, administered subcutaneously. This part of the study lasted 24 months. All patients enrolled in this study were also prescribed calcium (500–1000 mg) and vitamin D (600–800 IU) daily. Main endpoints were fractures at 12 and 24 months.
8. ***Concerning the Active-Controlled Fracture Study in Postmenopausal Women with Osteoporosis (ARCH study):***
   A. Recruited postmenopausal women aged between 55 and 90 years.
   B. T-score ≤−2.5 at the total hip or femoral neck.
   C. One moderate/severe OR two mild vertebral compression fractures.
   D. During the first year of the study, participants were allocated to either romosozumab one subcutaneous injection monthly or alendronate orally, 70 mg once a week.
   E. All of the above.

   Correct answer: E

Comments:

For the ARCH study, 4903 postmenopausal women with evidence of osteoporosis were recruited. They were randomly allocated to either romosozumab or alendronate. At the end of the first year they were all switched to alendronate 70 mg once a week for the remaining 2 years of the study.

9. ***Results of the ARCH study include:***
   - A. The number of vertebral compression fractures sustained during the study was about the same in both groups (romosozumab /alendronate: 2046 patients, alendronate/ alendronate: 2047 patients).
   - B. More patients in the alendronate/alendronate cohort sustained hip fractures than the romosozumab/alendronate group.
   - C. Patients included in the ARCH study were much younger and healthier than the general population with osteoporosis.
   - D. A and B.
   - E. B and C.

Correct answer: B

Comments:

Whereas 11.9% of the patients allocated to the alendronate group sustained a new vertebral compression fracture, only 6.2% of the patients in the romosozumab to alendronate group sustained a new vertebral compression fracture. Similarly, hip fractures occurred more frequently in the alendronate to alendronate group (13.0%) than in the romosozumab to alendronate group (9.7%). Finally, changes in BMD were larger in the romosozumab to alendronate group than on the alendronate to alendronate group: 13.7%, 15.2%, and 14.9% for increases at month 12, 24, and 36, respectively.[10]

10. ***The following is/are correct:***
    - A. The efficacy of romosozumab is higher in patients at high risk of sustaining fractures.
    - B. A second 12-month course of romosozumab leads to no further increases in BMD.
    - C. Romosozumab should not be administered to patients with impaired renal functions.
    - D. A and C.
    - E. B and C.

Correct answer: A

Comment:

The efficacy of romosozumab at reducing the fracture risk is higher in patients who are at an increased risk of sustaining fractures. In this study, fracture risk was determined by the FRAX score.[11]

A second course of romosozumab after a 12-month period on placebo (i.e., romosozumab then placebo then romosozumab) leads to increases in BMD of the lumbar vertebrae similar to those achieved after the first 12-month series: 12.4% and 12.0% increases in the first and second series, respectively. Less pronounced increases were achieved in the total hip BMD: 6.0% and 5.5%, respectively.

A second course after a month of denosumab (i.e. romosozumab then denosumab then romosozumab) leads to smaller increases in BMD than the first course: 2.3% in the lumbar vertebrae and no change at the total hip. This study was conducted on 167 participants.[12]

Key points

- Romosozumab is unique in that it stimulates bone formation and inhibits bone resorption.
- Romosozumab increases vertebral and nonvertebral bone density.
- Romosozumab reduces the vertebral and nonvertebral fracture risk.

References

1. Cy F, Romosozumab TJ. A review of efficacy, safety, and cardiovascular risk. *Curr Osteoporos Rep.* 2021;19:15–22.
2. Nealy KL, Harris KB. Romosozumab: a novel injectable sclerostin inhibitor with anabolic and anti-resorptive effects for osteoporosis. *Ann Pharmacother.* 2021;55(5):677–686.
3. Arceo-Mendoza, Camacho PM. Postmenopausal osteoporosis: latest guidelines. *Endocrinol Metab Clin N Am.* 2021;50:167–178.
4. Lewiecki EM. Romosozumab, clinical trials, and real world care of patients with osteoporosis. *Ann Transl Med.* 2020;8(15):974.
5. Rauner M, Taipaleenmaki H, Tsourdi E, Winter EM. Osteoporosis treatment with antisclerostin antibodies-mechanisms of action and clinical application. *J Clin Med.* 2021;10:787.
6. Kobayakawa T, Miyazaki A, Saito M, et al. Denosumab versus romosozumab for postmenopausal osteoporosis treatment. *Sci Rep Scientific Rep.* 2021;11:11801. PMID: 34083636.
7. Ebina K, Tsuboi H, Nagayama Y, et al. Effects of prior osteoporosis treatment on 12-month treatment response to romosozumab in patients with postmenopausal osteoporosis. *Joint Bone Spine.* 2021;105219.
8. Tominaga A, Wada K, Okazaki K, et al. Early clinical effects, safety, and predictors of the effects of romosozumab treatment in osteoporosis patients: one-year study. *Osteoporos Int.* 2021. PMID: 33770201.
9. Hassan N, Gregson C, Tobias JH. Anabolic treatments for osteoporosis in postmenopausal women. *Facul Rev.* 2021;10:44.
10. Saag KG, Petersen J, Karaplis AC, et al. Romosozumab or alendronate for fracture prevention in women with osteoporosis. *N Engl J Med.* 2017;377:1417–1427.
11. McCloskey EV, Johansson H, Harvey NC, et al. Romosozumab efficacy on fracture outcomes is greater in patients at high baseline fracture risk: a post hoc analysis of the first year of the FRAME study. *Osteoporos Int.* 2021;32:601–1608.
12. Kendler DL, Bone HG, Massari F, et al. Bone mineral density gains with a second 12-months course of romosozumab therapy following placebo or denosumab. *Osteoporos Int.* 2019;12:2437–2448.

CHAPTER 19

Parathyroid hormone analogs

Teriparatide/abaloparatide—Part I: Differences and similarities

Learning objectives

- Pharmacologic profile: efficacy and adverse effects of teriparatide and abaloparatide.
- Teriparatide and abaloparatide: differences and similarities.
- Impact of recent label changes.

The case study

Reason for seeking medical help

VO, a 71-year-old Caucasian woman, sustained a fragility hip fracture after slipping in her granddaughter's bedroom about a year ago. She underwent a successful hip replacement, responded well to physical therapy, and is now independent. Secondary causes of osteoporosis have been excluded; she is referred for the management of osteoporosis.

Past medical and surgical history

- Osteoporosis, diagnosed about a year ago, after she sustained a fragility hip fracture. She was prescribed oral bisphosphonates but developed severe upper gastrointestinal symptoms that she could not tolerate. After four doses, she decided to stop taking the bisphosphonate without notifying her treating physician. She also did not think she really needed any treatment: her hip fracture healed well; the range of lower limb movement is good. She is not in pain.

Diagnosis and Treatment of Osteoporosis. https://doi.org/10.1016/B978-0-323-99550-4.00023-X
Copyright © 2024 Elsevier Inc. All rights are reserved, including those for text and data mining, AI training, and similar technologies.

- Surgical menopause at age 37 years because of endometriosis. Good outcome. She has been on hormonal replacement therapy for about 3 years after the surgery. She then stopped taking it without notifying her primary care provider.
- No other relevant past medical history, no history of falls, no near-falls, no dizzy spells.

Lifestyle

- Physically independent, mentally good. She is a retired librarian.
- Sedentary lifestyle.
- Daily calcium intake about 1200 mg.
- No excessive sodium or caffeine intake, no cigarette smoking.

Medication

- Oral bisphosphonate, prescribed about a year ago, discontinued it after four doses because of gastrointestinal adverse effects.
- Multivitamin tablets, over the counter.
- Vitamin D, over the counter, 600 IU daily. She started taking these tablets after sustaining the fragility hip fracture, about a year ago. At that time her serum vitamin D level was within the normal range: 30 ng/mL.

Family history

- Mother sustained fragility hip fracture.

Clinical examination

- Weight 152 pounds, steady; height 62″, used to be 64″.
- Able to ambulate independently, steady. No orthostatic symptoms.
- Timed Get-up-and-Go test completed in 9.6 s.

Laboratory results

- CBC, comprehensive metabolic profile, serum 25-hydroxy-vitamin D all within normal limits.

DXA and radiologic results

- T-scores: L2–L4: −3.1; left femoral neck −2.8; left total hip −3.0.
- VFA: moderate biconcave compression fracture of T12 and L1, and severe wedge compression fracture of T7. VO denies any trauma to her back.

Multiple choice questions

1. ***After considering various treatment options, VO opted for teriparatide:***
   A. Teriparatide is recombinant human parathyroid hormone 1–84.
   B. Teriparatide is administered by daily subcutaneous injection.
   C. Patients' compliance with teriparatide is poor: adherence rate is less than 50%.
   D. A and C.
   E. B and C.
   Correct answer: B
   Comment:
   Teriparatide is a recombinant parathyroid hormone (first 34 amino acids). It is administered subcutaneously through a fixed-dose prefilled delivery device that contains 28 doses. Most patients self-administer the medication. After overcoming the initial trepidation about the need for daily injections, most patients adhere well: compliance has been reported to be as high as 89% at 6months and 82% at 18months.[1] It is nevertheless essential to motivate patients, and keep them motivated, to comply with the intake of the medication, especially if the patient is asymptomatic.
2. ***In VO's case, appropriate reasons for prescribing teriparatide include:***
   A. Diagnosis of established osteoporosis.
   B. Fragility fractures (hip and vertebrae).
   C. "Very high" fracture risk.
   D. A and B.
   E. A, B, and C.
   Correct answer: E
   Comment:
   The diagnosis of "established osteoporosis" is made when, at least, two criteria are met. First, is the densitometric evidence of osteoporosis. Second, in addition, the patient sustained 3 fragility fractures at T7, T12, ad L1 (i.e., a fracture occurring in the absence of any trauma or after trauma that ordinarily one would not expect to lead to a fracture).
   In VO's case, the fracture risk satisfies the criteria of "Very High Risk" of sustaining a fracture, as defined by the American Association of Clinical Endocrinologists (AACE), the American College of Endocrinology (ACE), the Endocrine Society, the European Society for Clinical and Economic Aspects of Osteoporosis and Osteoarthritis (ESCEO), and the International Osteoporosis Foundation (IOF). She has densitometric evidence of osteoporosis (lowest T-score −3.1 in the lumbar vertebrae), and in addition sustained a fragility hip fracture and three fragility vertebral compression fractures.[2,3]
   She also lost about 2″ in height, probably secondary to the vertebral compression fracture(s). Other risk factors for osteoporosis and fractures include Caucasian ethnicity; surgical menopause at age 37years, with no HRT, except for about 3years; and a positive family history of fragility hip fracture (her mother).

3. ***In postmenopausal women with osteoporosis, teriparatide* versus *placebo has been shown to reduce the fracture risk of:***
   A. Vertebrae.
   B. Hips.
   C. Ribs.
   D. All of the above.
   E. A and B.

   Correct answer: D

   Comment:

   Compared to placebo, teriparatide reduced the incidence of fragility and traumatic fractures of the vertebrae, hips, wrists, ankles, ribs, feet, and pelvis.[4] This trial was prematurely terminated to evaluate the clinical implications of toxicology animal studies. As a result, the mean duration of treatment in this study was only about 18 months. Notwithstanding, compared to placebo, the mean percent increase in BMD was 9.7%, 2.8%, 3.5%, and 2.6% at the lumbar vertebrae, femoral neck, trochanter, and total hip, respectively.[4]

4. ***Teriparatide and abaloparatide:***
   A. Can be administered for more than 2 years.
   B. Simultaneous administration of an antiresorptive, in addition to teriparatide, is advantageous.
   C. It should not be prescribed if the glomerular filtration rate is less than 35 mL/min.
   D. Once discontinued, an antiresorptive agent should be prescribed.
   E. A and D.

   Correct answer: E

   Comment:

   Teriparatide reduces the risk of vertebral and nonvertebral fractures in women with postmenopausal osteoporosis and glucocorticoid-induced osteoporosis.[5]

   Until recently the recommendation was to restrict the administration of teriparatide to 2 years because of the fear it might increase the risk of osteosarcoma. This was based on findings of an early study on experimental animals (Fischer 344 rats). A black box warning was issued by the US FDA (Food and Drug Administration). The 2-year limitation with teriparatide therapy was also justified by the observation that the initial robust increase in BMD tends to gradually taper off and that the readministration of teriparatide after a one-year hiatus does not replicate the robust initial increase in BMD.[6]

   In 2020 the results of a 15-year US postmarketing surveillance study became available and showed that teriparatide did not increase the risk of osteosarcoma.[7] The FDA withdrew the 2-year lifetime teriparatide treatment limit and the black box warning about the potential risk of osteosarcoma. This was followed by the removal of the two-year treatment limit for abaloparatide. Now, for how long therapy with teriparatide should be continued in individual patients is a clinical issue. Therefore patients with a "high" or "very high" risk of fracture may continue with this medication, as long as clinically indicated, beyond the two-year limit.

When teriparatide is discontinued, BMD gains are lost unless an antiresorptive is prescribed.[8,9] Starting bisphosphonate therapy immediately after discontinuing teriparatide induces further increases in BMD.[10]

As teriparatide is neither metabolized nor excreted by the kidneys, it can be administered if the patient's GFR is less than 35mL/min. Good hydration is, nevertheless, recommended and caution should be exercised because many patients with renal impairment have secondary hyperparathyroidism. Teriparatide is contraindicated in patients who have received radiation therapy.

A meta-analysis of nine randomized controlled trials (RCTs) which included 2990 postmenopausal women with osteoporosis (1515 treated with teriparatide and 1475 treated with bisphosphonates) showed that teriparatide reduced the vertebral and nonvertebral fracture risk and increased BMD to a greater extent than bisphosphonates.[11] Cyclic administration of teriparatide and denosumab was not superior to their sequential administration.[12]

5. ***Teriparatide increases bone formation by:***
   - A. Increasing the number of preosteoblasts.
   - B. Downregulating RANLK-ligand.
   - C. Stimulating osteoprotegerin secretion.
   - D. A and B.
   - E. A, B, and C.

   Correct answer: E

   Comment:

   Teriparatide administration increases the number of preosteoblasts, stimulates their differentiation into mature osteoblasts, and enhances their function.[13] Teriparatide also improves bone microarchitecture by increasing trabecular connectivity and cortical thickness, thus increasing bending and buckling strength. In addition, teriparatide downregulates RANK-Ligand expression and stimulates osteoprotegerin secretion resulting in reduced osteoclast formation, maturation, and stimulation, and therefore reduced bone resorption.[14]

6. ***Teriparatide administration after a fracture:***
   - A. Stimulates chondrogenesis in the callus.
   - B. Enhances chondrocyte maturation and mineralization.
   - C. Enhances fracture healing.
   - D. All of the above.
   - E. None of the above.

   Correct answer: D

Comment:

Teriparatide is also useful to reduce back pain and improve quality of life in patients who have sustained a vertebral compression fracture.[15] Studies on experimental animals document that teriparatide administration after a fracture enhances fracture healing by increasing the callus volume and enhancing endochondral bone formation through increased chondrogenesis, chondrocyte maturation and mineralization.[16] There is still a relative paucity of large studies on the effect of teriparatide on fracture healing in humans.[17]

7. ***Main adverse events of teriparatide include:***
   A. Postural hypotension.
   B. Nausea.
   C. Arthralgia.
   D. A and B.
   E. A, B, and C.

   Correct answer: E

   Comment:

   Adverse events after teriparatide administration include arthralgia (10.1% teriparatide versus 8.4% placebo) and nausea (8.5% teriparatide, 6.7% placebo), but no vomiting.[17] The latter is usually self-limited. In order to avoid it, many patients self-administer at night as they get ready for bed. As in most instances these symptoms occur late at night, when asleep, the patient may not notice them. Although symptomatic postural hypotension is rare (about 5%), it is nevertheless recommended that at least for the first few doses, teriparatide be administered under circumstances in which the patient can quickly sit or lie down should these symptoms arise.[17]

8. ***Teriparatide is contraindicated in patients with:***
   A. Hypercalcemia.
   B. Hypocalcemia.
   C. Nephrolithiasis.
   D. A and C.
   E. B and C.

   Correct answer: D

   Comment:

   As teriparatide may increase the serum and urinary calcium it should not be administered to patients with hypercalcemia or a history of renal calculi. It is also contraindicated in patients with bone metastases, metabolic bone diseases other than osteoporosis or a history of skeletal malignancies.

9. ***Osteosarcoma and teriparatide:***
   A. The risk of osteosarcoma is higher in patients on teriparatide.
   B. Toxicology studies showed an increased incidence of osteosarcoma in experimental rats.

C. Teriparatide should not be administered to patients who have received radiation therapy.
D. A and B.
E. B and C.

Correct answer: E

Comment:

Toxicology studies document that when teriparatide is administered to Fischer 344 rats in doses up to 60 times higher than those used in humans, the incidence of osteosarcoma is increased in a dose- and duration-dependent manner.[7] On the other hand, no bone tumors were detected after 18 months of teriparatide to mature oophorectomized monkeys, at doses 6 times higher than administered to humans.[7] Similarly, the risk of osteosarcoma is not increased in patients with hyperparathyroidism.[7]

Postmarketing surveillance showed that over a 15-year follow-up period the incidence of osteosarcoma in patients receiving teriparatide is not higher than in the general population.[7] Teriparatide, nevertheless, is not recommended in children and young adults with open epiphyses and those in whom the risk of osteosarcoma is increased such as patients who have received radiation therapy and those with Paget's disease of bone or unexplained increases in bony alkaline phosphatase levels.

10. ***Teriparatide is used for the treatment of:***
A. Women with postmenopausal osteoporosis at very high risk for fracture.
B. Men with primary or hypogonadal osteoporosis at very high risk for fracture.
C. Women and men with glucocorticoid-induced osteoporosis at very high risk for fracture.
D. A and B.
E. A, B, and C.

Correct answer: E

Comment:

Teriparatide is used for the treatment of all listed conditions. It is also used for treatment of patients who have failed or could not tolerate other medication for osteoporosis and for men and women with osteoporosis on daily doses of 5 mg or more prednisone.[18] It is also used to help healing of insufficiency fractures.[18,19]

Case summary

Analysis of data

Factors predisposing to bone demineralization/osteoporosis

- Multiple fragility fractures: hip and three vertebrae.
- Previously diagnosed osteoporosis, no medication.
- Surgical menopause at 37 years, no HRT.

- Positive family history for osteoporosis.
- Sedentary lifestyle.

Factors protecting against bone demineralization/osteoporosis

- Good daily calcium intake.
- Vitamin D supplements.
- No excessive sodium or caffeine intake; no cigarette smoking.

Factors increasing risk of falls/fractures

- Fragility fractures sustained.
- Positive family history.

Factors reducing risk of falls/fractures

- Physically independent.
- Timed Get-up-and-Go test completed in less than 14 s.

Diagnosis

- Established osteoporosis and high fracture risk.

Management recommendations

Treatment recommendation(s)/follow-up

- Six to eight weeks after initial outpatient visit to ensure adherence with teriparatide daily subcutaneous injections, answer any question the patient may have, and allay any anxiety. During this visit, other lifestyle issues such as adequate nutrition, adopting a physically active lifestyle, and possibly joining an exercise program could be discussed, especially as VO admitted to leading a sedentary lifestyle.
- Further pharmacologic management will depend on the results of this DXA scan and range from discontinuing teriparatide, to continuing it for another 2-year period. This could be accomplished after 4 years of treatment with teriparatide and repeating the DXA scan at that time.
- Antiresorptive medication when teriparatide is discontinued, 2–4 years after initiating pharmacologic therapy.

Medication(s)

- Given the degree of osteoporosis and high fracture risk, an osteoanabolic medication such as teriparatide, abaloparatide, or romosozumab is a good choice. Alternative choices include an antiresorptive medication such as denosumab or zoledronic acid. Oral bisphosphonates are not recommended as they may induce upper gastrointestinal adverse events that the patient could not tolerate.

Diagnostic test(s)

- None recommended at this stage. The diagnosis of osteoporosis has been made and secondary causes excluded.

Lifestyle

- An active physical lifestyle should be recommended, and, if possible, enrolling in a supervised exercise program.

DXA and radiologic

- DXA scan every 2 years.

Key points

- Teriparatide is an osteoanabolic medication.
- Teriparatide increases BMD and reduces fracture risk in patients at an increased risk of sustaining a fracture.
- Adherence with teriparatide is good once patients overcome their initial reservations.
- Depending on the patient's response teriparatide and abaloparatide can be continued for another 2-year period, or it can be discontinued and an antiresorptive administered.
- The 2-year limitation of teriparatide and abaloparatide therapy is no longer recommended. Therefore if the fracture risk is high/very high, the administration of teriparatide for longer periods may be appropriate.
- The concomitant administration of teriparatide and antiresorptives is not recommended at present. Sequential therapy is preferred to concomitant and cyclic therapy.

References

1. Adachi JD, Hanley DA, Lorraine JK, et al. Assessing compliance, acceptance, and tolerability of teriparatide in patients with osteoporosis. *Clin Ther*. 2007;29(9):2055–2067.
2. Arceo-Mendoza RM, Camacho PM. Postmenopausal osteoporosis: latest guidelines. *Endocrinol Metab Clin North Am*. 2021;50:167–178.
3. Camacho PM, et al. *Endocr Pract*. 2020;26(Suppl. 1):1–46.
4. Neer RM, Arnaud CD, Zanchetta JR, et al. Effect of parathyroid hormone (1-34) on fractures and bone mineral density in postmenopausal women with osteoporosis. *N Engl J Med*. 2001;344:1434–1441.
5. Hauser B, Alonso N, Riches PL. Review of current real-world experience with teriparatide as treatment of osteoporosis in different patient groups. *J Clin Med*. 2021;10:1403.
6. Finklestein JS, Wyland JJ, Leder BZ, et al. Effects of teriparatide retreatment in osteoporotic men and women. *J Clin Endocrinol Metab*. 2009;94(7):2495–2501.
7. Gilsenan A, Midkiff K, Harris D, et al. Teriparatide did not increase adult osteosarcoma incidence in a 15-year US post marketing surveillance study. *J Bone Miner Res*. 2021;36(2):244–251.
8. Miller PD, Lewiecki EM, Krohn K, Schwartz E. Teriparatide: label changes and identifying patients for long-term use. *Cleve Clin J Med*. 2021;88(9):489–493.
9. Leder BZ, Neer RM, Wyland JJ, et al. Effects of teriparatide treatment and discontinuation in postmenopausal women and eugonadal men with osteoporosis. *J Clin Endocrinol Metab*. 2009;94(8):2915–2921.

10. Kurland ES, Heller SL, Diamond B, et al. The importance of bisphosphonate therapy in maintaining bone mass in men after therapy with teriparatide. *Osteoporos Int.* 2004;15(12):992–997.
11. Ouyang Y, Chen S, Wan T, Zheng G, Sun G. The effects of teriparatide and bisphosphonates on new fractures in postmenopausal women with osteoporosis: a protocol for systematic review and meta-analysis. *Medicine.* 2021;100(7):o24839.
12. Cosman F, McMahon D, Dempster D, Nieves JW. Standard versus cyclic teriparatide and denosumab treatment for osteoporosis: a randomized trial. *J Bone Mineral Res.* 2020;35(2):219–225.
13. Canalis E, Giustina A, Bilezikian JP. Mechanisms of anabolic therapies for osteoporosis. *N Engl J Med.* 2007;357:905–916.
14. Resmini G, Iolascon G. New insights into the role of teriparatide. *Aging Clin Exp Res.* 2011;23(Suppl. 2):30–32.
15. Chen Z, Lin W, Zhao S, et al. Effect of teriparatide on pain relief, and quality of life in post-menopausal females with osteoporotic vertebral compression fractures, a retrospective cohort study. *Ann Palliat Med.* 2021;10 (4):4000–4007.
16. Kakr S, Einhom TA, Vora S, et al. Enhanced chondrogenesis and Wnt signaling in PTH-treated fractures. *J Bone Miner Res.* 2007;22:1903–1912.
17. Wang YK, Feb QSQ, Ma T, et al. Effects of teriparatide versus alendronate for treatment of postmenopausal osteoporosis: a meta-analysis of randomized controlled trials. *Medicine (Baltimore).* 2017;96(21):e6970. https://doi.org/10.1097/MD.
18. Zhang D, Potty A, Vyas P, Lane J. The role of recombinant PTH in human fracture healing: a systematic review. *J Orthop Trauma.* 2014.
19. Bovbjerg P, Hogh D, Froberg L, et al. Effect of PTH treatment on bone healing in insufficiency fractures of the pelvis: a systematic review. *EFFORT Open Ren.* 2021;6:9–14.

Subchapter

Abaloparatide/teriparatide—Part II: Differences and similarities

Abaloparatide is a second generation, osteoanabolic, synthetic molecular modification of PTH-related protein for the treatment of postmenopausal osteoporosis.[1–8] It has a 76% homology to PTHrP 1–34 and 41% homology to PTH 1–34.[9] This modification conveys abaloparatide receptors a different binding configuration than teriparatide. As a result, the subsequent osteoblastic stimulation is faster and of greater magnitude in bone mineral density than that with teriparatide.[10]

Multiple choice questions

1. ***The parathyroid hormone receptor type 1 (PTHR1):***
   A. Plays a key role in calcium homeostasis.
   B. Modulates proliferation and differentiation of bone cells.
   C. Acts through two distinct ligands.
   D. A and B.
   E. A, B, and C.
   Correct answer: E
   Comment:
   The parathyroid hormone receptor type 1 (PTHR1) maintains calcium homeostasis and a healthy skeleton through two separate, distinct, endogenous polypeptide ligands: PTH 1–34 (the first 34 amino acids of parathyroid hormone) and PTHrP 1–34 (the first 34 amino acids of PTH *related* protein), a paracrine-acting morphogenic factor that regulates cellular proliferation and differentiation in bones as well as other tissues. The genetic deletion of the PTH/PTHrP (PTH1R) receptor in mesenchymal stem cells results in low bone formation, elevated levels of RANK-Ligand, increased bone resorption, and elevated bone marrow adipose tissue.[11]

   PTH 1–34 plays a pivotal role in maintaining the serum calcium within a narrow range of normality and also directly stimulates osteoblasts to increase bone mass. PTHrP 1–34 regulates the bone mass by directly stimulating the osteoblasts to increase bone formation. It also, to a lesser extent, indirectly stimulates the osteoclasts by increasing the release of RANK-Ligand which triggers the recruitment, fusion, and differentiation of preosteoclasts to produce osteoclasts which then undergo maturation, and activation, leading to increased levels of RANK-Ligand, and rate of bone resorption. PTHrP therefore increases the rate of bone turnover in addition to maintaining calcium homeostasis.

   The effect of the two ligands (PTH 1–34 and PTHrP 1–34) is largely dependent on the frequency and duration of exposure of the receptors to the ligands: continuous versus intermittent. The continuous exposure of the receptors to the ligands leads to an increased bone resorption and hypercalcemia as seen in cases of primary hyperparathyroidism, whereas intermittent exposure to the ligand increases bone mass, but does not induce hypercalcemia.

PTH1R has two conformations: R^O and RG. The RG conformation induces a shorter intracellular signaling response than the R^O conformation and probably is the reason for its increased anabolic activity compared to the R^O conformation. Abaloparatide has a higher selectivity for the RG and a lower selectivity for the R^O conformation then teriparatide. This may explain the different potencies of the two anabolic agents.

These differences are thought to be, at least partly, due to the selective binding of the ligand to RG versus R^O PTHR1 receptors. PTHrP 1–34 has a greater selectivity for RG receptors and lesser affinity to bind to R^O receptors than PTH 1–34 and has been shown to be more effective at stimulating anabolic bone responses than PTH 1–34.[12] Both ligands are now commercially available as synthetic analogs and used for the management of osteoporosis: PTH 1–34 is known as teriparatide and PTHrP 1–34 is known as abaloparatide.

PTH 1–34 consists of the first 34 amino acids of the N-terminal end of parathyroid hormone. The entire molecule of PTH is made up of 84 amino acids. PTH 1–34 plays a pivotal role in maintaining the serum calcium within a narrow range of normality and also, to a lesser extent, and for a limited period of time, directly stimulates osteoblasts to increase bone mass. It, however, also stimulates the osteoclasts to increase bone resorption and therefore the release of calcium from bone tissue to the circulation. It also increases the renal calcium reabsorption in the distal renal tubules and increases the intestinal calcium absorption by stimulating the hydroxylation of 25-hydroxy-vitamin D at the 1-position, yielding the active 1,25-di-hydroxy-vitamin D metabolite.

PTHrP is produced by many tissues in addition to the parathyroid glands. It is a paracrine-acting morphogenic factor that regulates bone cellular proliferation and differentiation of osteoclasts and osteoblasts in bones as well as other tissues. It also regulates bone mass by directly stimulating the osteoblasts to increase bone formation. This effect, however, is short lived and referred to as the "anabolic window."

In addition, and to a lesser extent, PTHrP 1–34 indirectly stimulates the osteoclasts by increasing the release of RANK-Ligand which triggers the recruitment, fusion, and differentiation of preosteoclasts to produce osteoclasts which then undergo maturation and activation leading to an increased level of bone resorption. PTHrP therefore increases the rate of bone turnover in addition to maintaining calcium homeostasis. It is also involved in fetal calcium regulation, placental calcium transfer, and lactation.[13] Unlike PTH, PTHrP plays only a minor role in intestinal calcium absorption.

Abaloparatide has the same series of the first 21 amino acids as PTH 1–34, but several substitutions have been made to amino acids 22–34 to maximize its stability and bone anabolic activity, while having only a limited effect on bone resorption.[14]

2. ***The daily subcutaneous administration of teriparatide:***
   A. Reduces the risk of vertebral fractures.
   B. Reduces the risk of nonvertebral fractures.
   C. Increases the bone mineral density.
   D. A, B, and C.
   E. A and C.

Correct answer: D

Comments:

A randomized double-blind placebo-controlled clinical trial, the Fracture Prevention Pivotal Trial (FPT), was conducted on 1637 postmenopausal women who had evidence of prior vertebral fractures. They were randomly allocated to receive PTH 1–34 (subsequently referred to as teriparatide) subcutaneously daily 20μg (541 subjects), 40μg (552 subjects), or placebo (544 subjects). The clinical trial was terminated prematurely, by the sponsors, because of concern about the increased rate of osteosarcoma developing in Fischer 344 rats during a long-term toxicology study of PTH 1–34. The median duration of observation was 21 months.

This clinical trial, however, demonstrated that compared to placebo, PTH 1–34 reduced the risk of one or more new vertebral fractures by 65 and 69% in patients receiving 20 and 40μg doses, respectively, and the risk of two or more vertebral fractures by 77% and 86%, respectively. Similarly, the risk of at least one moderate or severe vertebral fracture was reduced by 90% and 78%, respectively. The risk of one or more new nonvertebral fractures was reduced by 35% and 40%, respectively. This clinical trial also documented that new or worsening back pain was reported by 23% of patients in the placebo group but only 17% and 16% in those receiving 20 μg and 40 μg PTH 1–34, respectively. The protective effect of parathyroid hormone became evident after 9–12 months of therapy. The main adverse effects were essentially benign and included nausea, dizziness, leg cramps, and mild hypercalcemia. Cancer developed in 4% of the subjects in the placebo group and 2% in the 20 μg and 40 μg groups.[15]

The ACTIVE (Abaloparatide Comparator Trial in Vertebral Endpoints) an 18-month phase III, double-blind, randomized clinical trial which included 2463 postmenopausal women, mean age 69 years (range 49–86) randomly allocated to abaloparatide, teriparatide, or placebo. The primary outcome was new morphometric vertebral fractures. There were 30 such fractures in the placebo group (4.2%) compared to six fractures in the teriparatide group (0.8%) and four in the abaloparatide group (0.6%). The relative risk of new vertebral fractures for abaloparatide compared to placebo was 0.14 (95% CI: 0.05–0.39). These differences were statistically significant: $P < .001$.[16]

Secondary outcomes included nonvertebral fractures: 33 in the placebo group (4.7%), 24 in the teriparatide group (3.3%), and 18 in the abaloparatide group (2.7%).[10] Similarly, the mean percentage increases in BMD at the total hip and femoral neck were significantly ($P < .001$) higher in the abaloparatide group than the placebo and the teriparatide group. Of note, over the 18 months course of the study there were two hip fractures in the placebo group and none in the teriparatide or abaloparatide group. Changes in BMD at the total hip, femoral neck, and lumbar vertebrae were also more marked in the abaloparatide than the teriparatide and placebo groups.[10]

An extension of the ACTIVE study "ACTIVExtend" compared the fracture relative risk reduction (RRR) of abaloparatide (ABL) versus placebo (PBO), i.e., the original ACTIVE Study followed by six months of alendronate therapy (ALN). At the end of the extended study period the RRR for new morphometric vertebral fractures was 87% ($P < .001$): 4.4% in those treated with placebo followed by alendronate (PBO/ALN) versus 0.55% in patients treated with abaloparatide followed by alendronate (ABL/ALN). The RRR of sustaining more than one nonvertebral fracture was 52% in patients treated receiving ABL/ALN versus PBO/ALN and the RRR of patients sustaining more than one major osteoporotic fracture was 58% in ABL/ALN patients compared to those receiving PBO/ALN: 4.7% in the PLO/ALN group versus 2.0% in the ABL/ALN group. Similarly, average gains for the ABL/ALN group compared to the PLO/ALN group were 12.8% for the lumbar vertebrae, 5.5% for the total hip, and 4.5% for the femoral neck. The group differences at all sites were $P < .001$.[6]

A bone histomorphometry study on transiliac bone in postmenopausal women with osteoporosis shows that the administration of abaloparatide for 3 months stimulates bone formation on cancellous, endocortical, intracortical, and periosteal envelopes.[17]

3. ***Comparing teriparatide to abaloparatide, the number of patients needed to be treated (NNT) for 18 months to prevent one fracture:***
   A. Is about the same for vertebral fractures.
   B. Is higher with teriparatide than abaloparatide for nonvertebral fractures.
   C. Is higher with teriparatide than abaloparatide for major osteoporotic fractures.
   D. B and C.
   E. A, B, and C.

   Correct answer: E

   Comments:

   Results of the ACTIVE clinical trial were used to compare the number of patients needed to treat (NNT) to prevent one fracture after an 18-month treatment course with teriparatide compared to abaloparatide. Fewer patients needed to be treated with abaloparatide than with teriparatide to prevent one nonvertebral fracture (55versus 92), one clinical fracture (37 versus 59), or one major fracture

(34 versus 75). The NNT for vertebral fractures was about the same in both groups: 28 in the abaloparatide and 30 in the teriparatide group. The fracture risk reduction appears to be independent of the baseline fracture risk as determined by the FRAX model.[18]

4. ***Comparing teriparatide to risedronate in postmenopausal women with new vertebral fractures:***
   A. The risk of sustaining new vertebral compression fractures was much lower in patients on teriparatide than in those patients on risedronate.
   B. Back pain was much worse in patients on teriparatide.
   C. Adverse events leading to withdrawal from study were significantly higher in the risedronate group.
   D. A and B.
   E. Arthralgia was much more common in the teriparatide group.

   Correct answer: A

   Comments:

   In the **VER**tebral fracture treatment comparisons in **O**steoporotic women (VERO), a multicenter, double-blind, double-dummy, randomized, controlled clinical trial, more patients in the risedronate group sustained new vertebral compression fractures 12% than in the teriparatide 5% group. Back pain was experienced in 11.2% of patients on teriparatide compared to 12.2% in those on risedronate. Among patients in the teriparatide group 9.9% developed adverse events that necessitated withdrawal from the study, compared to 7.1% in the risedronate group.[19]

5. ***Teriparatide and abaloparatide:***
   A. Can be administered for more than 2 years.
   B. Simultaneous administration of antiresorptives is advantageous.
   C. Should not be prescribed if the glomerular filtration rate is less than 35 mL/min.
   D. Once discontinued, an antiresorptive agent should be prescribed.
   E. A and D.

   Correct answer: E

   Comment:

   In 2020 the US FDA (Food and Drug Administration) approved changes to the label of teriparatide (Forteo): the two-year lifetime treatment limitation was removed as well as the boxed warning about the risk of osteosarcoma. The lifetime treatment limitation for abaloparatide now also has been removed. Clinicians now can prescribe both teriparatide and abaloparatide for period longer than 2 years to patients with “high” or “very high” fracture risk. When teriparatide is discontinued, BMD gains are lost unless an antiresorptive is prescribed.[4] Starting bisphosphonate therapy immediately after discontinuing teriparatide induces further increases in BMD.[20]

As teriparatide is not excreted by the kidneys, it can be administered if the eGFR is less than 35 mL/min. Caution should nevertheless be exercised as many patients with renal impairment have secondary hyperparathyroidism. The present evidence does not support the simultaneous use of teriparatide and antiresorptive agents.[21,22]

6. ***Teriparatide and abaloparatide increase bone formation by:***
   A. Increasing number of preosteoblasts.
   B. Downregulating RANLK-ligand.
   C. Stimulating osteoprotegerin secretion.
   D. A and B.
   E. A, B, and C.

   Correct answer: E

   Comment:

   In postmenopausal women with osteoporosis, the administration of abaloparatide for three months stimulates bone formation of cancellous, endocortical, intracortical, and periosteal envelopes in transiliac bone biopsies. These increases reflect the stimulation of both bone modeling and remodeling and elucidate mechanisms by which abaloparatide improves the bone mass and reduces the fracture risk.[17]

   Teriparatide administration increases the number of preosteoblasts, stimulates their differentiation into mature osteoblasts, and enhances their function.[23] Teriparatide improves bone microarchitecture by increasing trabecular connectivity and cortical thickness, thus increasing bending and buckling strength. In addition, teriparatide downregulates RANK-Ligand expression and stimulates osteoprotegerin secretion resulting in reduced osteoclast formation, maturation, and stimulation.[24]

   The increases in bone formation induced by teriparatide initially exceed the rate of bone resorption. This effect is nevertheless short-lived because the rate of bone resorption is also increased in time as a result of the increase in RANK-Ligand (receptor activator of nuclear factor kB ligand). In other words, the initial increased bone formation in excess of bone resorption is limited in time with teriparatide. It is also known as the "anabolic window" and is relatively short-lived when induced by teriparatide but not by abaloparatide which has been specifically engineered to overcome the loss of the anabolic window and hypercalcemia. Indeed, although the first 21 amino acids of PTH and PTHrP are identical, multiple substitutions have been made between amino acids 22 and 34 in the abaloparatide molecule to increase its stability and maintain an increased rate of bone formation versus bone resorption.[12]

7. ***Teriparatide administration after a fracture:***
   A. Stimulates chondrogenesis in the callus.
   B. Enhances chondrocyte maturation and mineralization.
   C. Enhances fracture healing.
   D. All of the above.
   E. None of the above.

   Correct answer: D

Comment:

Studies on experimental animals document that after a fracture, teriparatide administration enhances fracture healing by increasing callus volume and enhancing endochondral bone formation through increased chondrogenesis, chondrocyte maturation and mineralization.[25] There are, however, still a paucity of studies on the effect of teriparatide on fracture healing in humans.[26]

8. ***Main adverse events of teriparatide and abaloparatide include:***
   A. Orthostatic hypotension.
   B. Nausea.
   C. Arthralgia.
   D. A and B.
   E. A, B, and C.

   Correct answer: E

   Comment:

   Adverse events after teriparatide administration include arthralgia (10.1% teriparatide versus 8.4% placebo) and nausea, but not vomiting (8.5% teriparatide, 6.7% placebo).[26] The latter is usually self-limited. In order to avoid it, many patients self-administer at night as they get ready for bed. Although symptomatic orthostatic hypotension is rare (about 5%), it is nevertheless recommended that at least for the first few doses teriparatide and abaloparatide be administered under circumstances in which the patient can sit or lie down should symptoms arise.[26]

9. ***The following "Drug holiday" regimens are recommended in patients on teriparatide or abaloparatide:***
   A. One day, every week.
   B. One week, once a month.
   C. One month, once a year.
   D. Three months every 3 years.
   E. None of the above.

   Correct answer: E

   Comment:

   Drug holidays are not recommended for patients on teriparatide or abaloparatide. If there is a need to discontinue the medication, an antiresorptive medication may be prescribed to prevent any bone loss.

10. ***Osteosarcoma, teriparatide and abaloparatide:***
   A. The risk of osteosarcoma is significantly increased in patients on teriparatide.
   B. Teriparatide increased the incidence of osteosarcoma in Fischer 344 rats.
   C. Teriparatide should not be administered to patients who have received radiation therapy.
   D. A and B.
   E. B and C.

   Correct answer: E

Comment:

Toxicology studies documented that when teriparatide was administered to Fischer 344 rats in doses up to 60 times higher than those used in humans, the incidence of osteosarcoma was increased in a dose- and duration-dependent manner.[26] On the other hand, no bone tumors were detected after 18 months of teriparatide therapy to mature oophorectomized monkeys, at doses 6 times higher than administered to humans.[26]

The risk of osteosarcoma is not increased in patients with hyperparathyroidism and postmarketing surveillance showed that over a 7-year follow-up period the incidence of osteosarcoma in patients receiving teriparatide is not higher than in the general population. Teriparatide nevertheless is not recommended in children and young adults with open epiphyses and those in whom the risk of osteosarcoma is increased such as patients who have received radiation therapy and those with Paget's disease of bone or unexplained increases in bony alkaline phosphatase.

Although the convention has been to use antiresorptive medication, especially bisphosphonates as a first-line treatment for osteoporosis, the present data suggests that it may be more beneficial to use anabolic agents as first-line treatment in patients who are at high risk of sustaining a fracture.[27]

References

1. Pietrogrande L, Raimondo E. Abaloparatide for the treatment of postmenopausal osteoporosis. *Drugs Today.* 2018;54(5):293–303.
2. Eastman K, Gerlach M, Pliec I, et al. Effectiveness of parathyroid hormone (HRT) analogues on fracture healing: a meta-analysis. *Osteoporos Int.* 2021;32:1531–1546.
3. Thompson JC, Wanderman N, Anderson PA, Freedman A. Abaloparatide and the spine: a narrative review. *Clin Interv Aging.* 2020;15:1023–1033.
4. Leder BZ, Mitlak B, Hu M, et al. Effect of abaloparatide vs alendronate on fracture risk reduction in postmenopausal women with osteoporosis. *J Clin Endocrinol Metab.* 2019. https://doi.org/10.1210/clinem/doz162.
5. Leder BZ, Neer RM, Wyland JJ, et al. Effects of teriparatide treatment and discontinuation in postmenopausal women and eugonadal men with osteoporosis. *J Clin Endocrinol Metab.* 2009;94(8):2915–2921.
6. Cosman F, Miller PD, Williams GC, et al. Eighteen months of treatment with subcutaneous abaloparatide followed by 6 months of treatment with alendronate in ostmenopausal women with osteoporosis: results of the ACTIVExtend trial. *Mayo Clin Proc.* 2017;92(2):200–210.
7. Sahbani K, Cardozo CP, Bauman WA, Tawfeek HA. Abaloparatie exhibits greater anabolic response and higher CMP stimulation and B-arrestin recruitment than teriparatide. *Physiol Rev.* 2019;7(19):e14225.
8. Zhang C, Song C. Combination therapy of PTH and antiresorptive drugs on osteoporosis: a review of treatment alternatives. *Front Pharmacol.* 2021. PMID: 3358284.
9. Hattersley G, Dean T, Corbin BA, et al. Binding selectivity of abaloparatide for PTH-type-1-receptor conformations and effects on downstream signaling. *Endocrinology.* 2016;157:141–149.
10. Miller PD, Hattersley G, Riis BJ, et al. Effect of abaloparatide vs placebo on new vertebral fractures in postmenopausal women with osteoporosis: a randomized clinical trial. *JAMA.* 2016;316(7):722–733.

11. Fan Y, Le PT, Ruiye B, et al. Parathyroid hormone directs bone marrow mesenchymal cell fate. *Cell Metab.* 2017;25(3):661–672.
12. Battacharyya S, Pals S, Chattopadya. Abaloparatide, the second generation osteoanabolic drug: molecular mechanisms underlying its advantages over the first in class teriparatide. *Biochem Pharmacol.* 2019;166: 185–191.
13. Wysolmerski JJ. Parathyroid hormone-related protein: an update. *J Clin Endocrinol Metab.* 2012;97(9): 2947–2956.
14. Haas AV, LeBoff MS. Osteoanabolic agents for osteoporosis. *J Endocr Soc.* 2018;2(8):922–932.
15. Neer RM, Arnaud CD, Zanchetta JR, et al. Effect of parathyroid hormone (1-34) on fractures and bone mineral density in postmenopausal women with osteoporosis. *N Engl J Med.* 2001;344:1434–1441.
16. Boyce EG, Mai Y, Pham C. Abaloparatide: review of a next-generation parathyroid hormone agonist. *Ann Pharmacother.* 2018;52(5):462–472.
17. Dempster DW, Zhou H, Sudhaker DR, et al. Early effects of abaloparatide on bone formation and resorption indices in postmenopausal women with osteoporosis. *J Bone Miner Res.* 2021;36(4):644–653.
18. McCloskey EV, Johansson H, Oden A, et al. The effect of abaloparatide-SC on fracture risk is independent of baseline FRAX fracture probability: a post hoc analysis of the ACTIVE study. *J Bone Miner Res.* 2017;32(8): 1625–1631.
19. Geusens P, Marin F, Kendler DL, et al. Effects of teriparatide compared with risedronate on the risk of fractures in subgroups of postmenopausal women with severe osteoporosis: the VERO trial. *J Bone Miner Res.* 2018;33 (5):783–794. https://doi.org/10.1002/jbmr.3384.
20. Kurland ES, Heller SL, Diamond B, et al. The importance of bisphosphonate therapy in maintaining bone mass in men after therapy with teriparatide. *Osteoporos Int.* 2004;15(12):992–997.
21. Cusano NE, Bilezikian JP. Combination anti-resorptive and osteo-anabolic therapy for osteoporosis: we are not there yet. *Curr Med Res Opin.* 2011;27(9):1705–1707.
22. Uihlein AV, Leder BZ. Anabolic therapies for osteoporosis. *Endocrinol Metab Clin N.* 2012;41:507–525.
23. Canalis E, Giustina A, Bilezikian JP. Mechanisms of anabolic therapies for osteoporosis. *N Engl J Med.* 2007;357:905–916.
24. Resmini G, Iolascon G. New Insights into the role of teriparatide. *Aging Clin Exp Res.* 2011;23(Suppl. 2):30–32.
25. Kakr S, Einhom TA, Vora S, et al. Enhanced chondrogenesis and wnt signaliin PTH-treated fractures. *J Bone Miner Res.* 2007;22:1903–1912.
26. Zhang D, Potty A, Vyas P, Lane J. The role of recombinant PTH in human fracture healing: a systematic review. *J Orthop Trauma.* 2013;28.
27. Cosman F. The evolving role of anabolic therapy in the treatment of osteoporosis. *Curr Opin Rheumatol.* 2019;31(4):376–380.

CHAPTER 20

Atypical femoral fractures☆

Learning objectives

- Recognize the symptoms and presentation of atypical femoral shaft fractures (AFF).
- Understand the pathophysiology of AFF and the role of antiresorptive medication.

The case study

Reason for seeking medical help

- GL, 66years old, is complaining of pain in her left upper thigh that started insidiously about 8 weeks ago. Initially it was only a discomfort, but it gradually becomes worse. She now rates it as "7" on a scale of 1–10, with 10 being the worst possible pain. It is constant, occasionally throbbing, and often precipitated by exertion, especially walking or standing on the left leg.
- She had to stop jogging about 3 weeks ago because of the pain in her left hip. The pain is partly relieved by rest and local heat. It is not worse at night when she is in bed. It does not wake her up but is starting to interfere with her daily activities.

Past medical and surgical history

- Osteoporosis, diagnosed about 12 years ago: lowest T-score in the lumbar vertebrae was −3.0. She was prescribed alendronate. She still takes the tablets exactly as directed. She has not experienced adverse effects.
- Status postnatural menopause at age 43, no hormonal replacement therapy.

Lifestyle

- Daily dietary calcium intake estimated to be about 1200 mg.
- No excessive caffeine, sodium, or alcohol intake.
- No cigarette smoking.
- Physically active lifestyle; also, she jogs for about an hour every weekday.

☆ GL, 66 years old, Caucasian woman, 8 years on oral bisphosphonates, presents with pain in left thigh.

Diagnosis and Treatment of Osteoporosis. https://doi.org/10.1016/B978-0-323-99550-4.00010-1
Copyright © 2024 Elsevier Inc. All rights are reserved, including those for text and data mining, AI training, and similar technologies.

Medication(s)

- Alendronate tablets, 70 mg once a week, 12 years, good adherence.
- Cholecalciferol 400 units daily.

Family history

- Mother and older sister sustained fragility hip fractures.

Clinical examination

- Weight 153 pounds, steady, height 65″, used to be 66″.
- Some limitation in range of movement of the left hip.
- Pain in left upper thigh worse on standing up on left leg.
- Tenderness along the upper third of left femoral shaft.
- No evidence of localizing neurological lesions.
- No significant arthritic changes.
- No edema of the lower limbs.
- No evidence of peripheral arterial or venous insufficiency.

Laboratory results

- Comprehensive metabolic profile: no abnormality detected.
- Serum 25-hydroxy-vitamin D: 46 ng/mL.

DXA and radiological results

- T-scores: left femoral neck −2.4, left total hip −2.1, lumbar vertebrae −2.5.
- Compared to the baseline DXA scans, there has been an increase in the BMD: 6% in the total hip and 11% in the lumbar vertebrae. These changes exceed the least significant change of the center where the DXA scans were done.
- Vertebral fracture assessment: no evidence of vertebral compression fracture.

Multiple choice questions

1. ***GL's clinical presentation is compatible with:***
   A. Osteoarthritis left hip.
   B. Paget's disease of bone.
   C. Atypical femur fracture (AFF) left proximal femur.
   D. Any of the above.
   E. None of the above.
   Correct answer: C

Comments:

The presentation is suggestive of an atypical femoral shaft fracture (AFF).[1] About 70% of patients who sustain an AFF complain of pain and tenderness in the thigh or groin, at the site of the fracture.[1] The pain, sometimes throbbing, is worsened by movement and standing up on the affected leg.[2]

Atypical femoral fractures (AFF) are stress fractures. However, unlike typical stress fractures which start in the medial cortex, and then spread out, AFF usually originate in the lateral cortex and spread medially, hence their name "atypical."[3,4] The process starts by an accumulation of microscopic cracks that are usually resorbed by osteoclasts and replaced with new healthy bone laid by the osteoblasts, a process known as "targeted remodeling."

Antiresorptives, especially if administered over prolonged periods, may lead to the development of AFF. Bisphosphonates interfere with the removal of these microscopic cracks which then accumulate, enlarge, fuse, cause the bone to weaken. This in turn results in a fracture: a fracture that has the potential to increase in size to become a full transverse fracture, an atypical fracture.[4,5] The osteoclasts are normally steered by a receptor-activator of nuclear factor kappa-B ligand (RANKL) to areas of the bone where microcracks are present in order to start the clearing process.

Denosumab is an antibody to RANK-L and blocks the formation of osteoclasts. As a result of its long-term administration, however, the microcracks may not be resorbed, may accumulate, and may lead to a full fracture.[4,6,7]

The age-adjusted incidence of AFF increases with the increased exposure to antiresorptive agents.[8,9] It is estimated to be 1.8 per 100,000 person-years in patients who have been on bisphosphonates for less than 2years increasing to 118 per 100,000 person-years with more than 8years exposure.[5] AFF has also been seen in patients who have not been on bisphosphonates or other antiresorptive medications.[5]

The diagnostic features of AFF as developed by the American Society for Bone and Mineral Research (ASBMR) include a fracture located anywhere along the femoral shaft: from just distal to the lesser trochanter to just proximal to the supracondylar flare.[1,10]

In addition: 4 of the 5 following "**Major features**" should be present:

1. The fracture is preceded by only minimal or no trauma.
2. The fracture line originates at the lateral cortex and is substantially transverse in its orientation, although it may become oblique as it progresses medially across the femur.
3. Complete fractures extend through both cortices and may be associated with a medial spike.
4. Incomplete fractures involve only the lateral cortex.
5. The fracture is noncomminuted or minimally comminuted.
6. Localized periosteal or endosteal thickening of the lateral cortex at the fracture site: "beaking" or "flaring".

Minor features

Although often associated with AFF, none of the minor features are required to diagnose AFF. They include generalized increase in cortical thickness of the femoral diaphysis, unilateral or bilateral prodromal symptoms such as dull or aching pain in the groin or thigh, bilateral incomplete or complete femoral diaphysis fractures, and delayed fracture healing.

Criteria that have been removed with the 2014 ASBMR revision include:

Exclusion criteria

Exclusion criteria: fracture of the femoral head and neck, intertrochanteric fracture with spiral subtrochanteric extension, periprosthetic femoral fractures, and pathological fractures such as those associated with Paget's disease and fibrous dysplasia.

Comorbid conditions which have been removed from the ASBMR 2014 revision include vitamin D deficiency, rheumatoid arthritis, hypoparathyroidism, and hypophosphatasia. Pharmaceutical agents which may lead to atypical femoral fractures such as bisphosphonates, as well as glucocorticoids, hypoparathyroidism, and proton pump inhibitors.[10]

- Of interest:
  - Very occasionally, AFF are seen in patients who have not been on antiresorptive therapy.[11]
  - Severe suppression of bone turnover is not seen in most patients sustaining AFF.[11]
  - The geometry of the proximal femur may predispose to the development of AFF, specifically, bowed femurs and varus femoral neck/shaft angle.[11] Particularly vulnerable to AFF are patients with an increased femur bowing angle (>5.25 degrees) or a decreased femur neck/shaft angle (<125 degrees). The increased risk of AFF is such that it has been recommended to evaluate these 2 angles before prescribing bisphosphonates and to refrain from such a prescription if both angles are outside the "safe" zone.
  - It has also been recommended that if bisphosphonates cannot be avoided that they be given for shorter periods with timely "drug holidays" and that the angles of the 2 femurs be evaluated by X-rays at 6-monthly intervals and to be prepared to switch to another medication.[12]
  - Complete AFF needing surgical repair: intramedullary rods or other orthopedic hardware.
  - Although osteoarthritis is associated with hip pain, it is not associated with localized pain and tenderness in the femoral shaft. The range of movement of the affected joint is also often diminished or limited by pain. Other joints are also usually affected particularly the knees and hands.

- Pain associated with Paget's disease of bone is usually worse at night when the patient lies in a warm bed, as this increases the blood flow through the already congested bone. AFF have also been seen in patients with Paget's disease of bone.[13]

2. ***At this stage, the following imaging studies are indicated:***
   A. Plain X-ray, MRI, or CT scan left femur.
   B. Plain X-ray, MRI, or CT scan of both femurs.
   C. Technetium bone scan.
   D. A or C.
   E. B or C.

   Correct answer: B

   Comment:

   Anatomical visualization of the underlying pathology is necessary to develop an appropriate management strategy. Bilateral imaging studies are indicated because 50%–60% of patients who sustained an atypical femoral shaft fracture have, at almost the exact position on the contralateral femur, evidence of cortical thickening with or without an insufficiency fracture.[14] Although the diagnosis is usually quite obvious on X-rays, it is sometimes missed in early cases. In case of doubt an MRI is more sensitive.[3,15] The technetium scan shows a localized increased blood flow but will not identify the underlying pathology. Insufficiency fractures may not be visualized on a plain X-ray, but localized cortical swelling may be seen.

3. ***Given the radiological appearances, the following is/are recommended:***
   A. Discontinue alendronate.
   B. Initiate therapy with an osteoanabolic medication such as teriparatide or abaloparatide.
   C. Consider prophylactic placement of orthopedic software.
   D. A and B.
   E. A, B, and C.

   Correct answer: E

   Comment:

   The radiological appearances are compatible with an insufficiency fracture. If left untreated it may lead to a complete AFF. Alendronate should be discontinued as it may reduce the rate of bone resorption and possibly interfere with the normal healing process of insufficiency fractures. These patients should be closely monitored and may benefit from raloxifene, estrogen, tibolone, calcitonin, or a short course of bisphosphonates.[3,16]

   There are several reports of teriparatide being useful in the management of insufficiency fractures.[17] Orthopedic hardware could also be inserted prophylactically.[18]

   Patients should be investigated for secondary causes of osteoporosis including hypovitaminosis D and metabolic bone diseases such as hypophosphatasia.

4. ***Femoral shaft fractures:***
   A. Are also known as subtrochanteric fractures.
   B. Represent about 10% of all femoral fractures.
   C. Have a bimodal age distribution.
   D. A and B.
   E. A, B, and C.

   Correct answer: E

   Comment:

   Femoral shaft fractures, also known as subtrochanteric fractures, represent about 10% of all femoral fractures and have a bimodal age distribution, with an increased prevalence among young and older subjects.[19,20] About 75% are secondary to severe trauma, the remaining 25% are fragility fractures: atraumatic, low trauma, or low impact injuries and occur mostly in patients with osteoporosis.[21] They share common features with classical osteoporotic fractures: a steep increase in old age, more common in women than men, and occurring spontaneously or after low trauma that would not be expected to lead to a fracture.[22]

   In patients treated with antiresorptives there are three separate types of femoral shaft fractures: First, the "typical" fragility femoral shaft fractures due to mechanically weak osteoporotic bone. Second, the "atypical" femoral fragility shaft fractures which are the result of insufficiency fractures that have not healed, have spread across the femur shaft, and are possibly due to antiresorptive medication. Both types of fractures may occur spontaneously, in the absence of trauma or as a result of trauma that ordinarily would not be expected to induce a fracture.[1]

5. ***Prognosis of fragility femoral shaft fractures:***
   A. About 15% mortality at 12 months.
   B. About 50% of patients do not achieve their prefracture functional level.
   C. About 70% of patients need alternative accommodation.
   D. A and B.
   E. A, B, and C.

   Correct answer: E

   Comment:

   The prognosis of fragility femoral shaft fractures is similar to that of fragility hip fractures.[23] Hence the need to be alert to this potential complication of antiresorptive therapy. There is evidence that whereas the rate of hip and intertrochanteric fractures has significantly declined since the advent of bisphosphonates, the rate of subtrochanteric fractures has increased during this period, suggesting that it may be, at least partly, due to the antiresorptive medication.[24–27]

6. ***Mechanisms leading to AFF in patients on bisphosphonates:***
   A. Antiangiogenesis effect of bisphosphonates and impaired healing.
   B. Accumulation of microfractures and microarchitectural deterioration.
   C. Increased bone brittleness.

D. A and B.
E. A, B, and C.

Correct answer: E

Comments:

Data from experimental animals show that by suppressing bone turnover bisphosphonates may interfere with the healing process of bone microdamage, thus leading to microdamage accumulation, stress fractures, and eventually complete fractures.[28] Bisphosphonates also increase advanced glycation end products which are associated with more brittle bone and have an antiangiogenic effect.[29,30]

7. ***Match the following:***
   (a) Atypical femoral shaft fractures.
   (b) Osteoporotic femoral shaft fractures.
   (c) Both.
   (d) Neither.
      A. Usually comminuted.
      B. Transverse fracture line on the lateral cortex.
      C. Medial spike is often identified.
      D. Lateral cortical thickening.
      E. Short oblique configuration.

Correct answers: A (b); B (a); C (a); D (a); E (a)

Comment:

Atypical femoral shaft fractures originate as insufficiency or stress fractures and extend perpendicularly through the femur shaft. Unlike traumatic or osteoporotic fractures, they are noncomminuted and are transverse or have a short oblique configuration. As they approach the medial cortex, they may have a medial spike. Cortical thickening is often seen and represents an attempt to increase the mechanical strength of the bone in the presence of an insufficiency fracture that is unable to heal. The cortical thickening could be either localized (beaking or flaring) or generalized.[1]

Insufficiency fractures tend to originate in the lateral cortex which is subject to higher levels of tensile stress.[18,19,31,32]

Insufficiency fractures are due to an abnormally "weak bone" and a "normal or usual" load that should not ordinarily lead to a fracture. Stress fractures, on the other hand, are due to an abnormal load on a relatively healthy bone, as often occurs when a person who for years has led a sedentary lifestyle abruptly decides to go hiking, puts on a heavy load on his shoulders and back, and walks for a long distance. That person is likely to develop a stress fracture.

8. ***Fracture healing:***
   A. Complete fractures heal through callus formation.
   B. Stress fractures heal through a process of bone remodeling.
   C. Antiresorptives may interfere with the healing process of stress fractures.

D. A and B.
E. A, B, and C.

Correct answer: E

Comment:

Complete fractures heal through the formation of a soft callus which is gradually invaded by chondrocytes which subsequently ossify and undergo remodeling. Stress and insufficiency fractures heal through a process of bone remodeling: activated osteoclasts remove damaged bone, followed by osteoblasts depositing new healthy bone. Therefore, by interfering with the activity of osteoclasts, antiresorptive agents may interfere with the healing process of these stress and insufficiency fractures and may lead to a complete "atypical" fracture. It must be noted nevertheless that when bisphosphonates are administered to bisphosphonate naïve patients 2 weeks after a hip fracture, they do not interfere with fracture healing.[33]

9. ***The following medications have been associated with an increased risk of atypical femoral fractures:***
A. Bisphosphonates.
B. Teriparatide.
C. Denosumab.
D. A and C.
E. A, B, and C.

Correct answer: D

Comment:

Several studies have documented an increased rate of subtrochanteric fractures in patients on bisphosphonates, or denosumab, especially in patients who have been on these medications for more than 3 years.[9] Studies have also shown that longer treatment periods are associated with higher risks.[1] A study on 87,820 women between the ages of 45 and 84years shows that the risk of AFF is higher if they took bisphosphonates for 3 or more years compared to those who were on bisphosphonates for less than 3 years.[34] Discontinuation of bisphosphonates is associated with a rapid decrease in the risk of AFF.[8,35]

In patients on bisphosphonates, although the relative risk of an atypical femoral shaft fracture is increased, the absolute risk is very low: it is estimated to range from 3.2 to 50 cases per 100,000 person-years, and to increase to more than 100 per 100,000 person-years among patients on long-term bisphosphonate therapy.[1] This increased risk, however, must be weighed against the bisphosphonate-induced decrease in hip and intertrochanteric fracture.

A recent study based on 196,129 women has shown that after 3years of bisphosphonate therapy 149 hip fractures were prevented and only two bisphosphonate-associated AFF occurred. The authors also noted that the discontinuation of bisphosphonates was associated with a rapid decrease in the risk of AFF.[8]

10. ***The following increases the risk of atypical femoral shaft fractures:***
    - A. Glucocorticoids.
    - B. Hypovitaminosis D.
    - C. Rheumatoid arthritis.
    - D. A and B.
    - E. A, B, and C.

    Correct answer: E

    Comment:

    Glucocorticoids, antiresorptives (bisphosphonates and denosumab, calcitonin and raloxifene), omeprazole, and a number of medications increase the risk of subtrochanteric fractures. Active rheumatoid arthritis, a serum 25-hydroxy-vitamin D level below 16 ng/mL, prior low-energy fractures, and hypophosphatasia also increase the risk.[1,36]

Case summary

Analysis of data

The clinical presentation of an atypical femoral shaft fracture incudes ill-defined pain, tender points, and leg shortening.

Diagnosis

Atypical femoral fracture.

GL has been diagnosed with osteoporosis about 12 years ago and was prescribed alendronate. She adhered well to the medication and now presents with an insufficiency fracture in her left femur. Secondary causes of osteoporosis have been excluded. She is not vitamin D deficient. Her T-score is lower than −2.5.

Management recommendations

Treatment recommendation(s)

- Given the insufficiency fracture, which could be the precursor of a complete AFF, the bisphosphonate should be discontinued, and an osteoanabolic agent, teriparatide or abaloparatide, may be considered, especially as her lowest T-score is less than −2.5. Similarly, these patients may benefit from romosozumab which has both osteoanabolic and antiresorptive effects on the skeleton.
- Prophylactic femoral rod insertion, possibly bilateral.
- Follow-up clinic, 4–6 weeks to ensure she is adhering to teriparatide or abaloparatide therapy. If romosozumab is prescribed the follow-up visit could be postponed for about 2 months. This visit also will ensure the patient has adopted a healthy lifestyle and is getting a well-balanced diet.

Key points

- About 25% of AFF are stress fractures and can be due to:
  - Underlying osteoporotic process.
  - Extension of an insufficiency fracture, possibly related to antiresorptive therapy.
- Bisphosphonates administered for 3 or more years increase the risk of atypical femoral shaft fracture to a larger extent than if administered for less than 3 years.[34]
- Discontinuation of bisphosphonate therapy is associated with a rapid decrease in the risk of sustaining an atypical femoral shaft fracture.[8]
- About 1000 patients at risk of sustaining fractures need to be treated with bisphosphonates for 3 years to prevent 100 "typical" fractures. In this population, 1.25 AFF would be expected to develop within the given period.[37] Most patients will need more than 3 years of treatment with antiresorptives.[38]
- Several possible treatment models have been designed to minimize the risk of AFF including:
  - "Four-year plan": Osteoanabolic medication (teriparatide) for 2 years followed by denosumab for 2 years yielded much larger increases in BMD than denosumab for 2 years followed by teriparatide for 2 years.[39]
  - "Seven-year plan": 2 years anabolic medication followed by 5 years bisphosphonates.[11]
  - Use osteoanabolic agents as first-line treatment. Unfortunately, this strategy is not likely to be widely used because of their route of administration and their cost.[11]
  - The annual incidence of AFF is also decreasing possibly because of the decreasing number of bisphosphonate prescriptions.[40]
  - The reduction in the risk of sustaining an osteoporotic fracture as a result of bisphosphonate therapy grossly outweighs the risk of sustaining an atypical fracture as a complication of the administered therapy.[8]

References

1. Shane E, Burr D, Abrahamsen B, et al. Atypical subtrochanteric and diaphyseal femoral fractures: second report of a task force of the American Society for Bone and Mineral Research. *J Bone Miner Res.* 2014;29(1):1–23. https://doi.org/10.1002/jbmr.1998. Epub 2013 Oct 1. PMID: 23712442.
2. Kellar J, Givertz A, Matthias J, Cohen J. Bisphosphonate-related femoral shaft fracture. *Clin Pract Cases Emerg Med.* 2020;4(1):62–64.
3. Cheung AM, McKenna MJ, van de Laarschot DM, et al. Detection of atypical femur fractures. *J Clin Densitom.* 2019;22(4):506–516.
4. Tile L, Cheung AM. Atypical femur fractures: current understanding and approach to management. *Ther Adv Musculoskel Dis.* 2020;12:1–9.
5. Van de Laarschot DM, McKenna MJ, Abrahamsen B, et al. Medical management of patients after atypical femur fractures: a systematic review and recommendations from the European calcified tissue society. *J Clin Endocinol Metab.* 2020;105(5):1682–1699.
6. Aspenberg P. Denosumab and atypical femoral fractures. *Acta Orthop.* 2014;85(1):1.
7. Lewiecki EM, Dinavahi RV, Lazaretti-Castro M, et al. One year of romosozumab followed by two years of denosumab maintains fracture risk reductions: results of the FRAME extension study. *J Bone Miner Res.* 2019;34(3):419–428.
8. Black DM, Geiger EJ, Eastell R, et al. Atypical femur fracture risk versus fragility fracture prevention with bisphosphonates. *New Engl J Med.* 2020;383(8):743–753.

9. Khan AA, Kaiser S. Atypical femoral fracture. *CMAJ*. 2017;189(14):E542.
10. Troiano E, Giacche T, Facchini A, et al. Surgical and pharmacological management of periprosthetic atypical femoral fractures: a narrative literature review. *Geriatr Orthop Surg*. 2022;13:1–11.
11. Adler RA. Atypical femoral fractures: risks and benefits of long-term treatment: risks and benefits of long-term treatment of osteoporosis with anti-resorptive therapy. *Eur J Endocrinol*. 2018;178:R81–R87.
12. Papaioannou I, Pantazidou G, Baikousis A, et al. Femoral bowing and femoral neck-shaft angle evaluation can reduce atypical femoral fractures in osteoporotic patients: a scientific report. *Cureus*. 2020;12(10) e10771.
13. Nepal S, Jarusriwanna A, Unnanuntana A. Stress fracture of the femoral shaft in Paget's disease of bone: a case report. *J Bone Metab*. 2021;28(2):171–178.
14. Ing-Lorenzini K, Desmeules J, Platcha O, et al. Low-energy femoral fractures associated with long-term use of bisphosphonates. *Dru Saf*. 2009;32:775–785.
15. Seong YJ, Shin JK, Park WR. Early detected femoral neck insufficiency fracture in a patient treated with long-term bisphosphonate therapy for osteoporosis: a need for MRI. *Int J Surg Case Rep*. 2020;70:213–215. https://doi.org/10.1016/j.ijscr.2020.04.003.
16. Lewiecky ME, Anderson PA, Bilezikian JP, et al. Santa Fe Bone Symposium. Advances in the management of osteoporosis and metabolic bone diseases. *J Clin Densitom*. 2021. https://doi.org/10.1016/j.jocd.2021.10.001.
17. Carvalho NN, Voss LA, Almeida MO, et al. Atypical femoral fractures during prolonged use of bisphosphonates: short-term responses to strontium ranelate and teriparatide. *J Clin Endocrinol Metab*. 2011;96:2675–2680.
18. Ha YC, Cho MR, Park KH, et al. Is surgery necessary for femoral insufficiency fractures after long-term bisphosphonate therapy? *Clin Orthop Relat Res*. 2010;468(12):3393–3398.
19. Nieves JW, Bilzekian JP, Lane JM, et al. Fragility fractures of the hip and femur incidence and patient characteristics. *Osteoporos Int*. 2010;21:399–408.
20. Singer BR, McLauglan GJ, Robinson CM, Christie J. Epidemiology of fractures in 15,000 adults: the influence of age and gender. *J Bone Joint Surg Br*. 1998;80:243–248.
21. Salminen S, Pklajamakl H, Avikainen V, et al. Specific features associated with femoral shaft fractures caused by low energy trauma. *J Trauma*. 1997;43:117–122.
22. Weiss RJ, Montgomery SM, Al Dabbagh Z, Jansson KA. National data of 6409 Swedish inpatients with femoral shaft fractures: stable incidence between 1998 and 2004. *Injury*. 2009;40:304–308.
23. Bliuc D, Nguyen ND, Milch VE, et al. Mortality risk associated with low-trauma osteoporotic fracture and subsequent fracture in men and women. *JAMA*. 2009;301(5):413–421.
24. Wang Z, Bhattacharyya T. Trends in incidence of subtrochanteric fragility fractures and bisphosphonate use among the US elderly, 1996-2007. *J Bone Miner Res*. 2011;26:553–560.
25. Ng AC, Drake MT, Clarke BL, et al. Trends in subtrochanteric, diaphyseal and distal femur fractures, 1984-2007. *Osteoporos Int*. 2012;23:1721–1726.
26. Lee YK, Ha YC, Park C, et al. Bisphosphonate use and increased incidence of subtrochanteric fracture in South Korea. *Osteoporos Int E-pub*. 2012.
27. Girgis CM, Seibel MJ. Bisphosphonate use and femoral fractures in older women. *JAMA*. 2011;305:2068.
28. Li J, Mashiba T, Burr DB. Bisphosphonate treatment suppresses not only stochastic remodeling but also targeted repair of microdamage. *Calcific Tissue Int*. 2001;69:281–286.
29. Tang SY, Allen MR, Phipps R, et al. Changes in non-enzymatic glycation and its association with altered mechanical properties following 1-year treatment with risedronate or alendronate. *Osteoporos Int*. 2009;20:887–894.
30. Wood J, Bonjean K, Ruetz S, et al. Novel antiangiogenic effects of the bisphosphonate compound zoledronic acid. *Exp Ther*. 2002;302:1055–1061.
31. Koh JS, Goh SK, Png MA, et al. Distribution of atypical fractures and cortical stress lesions in the femur: implications on pathophysiology. *Singapore Med J*. 2011;52:77–80.
32. Donnelly E, Meredith DS, Nguyen JT, et al. Reduced cortical bone compositional heterogeneity with bisphosphonate treatment in postmenopausal women with intertrochanteric and subtrochanteric fractures. *J Bone Miner Res*. 2012;27:672–678.

33. Lyles KW, Colon-Emeric CS, Magaziner JS, et al. Zoledronic acid and clinical fractures and mortality after hip fracture. *N Engl J Med.* 2007;357:1799–1809.
34. Lo JC, Neugebauer RS, Ettinger B, et al. Risk of complete atypical femur fracture with oral bisphosphonate exposure beyond 3 years. *BMC Musculoskelet Disord.* 2020;21:801.
35. Park-Wyllie LY, Mamdani MM, Juurlink DN, et al. Bisphosphonate use and the risk of subtrochanteric or femoral shaft fractures in older women. *JAMA.* 2011;305:783–789.
36. Girgis CM, Sher D, Seibel MJ. Atypical femoral fractures and bisphosphonate use. *N Engl J Med.* 2010;362:1848–1849.
37. Black DM, Rosen CJ. Postmenopausal osteoporosis. *N Engl J Med.* 2016;374:254–262.
38. Adler RA, El-Hajj FG, Bauer DC, et al. Managing osteoporosis in patients on long-term bisphosphonate treatment: report of a task force on the American Society for Bone and Mineral Research. *JBMR.* 2016;31:16–35.
39. Tsai JN, Nishiyama KK, Lin D, et al. Effects of denosumab and teriparatide transitions on bone microarchitecture and estimated strength: the DATA-Switch HR-pQCT study. *J Bone Miner Res.* 2017;32:2001–2009.
40. Clout A, Narayanasamy N, Harris I. Trends in the incidence of atypical femoral fractures and bisphosphonate therapy. *J Orthop Surg.* 2016;24(1):36–40.

CHAPTER 21

Osteonecrosis of the jaw☆

Nonhealing cavity after tooth extraction

Learning objectives

- The definition, diagnosis, and staging of osteonecrosis of the Jaw (ONJ).
- Factors increasing the risk of ONJ.
- Developing a management plan tailored to individual circumstances of the patient.

The case study

Reasons for seeking medical help

- DD, 68 years old, has been diagnosed with osteoporosis about 12 years ago. She was prescribed alendronate and is taking it as directed. She has not experienced any adverse effect.
- Her dentist is concerned because she has a nonhealing cavity where a tooth was extracted about 4 months ago. DD is asymptomatic and did not know she had this cavity. Her dentist recommends multiple teeth extraction in the very near future.

Past medical and surgical history

- Natural menopause at 47 years, no HRT.
- Always enjoyed good health.

Lifestyle

- Daily dietary calcium intake about 1200 mg.
- No excessive sodium/caffeine intake.
- Observes meticulous dental hygiene.
- Exercises regularly: aerobic/resistive exercises, about 60 min, three times a week.

☆ DD, 68-year-old Caucasian woman, 12 years onsphosphonates.

Diagnosis and Treatment of Osteoporosis. https://doi.org/10.1016/B978-0-323-99550-4.00031-9
Copyright © 2024 Elsevier Inc. All rights are reserved, including those for text and data mining, AI training, and similar technologies.

Medication(s)

- Risedronate 75 mg once a week. Good adherence.

Family history

- Positive: her mother sustained a fragility hip fracture.

Clinical examination

- Weight 152 pounds, steady; height 64″.
- A cavity is present in the left mandible where the tooth was extracted, bone is visible, no signs of inflammation.
- No other relevant clinical signs.

Laboratory result(s)

- CBC, CMP, serum 25-hydroxy-vitamin D: all within normal limits.

DXA and radiologic result(s)

- T-scores: lumbar vertebrae −1.2, left femoral neck −1.1, left total hip −1.1.
- VFA: no evidence of vertebral compression fractures.
- FRAX scores: 1.3% and 9% for the 10-year risk of sustaining an osteoporotic hip or major fracture, respectively.

Multiple choice questions

1. ***DD's clinical presentation is suggestive of osteonecrosis of the jaw:***
   A. Stage 0.
   B. Stage I.
   C. Stage II.
   D. Stage III.
   E. None of the above; she has a posttooth extraction: a dry socket.
   Correct answer: B.
   Comment:
   The hallmark of ONJ is exposed mandibular or maxillary bone for at least 8 weeks as observed and recorded by a health care professional in a patient who has been on long-term antiresorptive medication (including bisphosphonates and denosumab), has not received radiation therapy to the craniofacial region, and does not have neoplastic lesions in the jaw.[1–4]

The American Association of Oral and Maxillofacial Surgeons developed a staging classification:

- Stage I: Exposed bone, no pain, no signs of inflammation.
- Stage II: Exposed bone, pain, and evidence of inflammation/infection.
- Stage III: Exposed bone, pain, and evidence of purulent discharge, fistulae and/or sinuses, and fractures.
- Stage 0 includes patients on bisphosphonates, with no exposed bone, but with nonspecific symptoms, clinical and/or radiological findings.[2,5]

The main underlying cause of ONJ is suppression of bone turnover by antiresorptive medications, inhibition of osteoclast activity, and apoptosis in conditions uniquely found in the mandible and maxilla. These include first, a very thin, easily breached mucosal barrier separating the mandible and maxilla from the oral cavity and the surrounding microflora. Second, infections, albeit superficial, frequently affecting the jaws. Third, surgery is often undertaken in this area, to extract teeth and manage periodontal infection.

Fourth, the rate of bone turnover may be higher in the mandible and maxilla than the rest of the skeleton. As a result, the jaw bones are exposed to a higher concentration of antiresorptive medication than the rest of the skeleton. In addition, the direct toxic effect on the epithelium and antiangiogenic properties of bisphosphonates may further interfere with wound healing.[6]

2. ***At this stage, the following investigation(s) is/are recommended:***

A. Panoramic X-ray, MRI, or CT scan of the mandible.
B. Technetium bone scan.
C. Bone markers.
D. A, B, or C.
E. None of the above.

Correct answer: A

Comment:

At this stage, although the diagnosis and staging are clinically obvious, it is possible that other lesions are present, hence the need for imaging studies of the mandible and maxilla. The absence of symptoms and leukocytosis makes an infectious process unlikely. The final diagnosis is therefore ONJ, stage I.[2] ONJ affects the mandible more frequently than the maxilla.[7] Radiological findings include[2,8]:

- Thickening of the lamina dura.
- Regional increased trabecular density of the alveolar bone.
- Alveolar bone loss not attributable to chronic periodontal disease.
- Widening of the periodontal space.
- The presence of a sequestrum.

CT scans allow the assessment of the following:

- Cortical integrity of the maxilla and mandible.
- Cortical and trabecular architecture of the maxilla and mandible.
- Thickening of the cortical outline.

- Periosteal bone reaction.
- Sequestrum formation.
- Early fistula track formation.
- Diffuse osteosclerosis and increased trabecular bone density.

Magnetic resonance imaging identifies early features of ONJ before the development of clinical features and includes a decrease in bone marrow signal intensity on T1-weighted images and increased signal intensity due to bone edema.[8] Although markers of bone resorption are sometimes assayed prior to undertaking dental work, especially invasive dental work, there is still no consensus as to their clinical usefulness.[9,10]

3. ***At this stage the following therapeutic intervention(s) is/are recommended:***
   A. Discontinue bisphosphonate.
   B. Prescribe teriparatide.
   C. Prescribe denosumab.
   D. A and B.
   E. A and C.

   Correct answer: A

   Comments:

   Although there is evidence to support that long-term oral bisphosphonate therapy is associated with delayed healing after tooth extraction, and a positive association has been documented between risk of ONJ and the dose and duration of bisphosphonate therapy, it is debatable whether the discontinuation of bisphosphonate or antiresorptive therapy significantly alters the course of ONJ in patients with osteoporosis, especially given the very long half-life of bisphosphonates.[11,12] On the other hand, several cases reported document that patients on antiresorptive therapy for osteoporosis who have developed ONJ (Stages 0, I, and II) heal spontaneously, even when the patients continue to take the bisphosphonates.[8]

   Notwithstanding, in DD's case, given her present marginally low T-scores (−1.1, −1.1, and −1.3), therefore low risk of sustaining a hip or major fracture and the duration of alendronate therapy (about 12 years), the oral bisphosphonate should be discontinued. There is no indication to prescribe denosumab. Although teriparatide or abaloparatide may be useful in ONJ, they are not recommended at this stage given DD's T-scores and low risk of sustaining a fracture or ONJ.[13]

4. ***Factors increasing the risk of ONJ include:***
   A. Dental procedures.
   B. Alcohol abuse.
   C. Cigarette smoking.
   D. A and B.
   E. A, B, and C.

   Correct answer: E

   Comment:

   Osteonecrosis of the jaw is believed to be due to a defect in the finely orchestrated bone remodeling process, whereby osteocytes send signals to the osteoclasts and osteoblasts to modulate bone resorption and bone formation.[14] Two main sets of factors increase the risk of ONJ: first, high doses of antiresorptive therapy and second, invasive dentoalveolar procedures especially in cancer patients. Although routine dental procedures are not associated with an increased risk of ONJ, they are the main triggers for ONJ in over 70% of the cases, and dental implants should be avoided in cancer patients exposed to high doses of bisphosphonates.[5,15,16] Dentures also increase the rate of ONJ in cancer patients.[17] There is no evidence that malocclusion increases the risk of ONJ in patients on bisphosphonates.[18] There is evidence that cigarette smoking and alcohol abuse increase the risk of ONJ in cancer patients treated with zoledronic acid.[16,19]

As much as possible, all invasive planned dental procedures should be completed before the initiation of bisphosphonate therapy, especially in the large doses needed by patients with neoplastic lesions.[8]

5. ***Medications predisposing to ONJ include:***
   A. Bisphosphonates.
   B. Denosumab.
   C. Teriparatide.
   D. A and B.
   E. A, B, and C.

Correct answer: D

Comments:

Although a definite causative relationship between bisphosphonates and ONJ has not yet been established, the circumstantial evidence is compelling, especially in cancer patients who receive larger doses of bisphosphonates.[2,5] Bisphosphonate therapy increases the risk of ONJ in a dose- and duration-dependent manner.[20,21] The mean time to developing ONJ in patients on denosumab is 23.83 ± 12.84 months.[1] For oral bisphosphonates that period is 21.9 months, and for zoledronic acid it is 33.8 months.[16] The incidence of ONJ among cancer patients prescribed intravenous bisphosphonates varies between 1% and 15%.[8,22] On the other hand, the risk in patients on bisphosphonates for osteoporosis varies between 1 in 10,000 and less than 1 per 100,000 patients.[1,8,15,23,24]

The increased risk of ONJ with bisphosphonates begins about 2 years after initiation of therapy and increases fourfold in the following 2 years.[15]

As bisphosphonates are not the only medications associated with an increased risk of ONJ, the American Association of Oral and Maxillofacial Surgeons adopted the term: MRONJ (Medication-Related Osteonecrosis of the Jaw).[2,25,26] The association of denosumab with ONJ suggests that ONJ is not a specific adverse event of bisphosphonates but of antiresorption therapy.[22,27–29]

As ONJ also may occur spontaneously, as in patients on placebo in clinical trials, antiresorptive therapy per se is therefore but one factor increasing the risk of ONJ. Glucocorticoids and cyclophosphamide also increase the risk of ONJ.[5,16,30,31]

6. ***Diseases increasing the risk of ONJ:***
   A. Neoplasia.
   B. Diabetes mellitus.
   C. Obesity.
   D. All of the above.
   E. A and B.

   Correct answer: D

   Comment:

   Many patients who develop ONJ have an underlying neoplastic condition treated with high doses of bisphosphonates. A number of other diseases also increase the risk of ONJ such as anemia, diabetes mellitus, hypertension, hypothyroidism, hypovitaminosis D, lupus erythematosus, malnutrition, obesity, pancreatitis, renal impairment, and renal dialysis.[16,19,31] Advanced age is another risk factor: it is estimated that the risk of ONJ is increased by about 10% for each decade.[16] Of interest, no case of ONJ has been reported in pediatric patients on iv bisphosphonates for osteogenesis imperfecta.[16]

7. ***The risk of ONJ may be reduced by:***
   A. Avoiding antiresorptive medication if the patient has evidence of gum disease.
   B. Educating the patient about ONJ and the importance of meticulous oral hygiene
   C. Anticipating dental interventions and, if possible, completing them prior to initiating antiresorptive therapy.
   D. B and C.
   E. A, B, and C.

   Correct answer: E

   Comment:

   All listed are useful measures to prevent ONJ.[5] Several preventive protocols have been developed to reduce the risk of ONJ and enhance its management.[32–34] Teriparatide has been shown to have a positive effect on MRONJ.[35] The sequential administration of antiresorptives: pamidronate/zoledronate and bisphosphonate/denosumab appears to increase the risk of MRONJ when compared to single **antiresorptive therapy**.[36]

   Thorough examination of the patient's gums prior to prescribing an antiresorptive medication is essential and can be done by the prescribing clinician. The need for good oral hygiene should be emphasized. If possible, dental procedures including tooth extraction should be performed and allowed to heal before prescribing antiresorptives.[37] For patients who are on antiresorptives and need to have a dental procedure done, it should be done by dental specialists with expertise in this area. Also, although there is no hard evidence, it is prudent to discontinue the antiresorptive therapy before the procedure and ideally until it heals. It is also important to ensure patients are vitamin D sufficient.

8. ***Long-term bisphosphonate therapy may increase the risk of ONJ by inhibiting:***
   A. Bone angiogenesis.

B. Osteoclastic activity.
C. Formation of new bone.
D. A and B.
E. A, B, and C.

Correct answer: E

Comment:

Several mechanisms explain the increased risk of ONJ in patients on long-term antiresorptive therapy including:

- The antiresorptive effect leads to reduced bone turnover, reduced bone formation, and suppression of bone turnover. As a result, microdamage, mature cross-links, and advanced glycation end products accumulate in the bone leading to an altered microarchitecture, impaired mechanical strength, and increased brittleness leading to microfractures and localized increased blood flow which attracts bisphosphonates, thus triggering a vicious cycle culminating in bone necrosis.
- The previously mentioned changes are possibly further aggravated by local inflammatory processes and associated pH changes which may trigger the release of bisphosphonates stored in the bones.[8]
- Bisphosphonates also have an antiangiogenic effect which is not limited to bone tissue but also affects endothelial cells.[20,38,39]
- Because of the jaw vascularity and exposure to repeated microtrauma, bisphosphonates are more concentrated in the jaw bones, especially when given parenterally in high doses.[20]
- Bisphosphonates also enhance the pathogenicity of periodontal bacteria through the promotion of interleukin-1-B.[40]
- There also may be a genetic susceptibility to developing ONJ with polymorphisms in cytochrome P450, CYP2C8 gene, or the farnesyl pyrophosphate synthase gene.[8,41]
- Vitamin D deficiency additionally may play a role in the development of ONJ: the resulting low serum calcium levels and elevated parathyroid hormone levels may trigger an immune response that leads to soft tissue destruction and interferes with bone healing.[42]

9. ***The management of ONJ includes:***

A. Scrupulous dental hygiene.
B. Frequent oral rinses with local antiseptic solution.
C. Surgical debridement/
D. A and B.
E. A, B, and C.

Correct answer: E

Comment:

In addition to discontinuing the antiresorptive medication, scrupulous dental hygiene, and frequent rinses with an oral antimicrobial solution such as chlorhexidine (0.15%), is recommended for all stages of ONJ. Long-term systemic antibiotics are recommended in ONJ stages II and III. Penicillin, quinolones, clindamycin, doxycycline, erythromycin, and metronidazole are good first choices. Microbial cultures and sensitivity tests should modulate the choice of antimicrobials. Analgesics are often required.

Debridement by clinicians experienced in ONJ is sometimes needed, and protocols for the surgical management of ONJ have been developed.[5,43] In stage III hyperbaric oxygen, medical ozone and resection of the affected area with reconstruction may be useful.[44,45]

10. ***Match the following:***
    (a) Inside-out theory.
    (b) Outside-in theory.
    (c) Both.
    (d) Neither.
    A. Infection starts in the oral mucosa and spreads to submucosa and bone.
    B. Process starts with bone necrosis and spreads to surrounding soft tissue.
    C. Supported by the microbiology of the oral cavity.
    D. Explains the increased risk among patients with neoplasia.
    E. Explains increased risk among cigarette smokers.

    Correct answers: A (b); B (a); C (a); D (c); E (b)

    Comment:

    Two main hypotheses have been put forward to explain the development of ONJ.[24] The outside-in hypothesis speculates that the oral mucosa sustains abrasions; infection sets in and gradually spreads to deeper tissue reaching the bones. Bisphosphonates also inhibit oral mucosal cell proliferation and healing.[46]

    The inside-out hypothesis speculates that the process is initiated in the bone as a direct result of antiresorptive therapy and then spreads to surrounding soft-tissues.[47] It is likely that the 2 mechanisms interact and potentiate each other leading to ONJ.

Case summary

Analysis of data

DD presents with a cavity where a tooth was extracted. She has been on oral bisphosphonates for about 12years and her present T-score is higher than −2.5. She has taken the medication as directed and now bone is visible at the bottom of the cavity. There is no evidence of inflammation. Her dentist states that the cavity has been evident for the past 4months. This is compatible with Stage I osteonecrosis of the jaw.

Diagnosis

- Osteonecrosis of the jaw, stage I, posttooth extraction.

Management recommendations

Treatment recommendation(s)

- Discontinue oral bisphosphonate.
- Given the degree of her bone demineralization, there is no need for any other medication for her low bone mass.
- Given the lack of inflammation or infection, there is no need for antibiotics or antiinflammatory medications.

Diagnostic test(s)

- None at this stage: there is no clinical evidence of inflammation, and her CBC is within normal limits.

Lifestyle

- Maintain scrupulous oral hygiene.
- Frequent mouth wash with oral antiseptics.
- Regular follow-up by dentist to ensure there is no inflammation/infection in the cavity.

DXA and radiological

- DXA scan in 2 years' time to monitor bone mass and fine-tune management strategy.

Key points

- ONJ is seen mostly in patients with neoplasia on bisphosphonates or denosumab. It also may occur spontaneously.
- The following stages are recognized: Stage I, II, III, and 0.
- Management varies according to the stage.

References

1. Khosla S, Burr D, Cauley J, et al. Bisphosphonate-associated osteonecrosis of the jaw: report of a task force of the American Society for Bone and Mineral Research. *J Bone Miner Res*. 2007;22(10):1479–1491.
2. Ruggiero SL, Dodson TB, Aghaloo LA, et al. American Association of Oral and Maxillofacial Surgeons' position paper on medication-related osteonecrosis of the jaws – 2022 update. *J Oral Maxillofacial Surg*. 2022;80:920–943.
3. Kawahara M, Kuroshima S, Sawase T. Clinical considerations for medication-related osteonecrosis of the jaw: a comprehensive literature review. *Int J Implant Dentis*. 2021;7:47.
4. Campisi G, Mauceri R, Bertoldo F, et al. Medication-related osteonecrosis of jaws (MRONJ) prevention and diagnosis: Italian consensus update 2020. *Int J Environ Res Public Health*. 2020;17:5998.
5. Ruggiero SL, Dodson TB, Assael LA, et al. American association of oral and maxillofacial surgeons position paper on bisphosphonate-related ONJ. *J Oral Maxillofacial Surg*. 2009;67(5 Suppl):2–12.

6. Mawardi HH, Treister NS, Woo SB. Bisphosphonate-associated osteonecrosis of the jaws. Primer of the Metabolic Bone Diseases and Disorders of Mineral Metabolism. 8th ed. John Wiley; 2013:929–940.
7. Woo SB, Hellstein JW, Kalmar JR. Systematic review: bisphosphonates and osteonecrosis of the jaws. *Ann Intern Med.* 2006;144(10):753–761.
8. Khan AA, Morrison A, Kendler DL, et al. Case-based review of osteonecrosis of the jaw and application of the international recommendations for management from the international task force on ONJ. *J Clin Densitom.* 2017;20(1):8–24.
9. Baim S, Miller PD. Assessing the clinical utility of serum CTX in postmenopausal women and its use in predicting ONJ. *J Bone Miner Res.* 2009;24(4):561–574.
10. Morris PG, Fazio M, Farooki A, et al. Serum N-telopeptide and bone-specific alkaline phosphatase levels in patients with ONJ receiving bisphosphonates for bone metastases. *J Oral Maxillofac Surg.* 2012;70 (12):2768–2775.
11. Shudo A, Kishimoto H, Takaoka K, Noguchi K. Long-term oral bisphosphonates delay healing after tooth extraction: a single institutional prospective study. *Osteoporos Int.* 2018;29(10):2315–2321. https://doi.org/10.1007/s00198-018-4621-7.
12. Jung S, Han S, Kwon H-Y. Dose-intensity of bisphosphonates and the risk of osteonecrosis of the jaw in osteoporosis patients. *Front Pharmacol.* 2018;9:796.
13. Chtioui H, Lamine F, Daghfous R. Teriparatide for ONJ. *N Engl J Med.* 2011;364(11):1081–1082.
14. George EL, Yi-Ling L, Saunders MM. Bisphosphonate related osteonecrosis of the jaw a mechanobiology perspective. *Bone Rep.* 2018;8:104–109.
15. Barasch A, Cunha-Cruz J, Curro FA, et al. Risk factors for osteonecrosis of the jaws: a case-control study from the CONDOR dental PBRN. *Tex Dent J.* 2013;130(4):299–307.
16. Palaska PK, Cartsos V, Zavras AI. Bisphosophonates and time to osteonecrosis development. *Oncologist.* 2009;14:1154–1166.
17. Vahtsevanos K, Kyrgidis A, Verrou E, et al. Longitudinal cohort study of risk factors in cancer patients of bisphosphonate-related ONJ. *J Clin Oncol.* 2009;27(32):5356–5362.
18. Edwards BJ, Hellstein JW, Jacobsen PL, et al. Updated recommendations for managing the care of patients receiving oral bisphosphonate therapy. *JADA.* 2008;139(12):1674–1677.
19. Wessel JH, Dodson TB, Zavras AI. Zoledronate, smoking and obesity are strong risk factors for ONJ. *J Oral Maxillofac Surg.* 2008;66(4):625–631.
20. Marx RE, Sawatari Y, Fortin M, Broumand V. Bisphoshonate-induced exposed bone of the jaws. *J Oral Maxillofac Surg.* 2005;63:1567–1575.
21. Khan AA, Sandor GK, Dore E, et al. Bisphosphonate ONJ. *J Rheumatol.* 2009;36(3):478–490.
22. Tofe VI, Bagan L, Bagan JV. Osteonecrosis of the jaws associated with denosumab: study of clinical and radiographic characteristics in a series of clinical cases. *J Clin Exp Dent.* 2020;12(7):e676–e681.
23. Compston J. Pathophysiology of atypical femoral shaft fractures and ONJ. *Osteoporos Int.* 2011;22 (12):2951–2961.
24. American Dental Association Council on Scientific Affairs. Dental management of patients receiving oral bisphosphonate therapy: expert panel recommendations. *J Am Dent Assoc.* 2006;137(8):1144–1150.
25. Ruggiero SL, Dodson TB, Fantasia J, et al. American association of oral and maxillofacial surgeons position paper on medication-related osteonecrosis of the jaw – 2014 update. *J Oral Maxillofac Surg.* 2014;72:1938–1956.
26. Bisphosphonate-Related Osteonecrosis of the Jaw. A mechanobiology perspective. *Bone Rep.* 2018;8:104–109.
27. Pendrys DG, Silverman SL. ONJ and bisphosphonates. *Curr Osteoporos Rep.* 2008;6(1):31–38.
28. Aljohani S, Gaudin R, Weiser J, et al. Ostenecrosis of the jaw in patients treated with denosumab: a multicenter series. *J Craniomaxillofac Surg.* 2018;1–11.
29. Voss PJ, Steybe D, Poxleitner P, et al. Osteonecrosis of the jaw in patients transitioning from bisphosphonates to denosumab treatment for osteoporosis. *Odontology.* 2018;106(4):469–480. https://doi.org/10.1007/s10266-018-0362-5.

30. Troeltzsch M, Woodlock T, Krielstein S, et al. Physiology and pharmacology of non-bisphosphonate drugs implicated in osteonecrosis of the jaw. *J Can Dent Assoc*. 2012;78:85–92.
31. Shannon J, Shannon J, Modelevsky S, et al. Bisphosphonates and ONJ. *J Am Geriatr Soc*. 2011;59 (12):2350–2355.
32. Romero-Ruiz MM, Romero-Serrano M, Serrano-Gonzalez A, Serrera-Figallo MA, Gutierrez-Perez JL, Torres-Lagares D. Proposal for a preventive protocol for medication-related osteonecrosis of the jaw. *Med Oral Patol Oral Cir Bucal*. 2021;26(3):e314–e326.
33. Varoni EM, Lombardi N, Villa G, Pispero A, Sardella A, Lodi G. Conservative management of medication-related osteonecrosis of the jaws (MRONJ): a retrospective cohort study. *Antibiotics*. 2021;10:195.
34. Drudge-Coates L, den Wyngaert TV, Schiodt M, van Muilekom HAM, Demnty G, Sven O. Preventing, identifying, and managing medication-related osteonecrosis of the jaw: a practical guide for nurses and other allied healthcare professionals. *Support Care Cancer*. 2020;28:4019–4029.
35. On SW, Cho SW, Byun SH, Yang BE. Various therapeutic methods for the treatment of medication-related osteonecrosis of the jaw (MRONJ) and their limitations. *Antioxidants*. 2021;10:680.
36. Srivastava A, Gonzales GMN, Geng Y, et al. Prevalence of medication related osteonecrosis of the jaw in patients treated with sequential antiresorptive drugs: systematic review and meta-analysis. *Support Care Cancer*. 2021;29:2305–2317.
37. Facon T, Bensadoun RJ, Blanc JL, et al. ONJ and bisphosphonates in oncology. *Bull Cancer*. 2008;95 (4):413–418.
38. Purcell PM, Boyd IW. Bisphosphonates and ONJ. *Med J Aust*. 2005;182:417–418.
39. Allegra A, Oteri G, Nastro E, et al. Patients with bisphosphonates-associated ONJ have reduced circulating endothelial cells. *Hematol Oncol*. 2007;25:164–169.
40. Deng X, Tamai R, Endo Y, et al. Alendronate augments interleukin-1-B release from macrophages infected with periodontal pathogenic bacteria through activation of caspase-1. *Toxicol Appl Pharmacol*. 2009;235:97–104.
41. Marini F, Tonelli P, Cavalli L, et al. Pharmacogenetics of bisphosphonate-associated osteonecrosis of the jaw. *Front Biosci*. 2011;3:364–370.
42. Chen L, Cencioni MT, Angelini DF, et al. Transcriptional profiling of gamma delta T cells identifies a role for vitamin D in the immunoregulation of the V Gamma9v Delta 2 response to phosphate-containing ligands. *J Immunol*. 2005;25:164–169.
43. Hauer L, Jabra J, Hrusak D, et al. Surgical therapy for medication-related osteonecrosis of the jaw in osteoporotic patients treated with anti-resorptive agents. *Biomed Pap Med Fac Univ Palacky Olomouc Czech Repub*. 2019;163:1–8.
44. Ripamonti CI, Cislaghi E, Mariani L, et al. Efficacy and safety of medical ozone delivered in oil suspension applications for the treatment of ONJ in patients with bone metastases treated with bisphosphonates. *Oral Oncol*. 2011;47(3):185–190.
45. Wutzl A, Pohl S, Sulzbacher I, et al. Factors influencing surgical treatment of bisphosphonate-related ONJ. *Head Neck*. 2012;34(2):194–200.
46. Landersberg R, Cozin M, Cremers S, et al. Inhibition of oral mucosal cell wound healing by bisphosphonates. *J Oral Maxillofac Surg*. 2008;66(5):839–847.
47. Otto S, Schreyer C, Hafner S, et al. Bisphosphonate-related ONJ. *J Craniomaxillofac Surg*. 2012;40 (4):303–309.

Drug holidays

Learning objectives

- "Drug holidays" refer to the discontinuation—temporary or permanent—of bisphosphonate therapy following a 3- to 5-year period of continuous therapy whether oral or IV.
- Determine whether to continue or discontinue long-term antiresorptive therapy.

Analysis of data

The efficacy of drug holidays is questionable. Rebound increase in bone turnover is sometimes seen. Patients on drug holidays should be monitored.

Multiple choice questions

1. ***The following is/are true about "drug holidays" in the management of osteoporosis:***
   A. They only apply to bisphosphonates.
   B. They apply to any medication used to treat osteoporosis.
   C. They do not apply to intravenously administered bisphosphonates.
   D. Patients should be closely monitored: three monthly DXA scans and monthly bone markers.
   E. A and D.

   Correct answer: A

   Comment:

   Bisphosphonates are effective medications for the management of osteoporosis. They have been repeatedly shown to increase the bone density and significantly reduce the fracture risk, including the much-dreaded hip fractures, which can be reduced by as much as 50% after a three-year period of continuous bisphosphonate administration.[1,2] With few exceptions, for the first 3–5 years of their administration, bisphosphonates are not associated with severe adverse effects apart from upper gastrointestinal adverse effects which, in most instances, can be easily managed. Furthermore, intravenously administered bisphosphonates such as zoledronic acid bypass the GI tract and eliminate the risk of upper GI adverse effects.

Diagnosis and Treatment of Osteoporosis. https://doi.org/10.1016/B978-0-323-99550-4.00014-9
Copyright © 2024 Elsevier Inc. All rights are reserved, including those for text and data mining, AI training, and similar technologies.

2. ***The following is/are true about drug holidays programs:***
   - A. The patient can take the orally administered medication with breakfast.
   - B. The patient can take the orally administered medication with any other medication.
   - C. The main purpose of the drug holidays program is to reduce the cost of treatment.
   - D. All of the above.
   - E. None of the above.

   Correct answer: E

   Comment:

   "Drug holidays" refer to the discontinuation, temporary or permanent, of bisphosphonate therapy following a three- to five-year period of continuous daily, weekly, or annual iv infusion therapy.[3] The rationale for this strategy is twofold: first, the assumption that benefits gained while the bisphosphonate was administered will persist after the medication has been stopped and second to reduce the risk of serious adverse effects of long-term bisphosphonate therapy such as atypical femoral fractures and osteonecrosis of the jaw. "Drug holidays" should only apply to bisphosphonates and not denosumab because the discontinuation of denosumab may be associated with multiple vertebral compression and other fractures.

3. ***The following is/are true about "Drug holidays":***
   - A. The BMD is maintained for at least the first 3 years of the "drug holiday."
   - B. The fracture risk remains at the preholiday level for at least 3 years.
   - C. They are associated with a decrease in BMD.
   - D. The fracture risk increases when the "drug holiday" starts.
   - E. C and D.

   Correct answer: E

   Comment:

   The long-term extension studies of alendronate (FIT/FLEX study) and zoledronic acid (HORIZON study) suggest that cessation of bisphosphonate administration (i.e., a "drug holiday") after completing a three- to five-year course of orally administered bisphosphonate or three-year course of zoledronic acid is associated with a decrease in BMD and an increased fracture risk during the no treatment phase of the study: vertebral fractures were about 50% higher in those who discontinued the bisphosphonate compared to those who continued with the medication. There was, however, no increase in nonvertebral or hip fracture, probably due to the studies not being powered to assess changes in fractures. Similar results were observed after examining longitudinal data from the Kaiser Permanente and data from Medicare.[3] It is also possible that had the duration of no bisphosphonate administration been shorter, i.e., about a year, the results would be different.

4. ***The following is/are correct:***
   - A. Bisphosphonates have a strong affinity to bone mineral hydroxyapatite in the bones.
   - B. They gradually dissociate themselves from hydroxyapatite and enter the activated osteoclasts.

C. In the osteoclasts they induce cellular apoptosis, mostly by inhibiting the farnesyl pyrophosphate enzyme and preventing essential protein synthesis.
D. All of the above.
E. None of the above.

Correct answer: D

Comment:

As the bisphosphonates slowly dissociate themselves from the hydroxyapatite crystals they continue to suppress bone turnover long after their intake is discontinued. In many instances, the fracture risk does not return to its original high level long after it has been discontinued. As such, therefore, bisphosphonates are ideal candidates for drug holidays, especially for patients with low to moderate risk of fracture. A popular regimen is 3–5 years of therapy followed by 2–3 years of "drug holiday," i.e., no medication. Patients at high risk of fracture may benefit from switching to another medication for osteoporosis.[4] Drug holidays are not recommended for patients on denosumab as its antifracture effect is short-lived and there may be a rebound increased fracture risk, especially vertebral fractures soon after discontinuing denosumab.

5. ***The main adverse effects of long-term bisphosphonate use include:***
A. Osteonecrosis of the jaw.
B. Atypical femoral fracture.
C. Oral mucosal ulceration.
D. Orbital inflammation.
E. All of the above.

Correct answer: E

Comment:

Ocular inflammation is a rare adverse effect in patients taking bisphosphonates. It usually presents with ocular and periocular pain, swelling, blurry vision, and photophobia. Whereas nonspecific conjunctivitis is usually benign, self-limited, and improves without specific therapy, uveitis and scleritis are serious complications, often preceded by chills, fever, fatigue, and malaise. It usually responds to high doses corticosteroid therapy.[5,6]
A case of severe oral mucosal ulceration associated with oral bisphosphonate use has been described: the patient stated that she was told she should keep the tablet in her mouth to be dissolved by saliva, then to sit upright for 45 min and then to drink water. After the first dose, she experienced sudden onset of gum pain associated with food intake and noticed a superficial ulcer about 1 cm on the hard palate. After the second dose the size of the ulcer had increased and she found it difficult to take any food. The ulcer extended to the upper gum. The ulceration progressed rapidly and involved the tongue and inside of the left lip. She responded well to prednisolone, antiseptic mouth rinse, and antiseptic gel. This case emphasizes the importance of giving clear instructions on how to take the oral bisphosphonate.[7]

Osteonecrosis of the jaw and atypical femoral fractures are discussed in separate chapters in this book.

6. ***The affinity of bisphosphonates for hydroxyapatite, in descending ranking:***
   A. Zoledronate, alendronate, ibandronate, risedronate, and etidronate.
   B. Alendronate, zoledronate, risedronate, ibandronate, and etidronate.
   C. Ibandronate, zoledronate, alendronate, risedronate, and etidronate.
   D. Etidronate, zoledronate, alendronate, risedronate, ibandronate.
   E. The affinity of a bisphosphonate to hydroxyapatite is essentially the same for all bisphosphonates.

   Correct answer: A

   Comment:

   The potency and affinity of the various bisphosphonates determine the duration between cycles of bisphosphonates and no medication.
7. ***The following is/are true about the "drug holidays" program:***
   A. The patient can take the orally administered medication with breakfast.
   B. The patient can take the orally administered medication with any other medication.
   C. The main purpose of the drug holidays program is to reduce the cost of treatment.
   D. All of the above.
   E. None of the above.

   Correct answer: E

   Comment:

   Drug holidays refer to the discontinuation, temporary or permanent, of bisphosphonate therapy following a three- to five-year period of continuous daily, weekly, or annual iv infusion therapy.[3] The rationale for this strategy is twofold: first, the assumption that benefits gained while the bisphosphonate was administered will persist after the medication has been stopped and second to reduce the risk of serious adverse effects of long-term bisphosphonate therapy such as atypical femoral fractures and osteonecrosis of the jaw. Drug holidays should only apply to bisphosphonates and not denosumab because the discontinuation of denosumab may be associated with multiple vertebral compression fractures.

Key points

- The benefits gained while the bisphosphonate was administered will persist after the medication has been stopped.
- Continuing antiresorptive therapy for more than 5 years increases the risk of rare complications such as osteonecrosis of the jaw and atypical femoral shaft fractures.
- "Drug holidays" should be considered after 5 years of completed antiresorptive medication. Caution, however, should be exercised with denosumab as its cessation may lead to a rebound increase in bone resorption and risk of fragility fractures, especially multiple vertebral fractures.

References

1. Black D, Cummings SR, Karpf DB, et al. Randomized trial of effect of alendronate on risk of fracture in women with existing vertebral fractures. Fracture Intervention Trial Research Group. *Lancet.* 1996;348:1535–1541.
2. Cummings SR, Black DM, Thompson DE, et al. Effect of alendronate on risk of fracture in women with low bone density but without vertebral fractures: results from the fracture intervention trial. *JAMA.* 1998;280:2077–2082.
3. Bauer DC, Abrahamsen B. Bisphosphonate drug holidays in primary care: when and what to do next? *Curr Osteoporos Rep.* 2021;19:182–188.
4. Hayes KN, Winter EM, Cadarette SM. Duration of bisphosphonate drug holidays in osteoporosis patients: a narrative review of the evidence and considerations for decision-making. *J Clin Med.* 2021;10:1140.
5. Rahimy E, Law SH. Orbital inflammation after zoledronate infusion: an emerging complication. *Can J Ophthalmol.* 2013;48(1):2013–2014.
6. Hamdy RC. Zoledronic acid: clinical utility and paytiet considerations in osteoporosis and low bone mass. *Drug Dsesign Dev Therapy.* 2010;4:321–335.
7. Chandran M, Zeng W. Severe oral mucosal ulceration associated with oral bisphosphonate use: the importance of imparting proper instructions on medication administration and intake. *Case Rep Med.* 2021;2021:6620489. https://doi.org/10.1155/2021/6620489.

SECTION 3

Select populations

CHAPTER 23

Osteoporosis in men☆

Learning objectives

Osteoporosis in men, as in women, is asymptomatic until a fracture occurs. It is very often underrecognized, underdiagnosed, and undertreated.

Osteoporosis is less frequent in men than in women, but its mortality and morbidity impact is worse in men.

- In men, osteoporosis tends to manifest itself about a decade later than women.
- As in women, once an osteoporotic fracture is sustained, the risk of sustaining further fractures is increased.
- With the exception of testosterone and estrogen, essentially the same medications used to treat osteoporosis in women can be used to treat men.
- In men, as in women, for best results, the pharmacologic management should be complemented by lifestyle changes and an adequate diet.

The case study

Reasons for seeking medical help

- JB, 71 years old, watched a documentary on falls and fractures in older people and is concerned he may have osteoporosis.
- He is asymptomatic; cognitively intact; physically independent; lives on his own; drives his own car; travels extensively; and denies dizzy spells, falls, or near-falls.

Past medical/surgical history

- Hyperlipidemia, well controlled.

Personal habits, lifestyle, daily routine

- JB is a retired school teacher but continues to be involved teaching English literature.
- He lives on his own and leads a sedentary lifestyle.

☆ JB, 71 years old, asymptomatic, enquiring about a DXA scan after watching a TV documentary on osteoporosis.

Diagnosis and Treatment of Osteoporosis. https://doi.org/10.1016/B978-0-323-99550-4.00008-3
Copyright © 2024 Elsevier Inc. All rights are reserved, including those for text and data mining, AI training, and similar technologies.

- Average daily caffeine intake: four cups, about 16 oz each cup.
- Daily calcium intake: average 1000 mg.
- Alcohol intake: at least two drinks every day, usually more during the weekend.
- Cigarette smoking: about 10 cigarettes a day, used to smoke more, plans to stop it altogether.
- Enjoys pickles, crisps, and salty food.

Medications

- Simvastatin 40 mg daily.
- Multivitamin tablets once a day.
- Over-the-counter sleep aids: on an as needed basis, not exceeding one tablet a week.

Family history

- Negative for osteoporosis.

Clinical examination

- Weight 186 pounds, steady, height 62.75″, used to be 66.5″.
- Mild kyphosis.
- No clinical signs suggesting an increased falls and fracture risk:
  - Sitting BP 136/85, standing BP 142/86, no orthostasis.
  - No clinical evidence of carotid stenosis, carotid sinus sensitivity, vertebrobasilar insufficiency.
  - No clinical evidence of fluid retention, heart failure, or pulmonary congestion.
  - No localizing neurological signs.
- No other significant clinical findings.

Laboratory investigations

- Comprehensive metabolic profile: no abnormal finding.
- Serum 25-hydroxy-vitamin D: 42 ng/mL.

DXA scan results

- **T-scores:** right femoral neck: −1.9, right total hip: −1.4, distal 1/3 radius: −1.3; L1–L4: cannot be reliably interpreted because of osteophytes.
  Vertebral fracture assessment: moderate wedge compression fractures of T7 (29.2%) and T8 (26.6%). He denies any history of back trauma or injury or pain.
- **FRAX score** (with BMD): hip fracture: 3.7%; major osteoporotic fractures: 22%.

Multiple choice questions

1. ***In JB's case the final diagnosis is:***
   A. Osteoporosis.
   B. Osteopenia.
   C. Morphometric vertebral compression fractures.
   D. A and C.
   E. B and C.
   Correct answer: D
   Comments:
   As mentioned earlier, osteoporosis in men is silent until a fracture occurs. It is underdiagnosed, undertreated, and associated with a worse prognosis than in women. Also, when compared to women, more men have secondary osteoporosis. A detailed medical history, thorough clinical examination, and laboratory profile are therefore recommended prior to initiating therapy.[1] As in women, the presence of vertebral compression fractures in the absence of significant trauma is, per se, characteristic of fragility fractures and establishes the diagnosis of osteoporosis, even if the BMD is not within the osteoporotic range.
   The indications for initiating pharmacologic treatment in men are the same as in women based on the following[2–4]:
   - **Clinical diagnosis:** the presence of fragility fracture(s), including morphometric (i.e. silent), vertebral compression fractures.
   - **Densitometric diagnosis**: lowest T-score in femoral neck, total hip, lumbar vertebrae, or distal 1/3 radius: −2.5 or lower.
   - **Increased fracture risk:** estimated by the 10-year probability of sustaining a hip fracture of 3% or more, or a major osteoporotic fracture of 20% or more, as determined by the FRAX algorithm and the threshold suggested by the National Osteoporosis Foundation.
2. ***At this stage, in JB's case, the following serum assays are recommended:***
   A. Parathyroid hormone.
   B. 1,25-Di-hydroxy-vitamin D.
   C. Testosterone.
   D. Estradiol.
   E. None of the above.
   Correct answer: E
   Comment:
   None of these tests are necessary at this stage. Unless secondary hyperparathyroidism is suspected, there is no need to assay the serum parathyroid hormone level because the serum calcium level is within the normal range. Similarly, there is no need to assay the serum 1,25-di-hydroxy-vitamin D because it only reflects the ability of the parathyroid

hormone to hydroxylate, in the kidneys, 25-hydroxy-vitamin D at the 1-position to produce 1,25-di-hydroxy-vitamin D which is the most active vitamin D metabolite produced when the serum calcium is about to fall. 1,25-di-hydroxy-vitamin D does not accurately reflect the overall vitamin D status and has a short half-life.

The preferred assay to determine vitamin D status is the 25-hydroxy-vitamin D assay, which includes 25-hydroxy-cholecalciferol and 25-hydroxy-ergocalciferol. The former is the result of the action of UV violet light, including sunlight, on the skin, and the intake of food rich in vitamin D: cholecalciferol or ergocalciferol. The latter (ergocalciferol) is derived from plants. Both cholecalciferol and ergocalciferol are metabolized through the same pathways.

Whether or not to routinely assay the serum testosterone level is debatable. It is likely to be low because of the expected age-related hypogonadism: andropause, similar to the menopause in women, albeit occurring about a decade or more, later than in women. Confirmation of low testosterone levels also will not affect the osteoporosis treatment strategy, because other medications, apart from testosterone, are effective at increasing bone mass and reducing the risk of fractures in men.

Furthermore, the administration of testosterone is associated with a number of adverse effects, including polycythemia, sleep apnea, benign prostate hypertrophy, and unmasking of prostate cancer. These adverse reactions outweigh the potential benefits of testosterone if used for the management of osteoporosis.

There is also a paucity of studies on the effects of testosterone in the management of osteoporosis in men with fractures as an end point.[5] In one placebo-controlled, double-blind study, the investigators randomly allocated 295 men, 65 years of age and older, with hypogonadism, as evidenced by two morning serum testosterone levels averaging less than 275 ng/dL, to either a testosterone gel or a placebo. One hundred and eighty-nine participants completed the one-year study.

At the end of this period, men allocated to receive testosterone gel, compared to those receiving placebo, showed significantly greater increases in mean spine trabecular, spine peripheral, hip trabecular, and peripheral volumetric BMD (vBMD) as determined by quantitative computed tomography. These increases were paralleled by increases in the mean estimated strength, as determined by finite element analysis of quantitative computed tomography at these bone sites, were more pronounced in trabecular than peripheral bone, and more in the spine than in the hip. As expected, the median serum concentrations of total testosterone, free testosterone, and estradiol increased in the testosterone gel group to within the normal ranges for young men. Changes in aerial BMD (aBMD) as assessed by bone densitometry (DXA) were much less than those seen by vBMD.[6] At present, these results must be tempered by the relative lack of long-term studies and the potential adverse effects associated with testosterone therapy in older men.

The serum estradiol level and sex hormone binding globulin (SHBG) are major factors affecting bone loss in older men. It has been suggested that whereas estrogen reduces the fracture risk by direct effects on bones, androgens in addition affect muscle bulk and may reduce the risk of falls and hence fractures.[7,8] The Endocrine Society Clinical Practice Guidelines emphasize that the diagnosis of hypogonadism be made only in men with symptoms and signs of testosterone deficiency and unequivocally and consistently low serum testosterone levels.[9]

3. ***In JB's case, the following medications are recommended as a first choice:***
   A. Bisphosphonates, teriparatide, abaloparatide, denosumab, romosozumab, raloxifene, or calcitonin.
   B. Bisphosphonates, teriparatide, abaloparatide, denosumab, or romosozumab.
   C. Bisphosphonates, teriparatide, abaloparatide, or denosumab.
   D. Bisphosphonates or denosumab.
   E. Bisphosphonates.

   Correct answer: D

   Comments:

   Most studies on the treatment of osteoporosis in men are much smaller than those conducted on postmenopausal women and with few exceptions, most do not have fractures as an end point. It is assumed that if the changes in BMD and bone turnover rates are similar to those observed in women then the effect on fracture risk is similar.[2] Therefore, as in this patient the hip fracture risk is elevated, medications that have been shown to effectively reduce the risk of hip fractures should be the first choice. Neither raloxifene nor calcitonin has been shown to be effective at reducing the risk of hip fractures.

   Teriparatide, abaloparatide, and romosozumab are osteoanabolic agents and have been shown to reduce the risk of fractures, including hip fractures. They are, however, not often used as first line of therapy for the management of osteoporosis because of their need to be administered parenterally and their cost. Up till recently the administration of teriparatide and abaloparatide was limited to 2 years because there was uncertainty about its possible carcinogenicity, as per findings of a study conducted on experimental rats. That restriction of 2 years for both teriparatide and abaloparatide has now been lifted. These medications are discussed in other sections.

   Bisphosphonates and denosumab have been shown to be effective in the management of osteoporosis in men either as monotherapy, consolidative therapy after a course of teriparatide/abaloparatide, or in combination with testosterone replacement therapy in men with osteoporosis secondary to hypogonadism.[10,11]

4. ***The following are also recommended in this patient:***
   A. Reducing the sodium and caffeine intake.
   B. Calcium and vitamin supplementation.
   C. Stop cigarette smoking.
   D. A, B, and C.
   E. A and C.

   Correct answer: E

Comments:

Reducing sodium and caffeine intake is important as both increase the renal calcium excretion and may induce a negative calcium balance resulting in secondary hyperparathyroidism and bone demineralization. Stopping cigarette smoking is an important integral part of the management of patients with osteoporosis. Cigarette smoking predisposes to osteoporosis and increases the risk of fractures in men more than in women.[12] The detrimental effect of cigarette smoking on bone mass during the growth period cannot be reversed once peak bone mass is reached.[13] There is no need to supplement the calcium and vitamin D intake as JB is already getting an adequate amount of calcium through food, and his serum 25-hydroxy-vitamin D level is within the normal range.

5. ***The following lifestyle and medication changes are recommended in JB:***
   A. Undertake regular weight-bearing physical exercise.
   B. Reduce alcohol consumption to no more than 2 drinks a day.
   C. Reduce and preferably discontinue use of over-the-counter sleep aids.
   D. B and C.
   E. A, B, and C.

Correct answer: E

Comment:

All the listed modalities are important in JB's case. There is, however, a paucity of well-designed and well-conducted long-term studies on the effects of physical exercise and lack of physical exercise on bone mass and fracture risk in older subjects. Nevertheless, given the available evidence, it seems reasonable to assume that physical exercise, especially weight-bearing exercises, may help improve bone mineral density, muscle bulk, postural reflexes, and reduce the risk of falls and fractures. The US Endocrine Society recommends weight-bearing activities for 30–40 min three to four times a week.[2] Lifting free weights, however, has a potential for physical injury. Similarly, high-resistance exercises may detrimentally affect neighboring joints especially in patients with arthropathies. Intuitively, supervised physical exercise programs should yield better results than nonsupervised ones, as it is possible to target and fine-tune exercise programs geared to the individual circumstances and needs of the patient.

Excessive alcohol intake is associated with bone demineralization, falls, and fractures.[14] With an alcohol consumption of more than 3 units a day, the relative hazard of hip fracture is almost double (RH 1.92, 95% CI 1.28–2.88) and for all fractures is 1.32 (95% CI 1.10–1.60).[2] Often, however, self-reported alcohol usage underestimates the true alcohol consumption.

Hypnotics, especially sleep aids available over the counter, increase the risk of unsteadiness, confusion, falls, and fractures and their effect is potentiated by the consumption of alcoholic beverages.

6. ***The following is/are true:***
   A. About a third of hip fractures occur in men.
   B. Posthip fracture mortality in men is much higher than in women.
   C. Most men who sustain fragility fracture also have a densitometric diagnosis of osteoporosis.
   D. A and B.
   E. A, B, and C.

Correct answer: D

Comment:

Osteoporosis in men remains underrecognized, underdiagnosed, and undertreated.[4,10,15–17] About a quarter of hip fractures occur in men.[18] The risk of sustaining a fragility fracture for men aged 50 and older is 13%–30%. Fragility fractures are, nevertheless, less frequent in men than in women for a variety of reasons, including that men tend to have larger bones than women, fall less frequently than women, and their life expectancy is shorter than in women. Notwithstanding, subsequent to a fragility hip fracture, mortality is two to three times higher in men than in women.[19]

Only about 20% of men who sustain a fragility hip or major osteoporotic fracture have a densitometric diagnosis of osteoporosis.[20] This could be due to changes in bone microarchitecture and increased cortical porosity which are not captured by DXA scans, hence the need for an assessment of the patient's fracture risk.[20]

There is also some controversy concerning the reference population used for the densitometric diagnosis of osteoporosis in men.[17] Whereas the International Osteoporosis Foundation recommends using a Caucasian female reference population to calculate the T-scores, the National Osteoporosis Foundation recommends a male reference population be used for this purpose and the International Society for Clinical Densitometry leaves it to the individual center to decide which reference population to use.[21]

The justification of using a female Caucasian reference population is that the risk of fracture is dependent on the bone's absolute BMD regardless of the patient's gender and ethnic group. This, nevertheless, may create problems when interpreting follow-up DXA scans done in different centers without knowing which reference population has been used to calculate the T-scores.

It also has important implications: if a female reference population is used to calculate the T-scores of a male patient, fewer patients will be diagnosed and hence treated for osteoporosis. On the other hand if a male reference population is used, more patients will be diagnosed with osteoporosis and may be unnecessarily treated.[21]

7. ***Men over the age of 50 years should be screened for osteoporosis if:***
   A. They have sustained a fragility fracture.
   B. They had a delayed puberty.
   C. They have evidence of hypogonadism.

D. B or C.

E. A, B, or C.

Correct answer: E

Comment:

It is estimated that one-third of fragility fractures occur in men and 20% of patients with osteoporosis or low bone mass are men.[22]

In men, as in women, a fragility fracture is diagnostic of osteoporosis. Therefore, although there is no need to screen these patients to diagnose osteoporosis, a DXA scan is still needed, not for diagnostic purposes, but to establish a baseline against which the patient's progress or lack thereof can be monitored.

Following a hip fracture, the mortality, morbidity, and loss of independence are more pronounced in men than in women.[17,23–25] Factors increasing the risk of sustaining a fall complicated by a hip or other bone fracture include: age: 70 years and older, low body weight, excessive alcohol consumption, impaired visual acuity, frailty, inability to perform daily activities, and low BMD.[2,26]

Repeated falls and fractures are also more likely to occur in patients who smoke cigarettes, have already sustained a fracture, experience falls or near-falls, have cataracts, impaired vision, cognitive impairment, or have been diagnosed with a number of medical conditions, including arrhythmias (especially atrial fibrillation, bradycardia, tachycardia, and tachy-bradycardia), hypertension, orthostatic hypotension, congestive cardiac failure, chronic obstructive pulmonary disease, diabetes mellitus, hypo/hyperthyroidism, myocardial infarction, Parkinson's disease, peripheral neuropathy, rheumatoid arthritis, strokes, and transient ischemic attacks. Reduced physical activity also increases the risk of sustaining a hip fracture by inducing muscle atrophy and sarcopenia.

A number of medications may predispose to falls and fractures, including benzodiazepines, antidepressants, anticonvulsants, psychotropics, beta-blockers, hypotensives, and hypnotics, including those available over the counter as they are likely to induce drowsiness, interfere with cognitive functions, and tend to have a long half-life.

The consensus is to screen men aged 70 years and older regardless of whether or not they have risk factors for osteoporosis and to screen men 50 years and older if they have risk factors for osteoporosis, including delayed puberty, hypogonadism, and hyperthyroidism.[2] Similarly, it is relevant to screen for osteoporosis in men taking medication that may increase the risk of falling as well as those whose lifestyle predisposes to bone demineralization such as cigarette smoking, sedentary lifestyles, and excessive sodium and caffeine intake.

Given the prevalence of osteoporosis in men, its prognosis, and silent nature until a fracture occurs, it has been suggested that screening for osteoporosis in men start at a younger age: 60 instead of 70 years.[27]

8. ***When assessing falls and fracture risks in men:***

A. A thorough clinical examination is essential to identify the cause(s) of repeated falls.

B. The Fracture Risk Assessment algorithm (FRAX) algorithm cannot be used in men.
C. The Garvan Fracture Risk Calculator cannot be used in men.
D. A and B.
E. A, B, and C.

Correct answer: A

Comment:

Assessing fracture risk is important to develop a comprehensive management strategy tailored to the individual circumstances of the patient which includes nonpharmacologic modalities and lifestyle modifications. Both the FRAX tool and the Garvan Fracture Risk Calculator can be used in men, although it has been suggested that FRAX underestimates the fracture risk in men.[28] The FRAX score, calculated without BMD, does not correctly identify men with densitometric evidence of osteoporosis.[29]

9. ***In aging men:***

A. Free estrogen rather than free testosterone levels correlates best with the BMD.
B. Sex Hormone Binding Globulin (SHBG) levels increase.
C. Free testosterone levels decrease.
D. B and C.
E. A, B, and C.

Correct answer: E

Comment:

In aging men, the decreases of serum testosterone (and estrogen) levels are more gradual and due to a more than twofold increase in Sex Hormone Binding Globulin which reduces the bioavailability of free testosterone and estrogen in older men by 64% and 47%, respectively.[30,31] In men, free estrogen rather than free testosterone levels correlates best with the BMD.[32] Testosterone also may reduce the fracture risk through its positive effect on balance, muscle bulk, and strength.[33]

10. ***In men with prostate cancer on androgen deprivation therapy:***

A. Lumbar vertebrae BMD decreases by about 4% in the first year of therapy.
B. Hip BMD decreases by about 6% in the first year of therapy.
C. Fracture risk is increased.
D. A and C.
E. A, B, and C.

Correct answer: D

Comment:

Decreases of 3%–4% in lumbar vertebrae BMD have been reported during the first year of androgen deprivation therapy in men with prostate cancer. The decreases in hip BMD are less pronounced, but the fracture risk is increased in this population.[34,35] Several medications have been shown to be effective to reduce bone loss in men on androgen deprivation therapy, including alendronate, zoledronic acid, pamidronate, denosumab, and raloxifene.[2] Over a 36-month period denosumab decreased the risk of vertebral fractures by 62% in men on androgen deprivation therapy.[36]

Case summary

Analysis of data

Factors predisposing to bone demineralization/osteoporosis

- Patient's age: 71 years.
- Sedentary lifestyle.
- High caffeine intake.
- Excessive alcohol intake.
- Cigarette smoking.
- High sodium intake (pickles, crisps, and salty food).

Factors reducing the risk of bone demineralization/osteoporosis

- Negative family history for osteoporosis.
- Good intake of vitamin D and calcium.

Factors increasing the risk of falls/fractures

- Over-the-counter sleep aids.

Factors reducing the risk of falls/fractures

- Physically active lifestyle.

Bone health diagnosis

- Osteoporosis, as evidenced by presence of fragility vertebral compression fractures of T7 and T8.
- Increased fracture risk as per FRAX: 10-year probability of sustaining a hip (3.7%) or major fracture (22%) exceeding National Osteoporosis Foundation threshold to initiate pharmacologic treatment.

Management recommendations

Further diagnostic tests

- None needed at present.

Treatment recommendations

Medications

- Bisphosphonates or denosumab.

Physical therapy/lifestyle changes

- Combination of aerobic and resistive exercises.
- Reduce sodium and caffeine intake.
- Stop cigarette smoking.
- Adopt a physically active lifestyle.

Follow-up

Outpatient clinic or telehealth encounter 4 to 6 weeks after initiating therapy:

- If the patient elected to go on oral bisphosphonate therapy this visit can be used to ensure the medication is taken exactly as directed, that no adverse effects developed, and that the patient is happy to continue taking the bisphosphonate. This also offers an opportunity to emphasize the importance of the recommended dietary and lifestyle changes including getting involved in a regular, preferably supervised, physical exercise program.
- If the patient elected to receive parenteral bisphosphonates or denosumab: an outpatient visit, 4–8 weeks later, to address any concern the patient may have and emphasize the importance of the recommended dietary and lifestyle changes including getting involved in a regular, preferably supervised, physical exercise program. In addition, if the patient decided to go on denosumab, this visit could be used to emphasize the importance of receiving the medication on the scheduled 6-month visit and of the risks involved should the next dose be postponed.
- Regardless, this follow-up visit is an opportunity to emphasize to the patient the seriousness of osteoporosis and the potentially good results anticipated provided the medication is taken regularly and exactly as directed.

Key points

- Osteoporosis is common in older men and its impact is worse than in women.
- The same diagnostic criteria, laboratory workup, and indications for treatment apply to men and women.
- As for women, the management strategy should not be limited to pharmacologic agents, but should be comprehensive and include lifestyle changes and nonpharmacologic modalities.

References

1. Vescini F, Chiodini IP, Falchetti A, et al. Management of osteoporosis in men: a narrative review. *Int JMol Sci.* 2021;22:13640.
2. Watts NB, Adler RA, Bilezikian JP, et al. Osteoporosis in men; an endocrine society clinical practice guideline. *J Clin Endocrinol Metab.* 2012;97(6):1802–1825.
3. Siris ES, Adler R, Bilezikian J, et al. The clinical diagnosis of osteoporosis: a position statement from the National Bone Health Alliance Working Group. *Osteoporos Int.* 2014;25:1439–1443.
4. Diab DL, Watts NB. Updates on osteoporosis in men. *Endocrinol Metab Clin North Am.* 2021;50:239–249.

5. Shigehara K, Izumi K, Kadono Y, Mizokami A. Testosterone and bone health in men: a narrative review. *J Clin Med.* 2021;10:530.
6. Snyder PJ, Kopperdahl DL, Stephens-Shields, et al. Effect of testosterone treatment on volumetric bone density and strength in older men with testosterone. *JAMA.* 2017;177(4):471–479.
7. Vanderschueren D, Laurent MR, Claessens F, et al. Sex steroid actions in male bone. *Endocr Rev.* 2014;35 (6):906–960.
8. Orwoll ES, Lapidus J, Wang PY, et al. The limited clinical utility of testosterone, estradiol and sex hormone binding globulin measurements in the prediction of fracture risk and bone loss in older men. *J Bone Miner Res.* 2017;32(3):633–640.
9. Bhasin S, Brito JP, Cunningham GR, et al. Testosterone therapy in men with hypogonadism: an endocrine society clinical practice guideline. *J Clin Endocrinol Metabol.* 2018;103(5):1715–1744.
10. Sim IW, Ebeling PR. Treatment of osteoporosis in men with bisphosphonates: rationale and latest evidence. *Ther Musculoskel Dis.* 2013;5(5):259–267.
11. Ruza I, Mirfakhraee S, Orwoll E, Gruntmanis U. Clinical experience with intravenous zoledronic acid in the treatment of male osteoporosis: evidence and opinions. *Ther Adv Musculoskel Dis.* 2013;5(4):182–198.
12. Kanis JA, Johnell O, Oden A, et al. Smoking and fracture risk: a meta-analysis. *Osteoporos Int.* 2005;16:155–162.
13. Yan C, Avadhani NG, Iqbal J. The effects of smoke carcinogens on bone. *Curr Osteoporos Rep.* 2011;9 (4):202–209.
14. Cawthon PM, Harrison SL, Barrett-Connor E, et al. Alcohol intake and its relationship with bone mineral density, falls and fracture in older men. *J Am Geriatr Soc.* 2006;54:1649–1657.
15. Bliuc D, Nguyen ND, Milch VE, et al. Mortality risk associated with low-trauma osteoporotic fracture and subsequent fracture in men and women. *JAMA.* 2009;301:513–521.
16. Sirufo MM, Ginaldi L, De Martinis M. Bone health in men: still suffer the gender gap. *Osteoporos Int.* 2021;32:791.
17. Chen W, Pocock N. Male osteoporosis awareness in the elderly: an analysis of dual energy X-ray absorptiometry use in Australia between 1995 and 2015. *J Clin Densitom.* 2016;21(1):105–109.
18. Kaufman JM. Management of osteoporosis in older men. *Aging Clin Exp Res.* 2021;33:1439–1452.
19. Haentjens P, Magaziner J, Colon-Emeric CS, et al. Meta-analysis: excess mortality after hip fracture among older women and men. *Ann Intern Med.* 2010;152:380–390.
20. Szulc P, Kaufman JM, Orwoll ES. Osteoporosis in men. *J Osteopor.* 2012;1–5.
21. Baim S, Binkley N, Bilezikian JP, et al. Official positions of the International Society for Clinical Densitometry and executive summary of the 2007 ISCD position development conference. *J Clin Densitom.* 2008;11:75–91.
22. Burge R, Dawson-Hughes B, Solomon DH, et al. Incidence and economic burden of osteoporosis-related fractures in the United States. *J Bone Miner Res.* 2007;22:465–475.
23. Khosla S, Amin S, Orwoll E. Osteoporosis in men. *Endocr Rev.* 2008;29(4):441–464.
24. Fransen M, Woodward M, Norton R, et al. Excess mortality or institutionalization after hip fracture: men are at greater risk than women. *J Am Geriatr Soc.* 2002;50(4):685–690.
25. Wright NC, Saag KG, Curtis JR, et al. Recent trends in hip fracture rates by race/ethnicity among older US adults. *J Bone Miner Res.* 2012;27(11):2325–2332.
26. Cauley JA, Cawthon PM, Peters KE, et al. Risk factors for hip fracture in older men: the osteoporotic fractures in men study (Mr OS). *J Bone Miner Res.* 2016;31(10):1810–1819.
27. Bhat KA, Kakaji M, Awasthi A, et al. High prevalence of osteoporosis and morphometric vertebral fractures in Indian males aged 60 years and above: should age for screening be lowered? *J Clin Densitom.* 2018;21 (4):517–523. https://doi.org/10.1016/j.jocd.2016.10.003.
28. Sandhu SK, Nguyen ND, Center JR, et al. Prognosis of fracture: evaluation of predictive accuracy of the FRAX algorithm and Garvan nomogram. *Osteoporos Int.* 2010;21:863–871.
29. Hamdy RC, Seier E, Whalen K, et al. FRAX calculated without BMD does not correctly identify Caucasian men with densitometric evidence of osteoporosis. *Osteoporos Int.* 2018;29:947–952.

30. Khosla S, Melton 3rd L, Atkinson EJ, et al. Relationship of serum sex steroid levels and bone turnover markers with bone mineral density in men and women: a key role for bioavailable estrogen. *J Clin Endocrinol Metab.* 1998;83(7):2266–2274.
31. Jardí F, Laurent MR, Claessens F, Vanderschueren D. Estradiol and age-related bone loss in men. *Physiol Rev.* 2018;98(1):1. https://doi.org/10.1152/physrev.00051.2017.
32. Drake MT, Khosla S. Male osteoporosis. *Endocrinol Metab Clin North Am.* 2012;41(3):629–641.
33. Ashe MC, dos Santos IK, Edwards NY, et al. Physical activity and bone health in men: a systematic review and meta-analysis. *J Bone Metab.* 2021;28(1):27–39.
34. Mittan D, Lee S, Miller E, et al. Bone loss following hypogonadism in men with prostate cancer treated with GnRH analogs. *J Clin Endocrinol Metab.* 2002;87:3656–3661.
35. Shahinian VB, Kuo YF, Freeman JL, Goodwin JS. Risk of fracture after androgen deprivation for prostate cancer. *N Engl J Med.* 2005;352:154–164.
36. Smith MR, Egerdie B, Hernandez TN, et al. Denosumab in men receiving androgen-deprivation therapy for prostate cancer. *N Engl J Med.* 2009;361:745–755.

CHAPTER 24

Premenopausal women with low bone mass ☆

Learning objectives

- There is no consensus on the diagnostic criteria of osteoporosis in premenopausal women.
- The relationship between BMD and fractures is not as well established in premenopausal as it is in postmenopausal women.
- In premenopausal women, the diagnosis of osteoporosis should be considered only if the patient has sustained one or more unequivocal fragility fractures.
- There are many causes of low bone mass in premenopausal women.

The case study

Reasons for seeking medical help

- FD is 32 years old. She is a full-time bank teller. She is experiencing sudden onset of severe pain in both hip joints anteriorly, in the groin, and the buttocks, the right side more than the left one. The pain is worse when she stands up, and weight bears, particularly on the right side. She ranks the pain as 7–8 on a scale of 1–10 with 1 being the mildest pain and 10 being the most severe excruciating pain.
- Initially it was felt that she fractured one or both hips, but plain X-rays revealed neither fractures, nor osteoarthritic changes, nor deformities of the hip joints, nor any abnormality of both femoral heads. There was nevertheless evidence of reduced bone density of both proximal femurs, more pronounced on the right side.
- The pain started spontaneously, got progressively worse, is now interfering with her daily activities, and causing her to be unsteady. She also now has to use a cane to ambulate. She fell a couple of times a week ago and had several near-falls. She was told that the pain will gradually subside, but it has not, it worsened.

☆ FD, 32 years old, sudden severe pain in both hips.

Diagnosis and Treatment of Osteoporosis. https://doi.org/10.1016/B978-0-323-99550-4.00006-X
Copyright © 2024 Elsevier Inc. All rights are reserved, including those for text and data mining, AI training, and similar technologies.

Past medical and surgical history

- She always enjoyed good health and until this present illness led a physically active lifestyle. For the past few weeks, she had to curtail her physical activities because of the pain she is experiencing. She is on no medication except for the occasional nonsteroidal antiinflammatory/analgesics she is getting over the counter. She is, however, reluctant to take them. The pain is more bearable when she uses hot/cold patches and transdermal nerve stimulation. She does not want to take opioids to relieve the pain.

Lifestyle

- She used to lead a physically active lifestyle and exercised regularly. She ran the marathon three times.
- She had a good appetite, and her weight was steady. Now both are decreasing.
- She used to sleep well, without any medication, but has not done so since the pain started.
- No cigarette smoking, no caffeine intake, no soda drinks, and no recreational drugs
- Her menstrual periods have always been regular.

Medication(s)

- None apart from NSAIDs and nonnarcotic analgesics, which now are no longer effective at controlling the pain.

Family history

- Negative for osteoporosis.
- She is happily married and has three children aged 12, 10, and 5 years. All are in good health.

Clinical examination

- Weight 120 pounds, height 62″.
- No significant clinical findings, except for marginal tenderness along the proximal end of both femurs, the right more than the left.
- No localizing neurologic findings. Range of motion of both hips maintained but painful. The pain is exacerbated by weight bearing. No sensory deficits. Evidence of mild muscle wasting in both legs, especially the right side and more so proximally. No fasciculations. Tendon reflexes preserved. Both plantar responses down-going. No clinical evidence of arthropathies.

DXA scan and radiological results

- Z-scores:
  - Left femoral neck −2.8, left total hip −2.6.
  - Right femoral neck −2.9, right total hip −2.7.
  - Upper 4 lumbar vertebrae −1.7.
- VFA: no evidence of vertebral compression fractures.
- FRAX: Not done given the patient's age and localized demineralization.
- Plain X-rays of both hips show localized, ill-defined areas of bone demineralization of the upper femurs, the right more than the left.
- There is no evidence of fractures. Femoral heads intact on both sides.

Multiple choice questions

1. ***FD's probable diagnosis is:***
   A. Osteoporosis of both proximal femurs.
   B. Osteopenia of the lumbar vertebrae.
   C. Idiopathic transient osteoporosis of the hips.
   D. Avascular necrosis of the femoral heads.
   E. Bilateral atypical femoral shaft fractures.
   Correct answer: C
   Comment:
   Unlike "Postmenopausal Osteoporosis" which is a well-established disease state with clear diagnostic criteria, well-defined trajectory, known complications, accepted thresholds to initiate therapy, multiple treatment modalities, and well-known anticipated treatment outcomes, premenopausal "low bone mass for given age" is rather nebulous.

   The term "osteoporosis" should not be applied to premenopausal women unless there is evidence of at least one fragility fracture or two trauma-induced fractures.[1,2] The International Society for Clinical Densitometry (ISCD) also recommends that the term "Osteopenia" not be used. Instead, the preferred terminology is based on the Z-score which compares the patient's BMD to that of a reference population matched for the patient's age, gender and, if available, ethnic group.

   A threshold Z-score of −2.0 is used to classify premenopausal patients into two categories: "Low bone mineral density for given age" if the Z-score is −2.0 or lower or "within expected range for given age" if the Z-score is higher.[2] The term "osteoporosis" therefore is not appropriate: FD sustained neither a fragility fracture, nor the required two traumatic fractures to qualify for the diagnosis of osteoporosis.[1] In this respect VFA can be a useful addition to DXA scans in young adults as it may identify previously undiagnosed fragility fractures.[3]

Transient osteoporosis of the hip is a rare, poorly understood cause of pelvic pain which affects both sexes. It is characterized by bone loss in the proximal femur on one or both sides. It may affect other joints in the leg. It usually presents as acute, severe sudden onset pain in the affected hip aggravated by standing on the affected leg and partially alleviated by lying down.

It is usually spontaneously relieved in most cases within 6–12 months. While the disease is active, bone loss takes place and may lead to fractures. In pregnant women, it tends to be more common during the last 3 months of pregnancy.

Its cause is not known. Bone marrow edema often can be visualized by imaging techniques, especially MRI. The diagnosis is one of exclusion: secondary causes of low bone mass must be first excluded. Given the transient nature of the illness, its real incidence is probably underestimated, and the diagnosis is often missed especially during pregnancy as the risks of radiographic imaging may deter clinicians from pursuing imaging studies.[4]

There are no evidence-based treatment modalities for idiopathic transient osteoporosis with fracture risk reduction as the outcome.[5] Its treatment is nonspecific and geared to minimizing symptoms and preventing injuries to the weakened bone. Weight bearing should be restricted or temporarily avoided. Walking aids help reduce weight bearing and may prevent falls and fractures from occurring. Water exercises relieve weight bearing and facilitate movement. NSAIDs may reduce any inflammation present and relieve the pain, at least partly. Physical therapy helps maintain strength and flexibility. A well-balanced diet with sufficient calcium and vitamin D also may help healing. Routine screening for idiopathic transient osteoporosis is not recommended in either premenopausal women or men under the age of 50 years.[2] Similarly, neither osteoanabolic, nor antiresorptive medications are recommended, especially in women in their child-bearing period.

2. ***Osteoporosis in premenopausal women:***
   A. Can only be diagnosed if the patient sustained a fragility fracture.
   B. Is usually due to secondary causes.
   C. Teriparatide or abaloparatide is the drug of choice for premenopausal osteoporosis.
   D. A and B.
   E. A, B, and C.

Correct answer: D

Comment:

Osteoporosis and fractures are rare in premenopausal women and are usually due to secondary osteoporosis.[6] Bone densitometry is seldom indicated unless the patient has sustained a fragility fracture or has a disease associated with bone demineralization.[5] In the absence of fractures, it is not recommended to use the terms osteoporosis and osteopenia in premenopausal women. The FRAX algorithm also has not been validated in people younger than 40 years.

Peak Bone Mass (PBM) reflects the maximum amount of bone accrued during skeletal growth and maturation and is a major factor affecting fracture risk.[5] Skeletal bone maturation goes through distinct phases. During childhood bone mass is driven by increasing bone size, and its accrual is steady with no significant differences between girls and boys.

Gender differences become obvious during puberty: male puberty is associated with accelerated periosteal apposition and endosteal expansion resulting in marked increases in bone diameter and in cortical thickness. Female puberty is associated with similar, but smaller, increases in cortical thickness and in bone diameter. Gender differences continue to be observed during late puberty with smaller increases in trabecular thickness and bone volume in girls compared to boys.[5]

By the end of puberty, bone strength is 30 to 50% higher in boys than in girls. Peak bone mass is achieved during the second or third decade of life and is site and gender dependent.[5] Multiple genetic factors are responsible for 60%–80% of the variability in bone mass accrual, including birth weight, timing of puberty, extent of pubertal growth spurt, general health status, height, and muscle mass. Optimal achievement of PBM largely determines future bone strength.

Fragility fractures must be present to diagnose osteoporosis in premenopausal women and men under the age of 40years. Several diseases may lead to a deficient bone mass and an increased fracture risk during childhood, including endocrine, neuromuscular, rheumatic, chronic inflammatory, nutritional, hematologic, and oncology diseases.[5]

A premenopausal woman who has sustained a fracture has a 35%–75% higher risk of sustaining another fracture after she reaches the menopause than a woman who has not sustained such a fracture.[6] This opens a window of opportunity to increase muscle and bone mass and strength before the menopause and reduce the risk of sustaining fractures by identifying those individuals at risk of sustaining a fracture. At this stage these interventions include changes in lifestyle habits, physical exercise, dietary food intake, an adequate vitamin D intake, and combined oral contraceptives.[6]

Bisphosphonates used to treat osteoporosis in postmenopausal women are not routinely used for premenopausal women because of their long half-life, the child-bearing potential, and the uncertain effect on the fetus.

3. ***Anorexia nervosa (AN):***
   A. Has a peak onset after the age of 30years.
   B. Patients are very conscious and particular of their body weight.
   C. The fracture risk is about twice that of the general population.
   D. B and C.
   E. A, B, and C.

   Correct answer: D

   Comment:

   AN has a peak onset between the ages of 15 and 19years. Although more common in girls it affects both sexes. Patients with AN have a low body weight, a distorted perception of their body weight and shape, and have an intense fear of gaining weight. They also often have amenorrhea. AN usually develops as a result of psychological trauma in individuals predisposed to it. Psychiatric problems are common. Overall mortality and suicide are increased,[6,7] BMD is decreased, and fracture risk is increased.

4. ***In anorexia nervosa (AN), the following contributes to bone loss:***
   A. Estrogen and progesterone deficiency.
   B. Reduced insulin-like growth factor-1 (IGF-1).
   C. Excess cortisol levels.
   D. A and B.
   E. A, B, and C.

   Correct answer: E

   Comment:

   Patients with AN lose weight and deplete their fat stores. A minimum of 10% fat stores is needed to maintain normal menstrual functions. When the total body fat mass drops below this level amenorrhea sets in. The resulting estrogen/progesterone deficiency arrests bone formation and vigorously promotes bone resorption as evidenced by the elevated markers of bone resorption (CTX and NTX) and the usually low markers of bone formation such as P1NP or bone-specific alkaline phosphatase. This "uncoupling" leads to significant bone loss. Other factors that further contribute to bone loss include low levels of IGF-1, excess cortisol secretion, and low testosterone levels.[8,9] Bone loss in AN occurs early, progresses rapidly during the disease process, and is not entirely reversible with weight restoration.[6]

5. ***The following are useful in the management of anorexia nervosa:***
   A. Estrogen/progesterone.
   B. Dehydroepiandrosterone (DHEA).
   C. Bisphosphonates.
   D. None of the above.
   E. A, B, and C.

   Correct answer: D

   Comment:

   Management of AN is notoriously difficult. Ideally the patient should very gradually increase her daily dietary intake to gradually increase her body weight to optimum levels for her given age and height. Unfortunately, this is rarely possible. The use of estrogen is controversial, and a meta-analysis and review of the literature failed to support its use for AN.[10,11]

   There is also concern that the resumption of menstrual periods induced by cyclical estrogen/progesterone may give the patient the impression that she is cured of AN and justify her stopping to restore her genetically determined body weight.[10,11] There is no convincing data to support the use of DHEA, testosterone, or fluoride.[10,11] The use of bisphosphonates in AN is also controversial given the child-bearing potential of most patients and the still not fully explored potential effect on the skeletal development of a child born to a patient who has been on bisphosphonates.

6. ***Contraceptives and bone mass:***
   A. Estrogen, in very low doses (Ethinyl estradiol (EE): 20 μg), provides contraception.
   B. Larger doses of estrogen increase the risk of thromboembolic disorders.
   C. Medroxyprogesterone acetate does not interfere with bone metabolism.
   D. A and B.
   E. A, B, and C.

   Correct answer: D

   Comment:

   Estrogen suppresses the release of follicular stimulating hormone from the anterior pituitary and therefore interferes with the recruitment of ovarian follicles and the production of endogenous estrogen. Progesterone prevents the release of luteinizing hormone from the pituitary and prevents ovulation. Estrogen/progesterone is an effective oral contraceptive. When the dose is sufficient, estrogen may have positive effects on bone metabolism. Unfortunately, higher doses of estrogen increase the risk of thromboembolic diseases and modern oral contraceptives contain the lowest effective dose for contraception, which often is not sufficient to maintain a neutral or positive effect on bone metabolism.

   By suppressing endogenous estrogen production, the nefarious effects of estrogen deprivation on bone mass manifest themselves: increased bone resorption and decreased bone mass, eventually leading to osteoporosis and fractures.[12] Medroxyprogesterone acetate administered parenterally at 3-month interval also is associated with a low bone mass.[13]

7. ***Celiac disease:***
   A. Affects about 1% of the population.
   B. Most patients are asymptomatic.
   C. The BMD is decreased even in asymptomatic patients.
   D. B and C.
   E. A, B, and C.

   Correct answer: E

   Comment:

   Celiac disease affects about 1% of the population. Most patients are asymptomatic and are unaware of the disease which is due to an immune response to dietary gliadins in genetically predisposed patients and results in malabsorption. Calcium and vitamin D malabsorption leads to hypovitaminosis D and secondary hyperparathyroidism. In addition, a number of immunological and inflammatory changes lead to a low bone mass, including an excessive production of RANK-L, interleukin-1, interleukin-6, and tumor necrosis factor-alpha. Hypogonadism may further contribute to bone loss.

Symptomatic cases present with weight loss, diarrhea, and bloating. Extra-intestinal manifestations include low bone mass, increased fracture risk, anemia, infertility, recurrent miscarriages, seizures, ataxia, peripheral neuropathies, dermatitis herpetiformis, enamel defects, and various vitamin deficiencies.[14] At present, plasma transglutaminase is the best serological screening test. If positive, a small-bowel biopsy is recommended. BMD and symptoms improve when patients adhere to a gluten-free diet and avoid wheat, rye, barley, and oats.

8. ***During pregnancy:***
   A. Bone turnover is increased.
   B. Intestinal calcium absorption is increased.
   C. Osteoporosis may present as severe low back or hip pain.
   D. A and B.
   E. A, B, and C.

Correct answer: E

Comment:

During pregnancy the fetus acquires about 30g of calcium; the maternal skeleton is protected by an increased intestinal absorption of calcium largely mediated through increased 1,25-di-hydroxy-vitamin D levels which nearly double early in pregnancy and remain at this level until delivery. The serum parathyroid hormone levels tend to be in the low normal range during the first trimester and gradually increase during pregnancy, reaching peak levels during the third trimester of pregnancy, but not exceeding normal values.

Pregnancy and lactation affect the mother's BMD: the BMD of the lumbar vertebrae may decrease by about 5% during normal pregnancy and there may be a further decline of 3%–10% after a 6-month period of lactation. A decline of 2%–4% in the hip BMD has been documented after 6months of lactation. It may take up to 1 year to reverse these losses.[3] Maternal rate of bone turnover is moderately increased and small decreases in BMD have been observed in the lumbar vertebrae, but not long bones.

Pregnancy-associated osteoporosis is rare, tends to affect primigravidae, affects mostly the vertebrae, and presents with back pain, often severe, which is often misdiagnosed as being due to ligamentous laxity induced by hormonal changes associated with pregnancy. Transient osteoporosis of the hip is rare, presents with unilateral or bilateral hip pain, and may be complicated by a fragility hip fracture. Patients with risk factors for bone demineralization are more likely to develop pregnancy-associated osteoporosis.

9. ***During lactation:***
   A. Bone turnover is increased.
   B. Intestinal calcium absorption is increased.
   C. Renal calcium resorption is increased.
   D. A and C.
   E. A, B, and C.

Correct answer: D

Comment:

Calcium metabolism is different in pregnancy and lactation. The average daily calcium in breast milk is about 200 mg, with the range varying between 280 and 1000 mg. During lactation the increased intestinal calcium absorption seen during pregnancy returns to the normal prepregnancy levels.

High prolactin levels induce a hypoestrogenic state which leads to increased bone resorption to mobilize calcium from bone to the circulation, to breast milk, and in the process, increase the risk of bone demineralization and reduced bone mass. Calcium reabsorption by renal tubules is also increased. Trabecular bones are affected more than cortical bones. Notwithstanding, BMD is usually restored 6 to 12 months after weaning. Epidemiological studies do not show a deleterious effect of lactation on bone mass and hip fracture risk.

10. ***The Female Athlete Triad includes:***
   A. Disordered/restrictive eating.
   B. Impaired ovarian functions.
   C. Bone demineralization.
   D. A and C.
   E. A, B, and C.

Correct answer: E

Comment:

The female athlete triad is characterized by[15]:

- Disordered/restricted eating, intense physical activity, low energy availability, and low body mass index (BMI).
- Ovarian dysfunction, associated with functional hypothalamic oligomenorrhea and amenorrhea as evidenced by low serum estradiol and gonadotrophins leading to an increased bone turnover and rapid bone loss.
- Decreased BMD and osteoporosis, eventually leading to fractures.[15]

Each element of the triad is a spectrum with a broad range.

Low energy availability may be due to dietary restrictions (intentional or inadvertent) or may be due to excessive energy expenditure. Notwithstanding, the imbalance triggers a cascade of physiologic and neuroendocrine adaptations including decreased frequency and pulses of gonadotrophin-releasing hormone from the hypothalamus leading to decreased pulsatile pituitary release of luteinizing hormone and follicle stimulating hormone, resulting in reduced production of estrogen and progesterone by the ovaries. Other hormones also may be involved, including cortisol, insulin, growth hormone, insulin-like growth factor-1, and leptin.[16]

The etiology of low BMD in the female athlete syndrome is also multifactorial and includes failure to achieve peak bone mass, bone loss resulting from estrogen deficiency, and other hormonal imbalances. Patients with the female athlete syndrome are more at risk of sustaining fractures.[17]

Management of the female athlete triad is difficult. The goal is to increase energy availability, restore menstrual functions, and normalize BMD. A multidisciplinary team approach is recommended. Nonpharmacologic means should be tried first. They include controlled physical activity, lifestyle changes, and weight regain by diet manipulation.

Bisphosphonates and denosumab are not routinely used because of the potential risk to future pregnancies. There is still no consensus as to how long medications for osteoporosis can/should be administered because their sudden cessation may lead to excessive bone loss and their continued long-term administration increases the risk of rare conditions such as osteonecrosis of the jaw and atypical femoral shaft fractures. Clinicians have to consider the potential benefit: essentially decreased fracture risk to the potential risks associated with the continuation of these medications, especially atypical femoral shaft fracture and osteonecrosis of the jaw. These issues are discussed in other sections.[18]

Teriparatide and abaloparatide are sometimes used for up to 2years in premenopausal women with very low BMD. At the end of the two-year course, however, bisphosphonates or denosumab should be prescribed to avoid bone loss. Ideally the female athlete triad should be treated as soon as possible to allow the patient to achieve her peak bone mass.[15]

Key points

- Osteoporosis is rare in premenopausal women and should be diagnosed only in the presence of at least one fragility fracture and two traumatic fractures.
- When interpreting DXA scans in premenopausal women, the *Z*-score, not T-score, should be considered, and the patient's BMD classified as either "below the expected range for the patient's age" if the *Z*-score is lower than −2.0 or "within the expected range for the patient's age" if the *Z*-score is above −2.0.
- Fifty to 90% of premenopausal women with low bone mass have secondary osteoporosis.[3]
- Main causes of "low bone mass for given age" in premenopausal women include:
  - Lifestyle habits: excessive alcohol intake, cigarette smoking, sedentary lifestyle.
  - Primary GI problems: malabsorption, malnutrition, celiac disease, anorexia nervosa.
  - The female athlete triad.
  - A number of diseases including hypogonadism, primary hyperparathyroidism, hyperthyroidism, Cushing's syndrome, diabetes mellitus, multiple myeloma, rheumatoid arthritis, HIV, liver and renal diseases.
  - Medications, including glucocorticoids, aromatase inhibitors, anticonvulsants, progesterone.
  - Inherited diseases: osteogenesis imperfecta and Marfan syndrome.
- Suggested laboratory tests for the evaluation of premenopausal osteoporosis include:
  - CBC.
  - Comprehensive metabolic profile.
  - Glomerular filtration rate.
  - Serum 25-hydroxy-vitamin D.
  - Serum transaminases.
  - Thyroid stimulating hormone.
  - 24-h urine for calcium, sodium, and creatinine.
  - Bone markers (CTx, P1NP, and bone-specific alkaline phosphatase isoenzyme).
- Low estrogen oral contraceptives may lead to bone demineralization.
- The impact of pregnancy and lactation on calcium homeostasis are different.

References

1. Baim S, Binkley N, Bilezikian JP, et al. Official positions of the ISCD position development conference. *J Clin Densitom.* 2007;11:75–91.
2. Lewiecki EM, Gordon CM, Baim S, et al. Special report on the 2007 adult and pediatric position development conferences of the International Society for Clinical densitometry. *Osteoporos Int.* 2008;19:1369–1378.
3. Conradie M, de Villiers T. Premenopausal osteoporosis. *Climacteric.* 2022;25(1):73–80.
4. Wright EV, Naqvi AZ, Syed S, Zaw H. Transient osteoporosis of the hip in pregnancy. *BMJ Case Rep.* 2021;14(3):e238659.
5. Rosenberg S, Bruyère O, Bergmann P, et al. How to manage osteoporosis before the age of 50. *Maturitas.* 2020;138:14–25.
6. Pepe J, Body J-J, Hadji P, et al. Osteoporosis in premenopausal women. *J Clin Endocrinol Metabol.* 2020;105 (8):2487–2506.
7. Arcelus J, Mitchell AJ, Wales J, et al. Mortality rates in patients with anorexia nervosa and other eating disorders. A meta-analysis of 36 studies. *Arch Gen Psychiatry.* 2011;68(7):724–731.
8. Mehler P, Cleary BS, Gaudiani JL. Osteoporosis in anorexia nervosa. *Eat Disord.* 2011;19:194–202.
9. Lawson EA, Miller KK, Bredella MA, et al. Hormone predictors of abnormal bone microarchitecture in women with anorexia nervosa. *Bone.* 2010;46:458–463.
10. Lim LA, McGovern L, Elamin MB, et al. Effect on bone health of estrogen preparations in premenopausal women with anorexia nervosa: a systemic review and meta-analysis. *Int J Eating Disord.* 2010;43:218–225.
11. Mehler PS. MacKenzie TD treatment of osteopenia and osteoporosis in anorexia nervosa: a systematic review of the literature. *Int J Eating Disord.* 2009;42:195–201.
12. Ziglar S, Hunter TS. The effect of hormonal oral contraception on acquisition of peak bone mineral density of adolescents and young women. *J Pharm Pract.* 2012;25(3):331–340.
13. Guilbert ER, Brown JP, Kaunitz AM, et al. The use of depot-medroxyprogesterone acetate in contraception and its potential impact on skeletal health. *Contraception.* 2009;79(3):167–177.
14. Fouda MA, Khan AA, Sultan M, et al. Evaluation and management of skeletal health in celiac disease: position statement. *Can J Gastroenterol.* 2012;26(11):819–829.
15. Zavatta G, Clarke BL. Premenopausal osteoporosis: focus on the female athlete triad. *Case Rep Women's Health.* 2021;29:e00276.
16. Warren MP. Endocrine manifestations of eating disorders. *J Clin Endocrinol Metab.* 2011;96(2):333–343.
17. Feingold D, Hame SL. Female athlete triad and stress fractures. *Orthop Clin North Am.* 2006;37(4):575–583.
18. Arceo-Mendoza RM, Camacho PM. Postmenopausal osteoporosis: latest guidelines. *Endocrinol Metab Clin North Am.* 2021;50:167–178.

CHAPTER 25

Osteoporosis in older adults☆

Learning objectives

- Osteoporosis is also common in very old age. It is often underrecognized, underdiagnosed, and undertreated.
- Osteoporosis is less frequent in older men than in women, but its mortality and morbidity are worse.
- As with younger patients, for best results, a comprehensive approach is recommended: the pharmacologic management should be complemented by lifestyle changes and an adequate diet.

The case study

Reason for seeking medical help

- Mr. WM, 89years old, is concerned he may have osteoporosis: about 2 weeks ago, while on a Mediterranean cruise, he tripped over a cable, slipped, fell, and sustained only superficial, albeit extensive bruises. A medical doctor among the passengers noticed the episode and recommended a medical examination. He is essentially asymptomatic. In about a month's time he is scheduled to go on a four-week "total immersion" tour in South Africa. He has been warned that this tour is quite demanding physically and mentally. He was offered the option to withdraw, but he is very keen to go on this adventure tour: "A once in a lifetime experience."

Past medical/surgical history

- Hyperlipidemia, well controlled.

Personal habits, lifestyle, daily routine

- Mr. WM is a widower, has no children, and no close relative alive. He lives on his own; is asymptomatic; cognitively intact; physically independent; drives his own car; travels

☆ Mr. WM, 94 years old, slipped and fell about 2 weeks ago. He sustained only superficial bruises, but is concerned about having osteoporosis.

Diagnosis and Treatment of Osteoporosis. https://doi.org/10.1016/B978-0-323-99550-4.00001-0
Copyright © 2024 Elsevier Inc. All rights are reserved, including those for text and data mining, AI training, and similar technologies.

extensively; and denies dizzy spells, falls, and near-falls. He has no hobby except reading and traveling.

- He is a retired college teacher and continues to be involved teaching Medieval History. He has written three books and is often invited to give talks to academic circles and the lay public.
- When not traveling, he leads a sedentary lifestyle.
- Average daily caffeine intake: 4 cups, about 16 oz each cup.
- Daily calcium intake: average 1000 mg.
- Alcohol intake: about two drinks most days, occasionally more when he is with friends.
- Cigarette smoking: about 10 cigarettes a day, used to smoke more. He is planning to stop smoking.
- Enjoys chocolates and salty food.

Medications

- Simvastatin 40 mg daily for "many years."
- Aspirin, 81 mg, once a day, also, for "many years."
- Multivitamin tablets once a day.
- Over-the-counter sleep aids, on an as-needed basis, not exceeding one tablet a week.

Family history

- Negative for osteoporosis.

Clinical examination

- Weight 186 pounds, steady, height 62.75″, used to be 66.5″, arm span 65.5″.
- Mild kyphosis, that, to a large extent, can be corrected by changing posture.
- No clinical signs suggesting an increased fracture risk:
  - Sitting BP 136/85, standing BP 142/86, no orthostasis.
  - No clinical evidence of carotid stenosis, carotid sinus sensitivity, and vertebrobasilar insufficiency.
  - No localizing neurological signs, cerebellar functions intact.
  - No clinical evidence of fluid retention, edema of the lower limbs, or heart failure. No evidence of pulmonary congestion. Lungs clear.

Laboratory investigations

- Comprehensive metabolic profile: no abnormal finding.
- Serum 25-hydroxy-vitamin D: 42 ng/mL.

DXA scan results

- **T-scores:** right femoral neck: −2.1, right total hip: −1.5, distal 1/3 radius: −1.3; L1–L4: cannot be reliably interpreted because of osteophytes. Left hip was not scanned.
- **Vertebral fracture assessment:** no evidence of vertebral compression fractures.
- **FRAX score** (with BMD): hip fracture: 3.7%; other major osteoporotic fractures: 22%.

Multiple choice questions

1. ***In Mr. VM's case, the final diagnosis is:***
   A. Densitometric diagnosis: osteoporosis.
   B. Densitometric diagnosis: osteopenia.
   C. Fracture risk exceeds NOF threshold to initiate therapy.
   D. B and C.
   E. A and C.
   Correct answer: D
   Comment:
   The densitometric diagnosis is osteopenia. It is nevertheless overridden by the fracture risk, as per the FRAX score, exceeding the threshold recommended by the National Osteoporosis Foundation Guidelines to initiate pharmacological therapy: 20% and 3% for the risk of major and hip fracture, respectively.
   Therefore, unless there are contraindications, this patient should be treated as if he had osteoporosis, including medications, reducing alcohol and caffeine intake, discontinuing cigarette smoking, and discontinuing the intake of hypnotics, especially those obtained over the counter as their half-lives are often long and may induce daytime sleepiness, disequilibrium, repeated falls and fractures.
   Other recommendations include adopting a physically active lifestyle and especially a combination of resistive and aerobic exercises. Several programs are now available in many public gymnasia. Old age should not be a hindrance to enroll in these programs.
2. ***The following laboratory tests are recommended:***
   A. Fasting serum C-TX.
   B. Fasting serum P1NP or alkaline phosphatase bony isoenzyme.
   C. Ionized serum calcium level.
   D. All of the above.
   E. A and B.
   Correct answer: E
   Comment:
   Bone markers are available to estimate the rate of bone formation and bone resorption. They therefore differentiate patients who may benefit from medication that stimulates bone

formation (osteoanabolics) from those who would benefit from medication that reduces the rate of bone resorption (antiresorptives).

The fasting serum carboxy-terminal collagen cross-link (Crosslaps, C-TX, serum cross-linked C-telopeptide of type 1 collagen) is a marker of bone resorption. The fasting serum Procollagen Type I intact N-terminal Propeptide (P1NP) and alkaline phosphatase bony isoenzyme are markers of bone formation.

Ideally therefore one should assay bone markers to select, fine tune, and monitor the management strategy. Patients whose rate of bone resorption is elevated, or are at the upper end of normality, are more likely to benefit from an antiresorptive and those with a reduced or at the lower end of normality are likely to benefit from an osteoanabolic medication.

A question that sometimes arises is whether it is appropriate to initiate pharmacological treatment in very old patients found to have an increased fracture risk. Given the potential impact of any fracture, especially hip fractures on morbidity and mortality, the answer should be a resounding YES! The impact of a hip fracture on patients similar to Mr. WM is such that quality of life and loss of autonomy with activities of daily living are likely to be severely affected. A study conducted in Europe shows that overall mortality in men, within 1 year of a hip fracture, increases from 15% before the age of 65 years to more than 30% after the age of 75 years. In women, one-year mortality rate is less than 10% before the age of 70 years but increases to 30% after the age of 90 years.[1]

3. ***The following medication(s) are most helpful at this stage:***
   A. Antiresorptives.
   B. Osteoanabolics.
   C. Vitamin supplementation.
   D. A and C.
   E. B and C.

Correct answer: B

Comment:

The skeletal mass goes through three distinct phases. First, a phase of bone accretion during childhood and adolescence. During this period the rate of bone formation exceeds the rate of bone resorption and the bone mass increases relatively quickly. During the second phase, the phase of consolidation, the rate of bone formation and bone resorption are about the same, the skeleton stops growing, but is continuously remodeled: old bone is resorbed and new bone, better able to meet various physical stressors, is formed. The bones get denser.

This is followed by the third phase when bone resorption exceeds bone formation and the skeletal mass decreases. In women this phase starts rather abruptly with the cessation of menstruation. The skeleton of men too goes through these phases albeit about a decade later than women.

Given the patient's age, 94 years, it is very likely that bone loss exceeds bone formation. An osteoanabolic agent therefore is likely to be more efficacious than an antiresorptive.

Finally, given that skeletal mass tends to respond better when it is first stimulated by the osteoanabolics and then resorption is inhibited, rather than being inhibited first by antiresorptives and then attempts made to stimulate bone formation. Notwithstanding, a medication that can be parenterally administered should be recommended to ensure the patient takes it as recommended. At present, several medications for osteoporosis can be parenterally administered and include: zoledronic acid intravenous infusion, once a year; denosumab, one injection subcutaneously every 6 months; and romosozumab, subcutaneous injection every month.

4. ***The incidence of fragility fractures:***
   A. Most fragility fractures occur before the age of 50 years.
   B. About half of the fractures occur after the age of 75 years.
   C. Affects about 20% of women aged 60 years.
   D. Affects about 50% of women aged 80 years.
   E. All of the above.

   Correct answer: B

   Comment:

   Osteoporosis in old age continues to be underdiagnosed and undertreated especially in older people.[2] And yet, the threshold between undertreatment and overtreatment is unclear especially in patients with limited life expectancy.[3]

   Concerning fragility fractures[1,4]:
   - Few fragility fractures occur before the age of 50 years.
   - About half of the fractures occur after the age of 75 years.
   - About 10% of women 60 years old sustain fractures.
   - About 20% of women aged 70 years old sustain fractures.
   - About 40% of women aged 80 years old sustain fractures.
   - Two-thirds of women aged 90 years and older sustain fractures.

     Similarly, a review of 377,561 female Medicare beneficiaries who sustained a fracture reveals that 10%, 18%, and 31% sustained another fracture within 12 months, 24 months, and 60 months of the original fracture, respectively.[5] Finally, a real-world cohort over the age of 65 years revealed that, regardless of the site of fragility fractures, mortality is increased for up to 6 years postfracture.[6]

5. ***Factors increasing the risk of fragility fractures:***
   A. Older age.
   B. Lower body weight.
   C. Greater height loss when compared to height at age 25 years.
   D. Hyperthyroidism.
   E. All of the above.

   Correct answer: E

   Comment:

   All the previously mentioned increase the risk of falls and fractures as per the Osteoporotic Fractures in Men Study. A prospective study on 5994 men, primarily White, 65 years of age or older, recruited at six US clinical centers. During a mean of 8.6 years, 97% completed follow-up, 178 men sustained a hip fracture. Other findings of this study include[7,8]:

- Almost 30% of hip fractures occur in older men.
- Mortality, morbidity, and loss of independence after a hip fracture are greater in men than in women.
- Although assessment protocols are available to identify patients likely to sustain an initial or first fragility fracture, scarce information is available about predicting the sequelae of second and subsequent fractures.[9]

6. ***Osteosarcopenia:***
   A. Is a benign, age-associated, loss of skeletal and muscle mass.
   B. Affects about 70% of adults aged 70 years or more.
   C. Increases the fracture risk.
   D. B and C.
   E. A, B, and C.

   Correct answer: C

   Comment:

   Osteosarcopenia is characterized by the simultaneous loss of muscle and bone density, culminating in functional decline, physical disability, increased falls and fracture risk, and poor quality of life.[10,11] It is estimated to affect more than 40% of patients aged 70 years or older.[11]

7. ***Factors affecting ability to conduct activities of daily living after a hip fracture include:***
   A. Age.
   B. Depression.
   C. Prefracture ability to conduct activities of daily living.
   D. Nutritional status.
   E. All of the above.

   Correct answer: E

   Comment:

   All listed factors affect functional recovery outcome after sustaining a hip fracture.[10–12]

   If the patient is to be discharged back home, an evaluation of the home/institution conditions would help ensuring the patient is safe and able to cope with activities of daily living, including the intake of medications. Often older people find it difficult to open the tablet containers and may not be able to read the directions as to when to take the medication.

   The need for long-term care following a hip fracture increases significantly with age from 4% in those aged 70–79 years, to 14% for those aged 80–89 years, and 35.3% in those between the ages of 90 and 100 years.[1]

   Hip fractures are life-changing events, hence the urgency of treating patients who are at high risk of sustaining a hip fracture. Similarly, as soon as possible after the surgery is completed, these patients should be thoroughly evaluated and enrolled in a rehabilitation program tailored to the individual deficits and needs of the patient.

8. ***Factors increasing the risk of falls and fractures include:***
   A. Age.
   B. Comorbidities.
   C. Decreased mental alertness.
   D. Balance and gait abnormalities.
   E. All of the above.

   Correct answer: E

   Comment:

   All listed factors affect functional recovery outcome after sustaining a hip fracture.[13] Other factors include low femoral neck BMD, current smoking, greater height, height loss since age 25 years, use of tricyclic antidepressants, history of myocardial infarction, hyperthyroidism, Parkinson's disease, and low protein intake.[14]

9. ***The initial evaluation of older men after a fracture is sustained should include:***
   A. An assessment of the clinical impact of the disease.
   B. An evaluation of the patient's cognitive functions.
   C. An evaluation of the risks of falling.
   D. The presence of comorbidities.
   E. All of the above.

   Correct answer: E

   Comment:

   An initial systematic thorough evaluation is necessary once the diagnosis of osteoporosis is established. This should include the potential impact on the risk of falling and fractures, as well as the ability to live in the prefall/prefracture environment.

   An assessment of cognitive functions is also important to determine whether the patient is able to make medical and financial decisions. An often overlooked issue is whether the patient is mentally and physically capable to self-administer prescribed medication. The home environment also should be assessed, including the patient's safety and ability to call for help.[15]

10. **Frailty:**
    A. Has definite, clear-cut parameters to establish a diagnosis.
    B. Is responsible for negative health events.
    C. Is more common among individuals who have sustained a fracture.
    D. B and C.
    E. A, B, and C.

    Correct answer: D

    Comment:

    Frailty is considered to be a state of vulnerability and poor adaptability to pathological, psychological, social, or pharmacological assaults. It is responsible for negative health events, including disability, institutionalization, and death.[1,6] It could be an effective predictor of osteoporotic fracture, but unfortunately lacks a clear definition and quantification.

Other factors increasing the risk of subsequent hip fracture include older age, male sex, degree of autonomy, femoral neck and total hip bone mineral density. Several diseases increase the risk of fracture after a hip fracture, including neurological diseases, chronic obstructive pulmonary disease, diabetes mellitus, and heart failure.

Case summary

Analysis of data

Factors predisposing to bone demineralization/osteoporosis in WM's case

- Sedentary lifestyle, when not traveling.
- Living on his own since his wife died. In this cohort, the risk of malnutrition is increased and may lead to loss of bone and muscle bulk, weakness, unsteadiness, and increased falls and fractures risk.
- Cigarette smoking.
- Alcohol intake.

Factors reducing the risk of bone demineralization/osteoporosis

- The physical exercises undertaken while traveling.
- Intact cognition.

Factors increasing the risk of falls/fractures

- Alcohol intake.
- Living alone.

Factors reducing the risk of falls/fractures

- Active lifestyle.

Bone health diagnosis

1. Densitometric diagnosis:

Osteopenia, as manifested by the lowest T-score (−2.1) of the right total hip, right femoral neck, right total hip, or distal radius. The lumbar vertebrae BMD could not be appropriately analyzed because of the presence of osteophytes and osteoarthritic changes.

2. Increased fracture risk:
   According to the Fracture Risk Assessment algorithm (FRAX Score), the 10-year probability of sustaining a fracture is 3.7% and 22% for the risk of a hip and major fracture. These probabilities exceed the threshold recommended by the National Osteoporosis Foundation to initiate pharmacological treatment to reduce the fracture risk.

   The final diagnosis therefore is osteopenia, with fracture risk exceeding the NOF threshold to initiate pharmacologic treatment.

Management recommendations

Further diagnostic tests

Markers of bone resorption and bone formation to determine whether an antiresorptive or an osteoanabolic should be the first medication to be offered. The results of these tests will also determine whether the prescribed medication is the most efficacious in this particular patient at this point in time and can be used to monitor the patient's response to the prescribed medication.

Treatment recommendations

Medications

- Osteoanabolic agent.

Physical therapy/lifestyle changes

Ideally the patient should be enrolled in an exercise program supervised by an experienced physical therapist/occupational therapist and tailored to the specific needs of the individual patient. The goal is for the patient to reach confident independence to perform all the needed Activities of Daily Living (ADL).

Follow-up

A visit or telehealth encounter 4–6 weeks after starting therapy is appropriate to ensure the patient is taking the medication as directed and has not encountered any difficulty. This visit also emphasizes the importance of osteoporosis and its pharmacological treatment as well as the prescribed lifestyle changes.

Further follow-up visits will depend on the patient' condition and circumstances.

Key points

- Osteoporosis is less frequent in older men than older women, but its negative impact on morbidity and mortality is higher in men than in women.
- Bone markers can be used to identify the most appropriate medication for a given patient.
- If alcohol intake is essential for a given person, it should not exceed two drinks a day for men and one drink for women.
- Over-the-counter hypnotics should be avoided.
- Whether or not to prescribe a medication for low bone mass should be based on the presence of fragility fractures, the densitometric findings (T-scores), and the FRAX score.
- Regular follow-up is important to ensure the patient is compliant with the intake of the prescribed medication and lifestyle changes. This follow-up could be done by telehealth.

References

1. Bouvard B, Annweiler C, Legrand E. Osteoporosis in older adults. *Joint Bone Spine*. 2021;1297–1319.
2. Vandenbroucke A, Luyten EP, Flamaing J, Gielen E. Pharmacological treatment of osteoporosis in the oldest old. *Clin Interv Aging*. 2017;12:1065–1077.
3. Gosch M, Bail HJ, Grueninger S, et al. What is a reasonable rate for specific osteoporosis drug therapy in older fragility fracture patients? *Arch Osteoporos*. 2020;15:20.
4. Borgstrom F, Karlsson L, Ortsater G, et al. Fragility fractures in Europe: burden, management and opportunities. *Arch Osteoporos*. 2020;15:59.
5. Balasubramanian A, Zhang J, Chen L, et al. Risk of subsequent fracture after prior fracture among older women. *Osteoporos Int*. 2019;30:79–92.
6. Brown JP, Adachi JD, Schemitsch E, et al. Mortality in older adults following a fragility fracture: real-world retrospective matched-cohort study in Ontario. *BMC Musculoskelet Disord*. 2021;22:105–116.
7. Khosla S, Amin S, Orwoll E. Osteoporosis on men. *Endocr Rev*. 2008;29(4):441–464.
8. Cauley JA. Public health impact of osteoporosis. *J Gerontol A Biol Sci*. 2013;68(10):1243–1251.
9. Ganhao S, Guerra G, Lucas R, et al. Predictors of mortality and refracture in patients older than 65 years with a proximal femur fracture. *J Clin Rheumatol*. 2020.
10. Pizzonia M, Casabella A, Natali M, et al. Osteosarcopenia in very old age adults after hip fractures: a real-world therapeutic standpoint. *Front Med*. 2021;8:612506.
11. Teng Z, Zhu Y, et al. The analysis of osteosarcopenia as a risk factor for fractures, mortality and falls. *Osteoporos Int*. 2021;32(11):2173–2183.
12. Ramirez-Garcia E, Garcia de la Torre GS, Reyes R, et al. Factors associated with recovered functionality after hip fracture in non-institutionalized older adults: a case-control study nested in a cohort. *Clin Interv Aging*. 2021;16:1515–1525.
13. Kaufman JM. Management of osteoporosis in older men. *Aging Clin Exp Res*. 2021;33:1439–1452. 1s4.
14. Cauley JA, Cawthon PM, Peters KE, et al. Risk factors for hip fracture in older men: the osteoporotic fractures in men study (Mr. OS). *J Bone Miner Res*. 2016;31(10):1810–1819.
15. Lampshire Z, Tingley D, Jarvis A, et al. Fracture risk is under-recognized and under-treated in memory clinic attendees. *Maturitas*. 2019;123:37–39.

CHAPTER 26

Low bone mass and osteoporosis in young adults

Learning objectives

- The diagnosis of low bone mass in young adults.
- Factors affecting peak bone mass.

The case study

Reason for seeking medical help

Mrs. RT, 24 years old, is referred because, about 6 months ago, she sustained a right Colles' fracture of the distal radius while playing table tennis with her husband: she tripped and her right hand hit the table. The fracture was not displaced and healed well. She nevertheless is concerned she may have osteoporosis. She is essentially asymptomatic, has a free range of movement of the right wrist, and has no pain.

Past medical/surgical history

- No relevant medical or surgical history.
- Menarche at age 13 years, regular menstrual periods.
- Her weight has been steady. Her appetite is good. Her diet is well balanced.
- Good daily calcium intake from food, estimated at about 1200 mg daily.

Personal habits, lifestyle, daily routine

- She leads a healthy lifestyle: exercises regularly at least 1 h three times a week in a gymnasium. She has a personal trainer.
- No cigarette smoking. She consumes alcohol only in moderation, not exceeding an occasional glass of wine with dinner, once or twice a week.
- Drinks neither coffee, nor soda drinks.

Diagnosis and Treatment of Osteoporosis. https://doi.org/10.1016/B978-0-323-99550-4.00022-8
Copyright © 2024 Elsevier Inc. All rights are reserved, including those for text and data mining, AI training, and similar technologies.

Medication

- No medication intake, except for the occasional multivitamin tablet, when she remembers to take it!
- She stopped taking the ibuprofen and acetaminophen tablets prescribed after she sustained the Colles' fracture.
- No over-the-counter medication.

Family history

- Negative for osteoporosis and fractures.
- Negative for bone diseases.

Clinical examination

- She is 5′4″ tall, weighs 128 pounds.
- BP 112/72 sitting and 116/74 on standing up. No clinical evidence of orthostasis.
- No relevant clinical signs.

Laboratory investigations

- CBC and CMP within normal limits.
- Serum vitamin D: 44 ng/mL.
- Serum thyroid stimulating hormone: within the normal range.

DXA scan

- Low bone mineral density for given age: lowest Z-score: −2.3 in upper 4 lumbar vertebrae.

Multiple choice questions

1. ***The diagnosis of osteoporosis in young adults:***
   A. There are clear, well-defined clinical criteria to diagnose osteoporosis in young adults.
   B. Imaging studies are available to confirm the diagnosis of osteoporosis in young adults.
   C. Specific laboratory tests are available to confirm the diagnosis of osteoporosis in young adults.
   D. A and B.
   E. None of the above.
   Correct answer: E

Comment:

Unlike osteoporosis in postmenopausal women and older people, the diagnosis of osteoporosis in young adults is nebulous, ill-defined, largely subjective, and open to misinterpretation.[1] There is nevertheless consensus that a fragility fracture occurring in any age group is, per se, diagnostic of osteoporosis and is a required event to diagnose osteoporosis in young people. The definition of a fragility fracture is a fracture resulting from trauma that ordinarily would not be expected to cause a fracture, or occurring spontaneously, in the absence of trauma: atraumatic fracture. These issues are discussed in the section discussing the diagnosis of osteoporosis.

2. ***A low bone mass in young adults could be due to:***
   A. A number of chronic diseases preventing the expected peak bone mass from being reached.
   B. A number of lifestyle issues preventing the expected peak bone mass from being reached.
   C. A genetically determined low peak bone mass.
   D. All of the above.
   E. None of the above.

   Correct answer: D

   Comment:

   A number of factors may prevent an individual person from reaching the genetically predetermined peak bone mass, including diseases and lifestyle choices that may lead to secondary osteoporosis. Some of these are discussed in a different section. Once peak bone mass is reached and the epiphyses fuse, there is little subsequent bone growth, although through the processes of bone turnover, i.e. bone resorption and bone formation, the bone mineral content (BMC) and bone mineral density are constantly changing to strengthen individual bones, maintain their integrity, and prevent fractures, in spite of the exposure to an increased work load.

   It is well known that bones in the dominant arm of tennis players are denser than the same bones in the nondominant arm. Similarly, the bones of hemiplegic patients tend to be less dense in the paralyzed than nonparalyzed side.

3. ***Common causes of secondary osteoporosis include:***
   A. Vitamin D deficiency.
   B. Hyperparathyroidism.
   C. Juvenile rheumatoid arthritis.
   D. Any of the above.
   E. A and C.

   Correct answer: D

   Comment:

   Any of the above mentioned can lead to secondary osteoporosis.

4. ***Diseases affecting bone mass include:***
   A. Inflammatory bowel diseases.

B. Type I diabetes mellitus.
C. Secondary amenorrhea.
D. All of the above.
E. A and B.

Correct answer: D

Comment:

All of the diseases mentioned before affect bone mass, especially if they develop before the epiphyses fuse. Approximately 50%–80% of the variation in bone mass and structure among individuals is governed by heredity.[2]

The major causes of secondary osteoporosis can be grouped into 4 major categories: First, chronic inflammatory conditions such as inflammatory bowel disease, Celiac disease, juvenile rheumatoid arthritis, systemic mastocytosis, and HIV. Second, endocrinal diseases including type I diabetes mellitus, Cushing's syndrome, hyperparathyroidism, hypoparathyroidism, hyperthyroidism, and hypogonadism. Third, medications such as glucocorticoids, proton-pump inhibitors, and anticonvulsants. Fourth, lifestyle choices including sedentary lifestyles and inadequate diet with low daily calcium and mineral intake, vitamin D deficiency, alcoholism, and cigarette smoking.

5. ***Idiopathic osteoporosis in young people:***

A. Affects young men and women.
B. Is due to a defect in bone formation.
C. Can be diagnosed only after excluding common secondary causes of osteoporosis.
D. A and C.
E. A, B, and C.

Correct answer: E

Comment:

Idiopathic osteoporosis of the young affects both genders. Common secondary causes of osteoporosis, especially hypogonadism, alcoholism, and medication-inducing osteoporosis, have to be excluded before making a diagnosis. The defect in bone formation leads to decreased bone mass acquisition and a higher bone turnover rate. Idiopathic osteoporosis is also seen in premenopausal women. Its pathophysiology is not yet fully understood.[3]

6. ***The following is/are true:***

A. Pregnancy-associated osteoporosis affects about 25% of pregnant women.
B. Pregnancy is associated with an increased intestinal calcium absorption.
C. Lactation is associated with an increased intestinal calcium absorption.
D. B and C.
E. A, B, and C.

Correct answer: B

Comment:

Pregnancy-associated osteoporosis and fractures are rare and can cause severe back pain, fractures, loss of height, and disability.[4] The etiology, pathogenesis, natural history, and management are not clearly defined. During pregnancy the mother's intestinal calcium absorption is increased. It tends to return to normal levels during lactation. The mother's body adjusts by increasing intestinal bone resorption and decreasing renal calcium excretion.[5] It seems to respond well to denosumab.[5]

7. ***Postpregnancy osteoporosis may lead to:***
   A. Fractures.
   B. Height loss.
   C. Severe back pain.
   D. All of the above.
   E. None of the above; it is a benign, physiologic, self-limited condition.

   Correct answer: D

   Comment:

   In addition to the above mentioned, postpregnancy osteoporosis may present as transient osteoporosis of the hip(s), sometimes complicated by fragility fractures of one or both hips.
8. ***Management of osteoporosis in the young should include:***
   A. Correcting any underlying nutritional deficiency, especially vitamin D.
   B. Adequate calcium and protein intake.
   C. Increasing level of physical activity.
   D. Treating any underlying condition.
   E. All of the above.

   Correct answer: E

   Comment:

   These are the sine qua non for the appropriate management of diseases and are discussed in various sections.
9. ***The following diseases increase the risk of osteoporosis in young people:***
   A. Inflammatory bowel disease.
   B. Type I diabetes mellitus.
   C. Hyperthyroidism.
   D. Rheumatoid arthritis.
   E. All of the above.

   Correct answer: E

   Comment:

   All of the above-mentioned diseases increase the risk of osteoporosis in young people.
10. ***The following is/are correct:***
   A. The FRAX algorithm is valid for all ages, including young adults.
   B. The relationship between BMD and fracture risk is well established in young adults.
   C. Bone turnover markers are not useful while developing a management strategy for young people with osteoporosis.

D. Vertebral fractures are rare in men with idiopathic osteoporosis.
E. None of the above.

Correct answer: E

Comment:

All these statements are incorrect and are discussed in other sections.

Case summary

Analysis of data

Osteoporosis is rare in young people and is usually associated with a number of diseases. Postpregnancy associated osteoporosis may present with back pain and lead to increased fracture risk.

Diagnosis

- Low bone mass for given age.
- Status post right Colles' fragility fracture.

Management recommendations

Further diagnostic tests

- None indicated at this stage.

Pharmacological treatment recommendations

- None indicated at this stage.

Follow-up recommendations

- A repeat DXA scan in 2–3 years to monitor the bone mass.

Key points

- The diagnosis of osteoporosis in young adults is nebulous, ill-defined, largely subjective, and open to misinterpretation.[1]
- A fragility fracture occurring in any age group is, per se, diagnostic of osteoporosis and is a required event to diagnose osteoporosis in young people.
- A number of factors may prevent an individual person from reaching the genetically predetermined peak bone mass, including diseases and lifestyle choices that may lead to secondary osteoporosis.

References

1. Ferrari S, Bianchi ML, Eisman JA, et al. Osteoporosis in young adults: pathophysiology, diagnosis and management. *Osteoporos Int*. 2012;23:2735–2748.
2. Ferrari S. Human genes and osteoporosis. *Best Pract Res Clin Endocrinol Metab*. 2008;22:723–735.
3. Yun KY, Han ES, Kim SC, et al. Pregnancy-related osteoporosis and spinal fractures. *Obstet Gynecol Sci*. 2017;60(1):133–137.
4. Bazgir N, Shafiei E, Hashemi N, Nourmohamadi H. Woman with pregnancy and lactation associated osteoporosis. *Case Rep Obstet Gynecol*. 2020; [Article ID 8836583].
5. Sanchez A, Zanchetta MB, Danilowicz K. Two cases of pregnancy and lactation associated osteoporosis successfully treated with denosumab. *Clin Cases Miner Bone Metab*. 2016;13(3):244–246.

Iatrogenic osteoporosis☆

Learning objectives

- Glucocorticoids induce bone loss, lead to osteoporosis, and increase the patient's fracture risk.
- Glucocorticoid-induced bone loss and increased fracture risk can be reduced.

The case study

Reason for seeking medical help

- Mrs. GOI, 57 years old, has been diagnosed with giant cell arteritis about 4 weeks ago. She responded only to very high doses of corticosteroid therapy and is referred because of concerns about her bone health: the plan is to continue with high doses of prednisone: 60–120 mg daily for at least 6, probably 12 months.

Past medical and surgical history

- No relevant past medical history except for a bout of giant cell arteritis (GCA) about 3 years ago which was successfully treated with very large doses of prednisone.
- Mrs. GOI always enjoyed good health and led a physically active lifestyle.
- Menarche at age 13 years, regular menstrual periods.
- Natural menopause at age 46 years, no hormonal replacement therapy.
- Three children aged 39, 37, and 32 years, all in good health.

Lifestyle

- Mentally good and physically independent, drives her own car.
- Lives on her own since the death of her husband about 4 years ago.
- Retired dietitian works on a part-time basis 3 days a week in the local hospital and as a volunteer in the town visitors' center during weekends.

☆ Mrs. GOI, 53 years old, prescribed prednisone in large doses for giant cell arteritis.

Diagnosis and Treatment of Osteoporosis. https://doi.org/10.1016/B978-0-323-99550-4.00034-4
Copyright © 2024 Elsevier Inc. All rights are reserved, including those for text and data mining, AI training, and similar technologies.

- Good appetite, well-balanced, nutritious diet. No weight loss.
- No cigarette smoking, no alcohol intake, no caffeine intake, no excessive sodium intake.

Medication(s)

- Prednisone 80 mg daily, this is the lowest dose that controlled the giant cell arteritis.
- Vitamin D3 1000 units daily.
- Multivitamins 1 tablet daily.

Family history

- Negative for osteoporosis.

Clinical examination

Weight 115 pounds, steady; height 65″, no height loss.

Fading clinical evidence of giant cell arteritis.

Sitting BP 126/78, no postural drop, no orthostasis. No cushingoid features. Mild osteoarthritic changes in knees and hands, not interfering with daily activities. No clinical evidence of heart failure, good peripheral circulation, no significant clinical signs.

Laboratory results

She recently had the following laboratory tests done as part of her annual physical examination: comprehensive metabolic profile, complete blood count, serum TSH, and serum vitamin D. All were within the normal range. Erythrocyte sedimentation rate: 38 mm in first hour was much higher when the GCA was active.

DXA and radiologic results

T-scores: −1.0 in the upper four lumbar vertebrae; −0.8 and −0.6 in the right and left femoral necks, respectively; and −0.9 in the distal nondominant one-third radius. FRAX scores 1.2% and 9% for the 10-year risk of hip and major osteoporotic fractures, respectively.

Multiple choice questions

1. ***In Mrs. GOI's case, the following is/are correct:***
   A. The diagnosis is osteopenia.
   B. The fracture risk is not increased.
   C. There is no need for any medication for her bone health.

D. All of the above.

E. None of the above.

Correct answer: E

Comment:

The lowest T-score is −1.0, which is within the normal range. There is therefore densitometric evidence of neither osteopenia nor osteoporosis. Glucocorticoids, however, per se, increase the risk of fracture through a variety of mechanisms that are discussed later. Therefore, even though the bone density is within the normal range, Mrs. GOI is at an increased risk of fractures because of the glucocorticoids she has been prescribed, especially in large doses and the need to continue with this therapy.

She therefore should be aggressively treated to maintain her bone mass. There is some urgency in the pharmacological management of Mrs. GOI because she is on a high dose of glucocorticoids, which she needs to treat her giant cell arteritis. This is discussed further later.

2. ***Bone loss associated with glucocorticoids:***

A. Is accentuated during the first 3 months of therapy.

B. Peaks at about 6months of therapy, then continues to increase, but at a slower rate.

C. Increased fracture risk is related to the daily and cumulative dose of glucocorticoids.

D. A and B.

E. A, B, and C.

Correct answer: E

Comment:

Glucocorticoid-induced osteoporosis is the most frequent type of secondary osteoporosis. Bone loss is accentuated during the first 3months of therapy, peaks at about 6months of continuous use, and then continues at a slower rate but remains elevated for the duration of glucocorticoid therapy. During the first year of therapy, 6%–12% of the BMD may be lost; the annual rate of decrease thereafter is about 3%. Although both cortical and cancellous bones are affected, the latter is more severely affected.[1] High daily doses and high cumulative doses increase the risk of fractures. The rate of bone loss declines once glucocorticoid therapy is discontinued, but it is not clear whether it reverts to the baseline preglucocorticoid therapy level.

Glucocorticoids are frequently prescribed to older people for a variety of reasons. More than 10% of patients on long-term glucocorticoid therapy sustain a clinical fracture and 30%–40% have evidence of morphometric vertebral compression fractures.

The increased fracture risk parallels the decrease in BMD, is seen as early as the first 3months of therapy, and is also modulated by other effects of glucocorticoids, including osteoblastic inhibition and apoptosis (therefore decreased bone formation), osteoclastic stimulation leading to an increased expression of Receptor Activator of Nuclear Factor Kappa-ß (RANK-L) ligand (therefore increased bone resorption), and a decreased osteoprotegrin expression and reduced osteoclastic apoptosis. Glucocorticoids also impair osteocyte function and increase their apoptosis.[1,2]

A number of guidelines and algorithms are available to help clinicians decide when and how to treat patients on long-term glucocorticoid therapy including the FRAX and NOGG (National Osteoporosis Guideline Group), the International Osteoporosis Foundation, and the European Calcified Tissue Society algorithms and the American College of Rheumatology.[1]

In addition, glucocorticoids reduce gastrointestinal calcium absorption, increase renal calcium excretion, and reduce gonadal hormones, which induce myopathy and muscle atrophy leading to impaired neuromuscular functions and thus an increased risk of sustaining repeated falls and fracture(s). Alternate day regimens, intermittent therapy, and inhaled glucocorticoids are also associated with nefarious skeletal effects.

3. ***Assessing fracture risk in patients on glucocorticoids:***
   A. The FRAX tool overestimates the risk of fractures in patients on $\leq$2.5 mg prednisone daily.
   B. The FRAX tool underestimates the risk of fractures in patients on $\geq$7.5 mg prednisone daily.
   C. A number of algorithms are available to assess the patient's fracture risk.
   D. A and B.
   E. A, B, and C.

   Correct answer: E

   Comment:

   A number of algorithms are available to assess the fracture risk of patients on glucocorticoid therapy. The FRAX algorithm, however, is of limited use in patients on glucocorticoids because it considers neither the daily dose, nor the cumulative dose, nor the duration of treatment. Adjustments, nevertheless, can be made to the FRAX algorithm to better reflect the fracture risk in patients on glucocorticoid therapy. Because fracture risk is modulated by the dose of glucocorticoids, many algorithms classify the patient population on daily glucocorticoid therapy into those on high doses, i.e., those on 7.5 mg or more of prednisone or equivalent and those on smaller doses: 2.5 mg daily or less. It is possible, however, that even this classification underestimates the fracture risk in patients on very high-dose glucocorticoids as is the case in patients with giant cell arteritis, dermatomyositis, lupus, and vasculitis. Patients on high doses, i.e., exceeding 30 mg/day, even in those receiving that dose intermittently, are particularly at risk of sustaining hip and vertebral fractures.

   Glucocorticoid-induced osteoporosis is potentially reversible: once glucocorticoids are discontinued the BMD gradually increases and the increased fracture risk gradually declines.[3]

4. **The initial assessment of patients on glucocorticoid therapy includes:**
   A. An assessment of the fracture risk.

B. An assessment of the risk of falling.
C. A review of the glucocorticoid daily dose, frequency, and cumulative dose.
D. A, B, and C.
E. A and C.

Correct answer: D

Comment:

The initial fracture risk assessment should be made as soon as possible after initiating long-term glucocorticoid therapy. It should include an assessment of the fracture risk. If the FRAX tool is to be utilized, it first should be corrected for the intake of glucocorticoids.[4] As the FRAX does not include the risk of falling and as fractures are usually preceded by falls it is important to also determine the patient's risk of falling as this may alter the overall management strategy.

A thorough review of the patient's medication should be done with particular emphasis on medication that can affect cognitive functions and increase the risk of falling. As much as possible sedatives, tranquilizers and hypnotics should be avoided. The daily dose, frequency, and cumulative dose of glucocorticoids are also important as they affect the fracture risk.

5. **Direct effects of glucocorticoids on bone cells and bone turnover include:**

A. Increase bone resorption.
B. Decrease bone formation.
C. Induce osteocytes apoptosis.
D. A and C.
E. A, B, and C.

Correct answer: E

Comment:

Glucocorticoids increase the rate of bone resorption through a variety of mechanisms including[5]:

- Effect on osteoclasts:
  - Stimulating the synthesis and release of RANK-L, thus increasing the recruitment and activation of osteoclasts.
  - Decreasing osteoprotegerin expression by osteoblasts, thus increasing the impact of RANK-L on preosteoclasts and their precursors.
  - Decreasing osteoclast apoptosis, thus further enhancing bone resorption.
- Effect on osteoblasts:
  - Suppress osteoblast differentiation.
  - Induce osteoblast apoptosis, thus reducing the rate of bone formation. Decreases in the serum levels of markers of bone formation have been documented almost immediately after the initiation of glucocorticoid therapy. Stimulate bone marrow stromal cells to differentiate into adipocytes rather than osteoblasts, thus reducing the number of functional osteoblasts and rate of bone formation.

- Effect on osteocytes:
  - Induce apoptosis of osteocytes, thus reducing their number.
  - Impair the osteocyte ability to increase local bone remodeling.

6. ***Glucocorticoid-induced changes in BMD and bone architecture include:***

A. Lower total, cortical, and trabecular volumetric BMD.
B. Increased trabecular separation and reduced trabecular number.
C. Lower trabecular bone score.
D. A and C.
E. A, B, and C.

Correct answer: E

Comment:

In addition to loss of bone mass, glucocorticoids induce profound changes in bone microarchitecture and strength which increase the fracture risk. Trabecular bone is affected more than cortical bone. This explains the high prevalence of vertebral compression fractures, most of which are asymptomatic because of the antiinflammatory effect of glucocorticoids. The risk of vertebral fractures is increased even in patients on very small doses of glucocorticoids such as 2.5 mg daily. The glucocorticoid increased risk of vertebral compression fractures is independent of the observed decreases in BMD.

7. ***Glucocorticoids also induce bone demineralization by:***

A. Reducing intestinal calcium absorption.
B. Increasing renal calcium loss.
C. Reducing gonadal hormone.
D. A and B.
E. A, B, and C.

Correct answer: E

Comment:

Glucocorticoids increase bone loss through a number of factors, in addition to the direct effect on osteocytes, osteoblasts, and osteoclasts. These include:

- Reducing the intestinal calcium absorption by inhibiting vitamin D action and down-regulating the expression of calcium receptors in the duodenum. Increasing the renal calcium loss by down-regulating the expression of tubular calcium receptors in the kidneys.
- Increasing the release of parathyroid hormone as a result of the tendency for the serum calcium level to fall secondary to the low intestinal absorption of calcium and increased renal calcium loss.
- Decreased production of growth hormone, insulin-like growth factor 1 (IGF1), and IGF1 binding protein.
- Interfering with the hypothalamus-pituitary-adrenal-gonadal axis reducing the synthesis and release of gonadotropin-releasing hormone, luteinizing hormone, and follicle-stimulating hormone in the hypothalamus and inducing hypogonadism.

- Glucocorticoids also increase the risk of falls and subsequent fractures by inducing a myopathy due to:
- Increased muscle proteolysis.
- Reduced protein synthesis.
- The production of myostatin which inhibits myogenesis.

Other extrinsic factors leading to bone demineralization include reduced physical activity and the underlying disease state for which glucocorticoids are prescribed.

8. ***Other adverse effects of glucocorticoid therapy include:***

A. Hypertension, hyperlipidemia, and hyperglycemia.
B. Cataracts and glaucoma.
C. Easy bruisability.
D. A and C.
E. A, B, and C.

Correct answer: E

Comment:

Glucocorticoid therapy is associated with a number of adverse events in addition to the listed one, including weight gain, fluid retention, increased susceptibility to infections, hypokalemia, depression, neuropsychiatric disorders, and osteonecrosis. Notwithstanding, in some patients the risk/benefit ratio is such that glucocorticoids, sometimes in large doses, have to be prescribed for prolonged periods as in cases of giant cell arteritis, other vasculitis, status asthmaticus, and inflammatory bowel diseases. In these instances, it behooves the prescribing clinician to ensure the patient is informed and that adequate measures are taken to minimize the associated risks and that patients are adequately followed up.

9. ***Nonpharmacologic management of patients on glucocorticoids ≥2.5 mg/day for 3 or more months includes:***

A. A daily calcium intake of 1000–1200 mg.
B. A daily vitamin D intake of 600–800 IU.
C. Lifestyle modification, including weight-bearing exercises.
D. A and B.
E. A, B, and C.

Correct answer: E

Comment:

Nonpharmacologic management of patients on glucocorticoids ≥2.5 mg/day for 3 or more months includes an adequate daily calcium and vitamin D intake, preferably from food sources, but failing this from supplements. Patients who have laboratory evidence of vitamin D deficiency may need larger doses of vitamin D. Vitamin D supplementation is discussed in another chapter.

Lifestyle modification is an integral part of the management of all patients at risk of fractures and includes balanced diet, weight-bearing exercises, limited alcohol intake, and smoking cessation.

10. ***Pharmacologic management of glucocorticoid-induced osteoporosis includes:***
    A. Oral or iv bisphosphonates.
    B. Teriparatide or abaloparatide.
    C. Denosumab.
    D. Raloxifene.
    E. A, B, C, or D.

    Correct answer: E

    Comment:

    A number of guidelines are available to help clinicians develop a treatment strategy geared to the particular needs and circumstances of the patient in question.[1] Oral bisphosphonates are frequently recommended as a first-line treatment and prevention of glucocorticoid-induced osteoporosis in patients on 2.5 mg or more prednisone daily for 3 or more months. If the patient cannot tolerate them or cannot adhere to the intake of oral bisphosphonates, all the previously listed medications are effective at increasing BMD and reducing fracture risk. It is also important to emphasize the importance of a well-balanced diet, adequate calcium, vitamin D intake, and lifestyle changes to maximize the impact of the medication prescribed.

References

1. Cho SK, Sung YK. Update on glucocorticoid induced osteoporosis. *Endocrinol Metab.* 2021;36:536–543.
2. Wang L, Heckmann BL, Yang X, Long H. Osteoblast autophagy in glucocorticoid-induced osteoporosis. *J Cell Physiol.* 2019;234(4):3207–3215.
3. Buckley L, Humphrey MB. Glucocorticoid-induced osteoporosis. *N Engl J Med.* 2018;379:2547–2556.
4. FRAX. www.shef.ac.uk/FRAX/tool.jsp.
5. Deng J, Silver Z, Huang E, et al. Pharmacologic prevention of fractures in patients undergoing glucocorticoid therapies: a systemic review and network meta-analysis. *Rheumatology.* 2021;60:649–657.

CHAPTER 28

Primary hyperparathyroidism☆

Learning objectives

- Appreciate the presentation, diagnosis, and management of primary hyperparathyroidism.
- Know the differences between primary and secondary hyperparathyroidism.
- Recognize the main causes of hypercalcemia.

The case study

Reason for seeking medical help

Mrs. TW, 56-year-old Black woman, sustained a fragility fracture of her right radius about 3 weeks ago. Hypercalcemia was noted on routine CMP. Subsequently the serum parathyroid hormone level was elevated, and serum 25-hydroxy-vitamin D level was within normal range. She is asymptomatic except for a worsening "low energy level" and depression. She refuses to consult a psychiatrist and refuses to take any antidepressant medication. She works as a primary school teacher.

Past medical/surgical history

- Natural menopause, at age 51 years, no HRT.
- Renal calculi 5 and 2 years ago.

Personal habits

- Sedentary lifestyle.
- Daily calcium intake: about 400 mg: has been restricting calcium intake because of renal calculi.
- No cigarette smoking.
- No excessive sodium, caffeine, or alcohol intake.

☆ Mrs. TW, 56-year-old Black woman, with osteoporosis and hypercalcemia.

Diagnosis and Treatment of Osteoporosis. https://doi.org/10.1016/B978-0-323-99550-4.00035-6
Copyright © 2024 Elsevier Inc. All rights are reserved, including those for text and data mining, AI training, and similar technologies.

Medication

- No medication.

Family history

- Negative for osteoporosis.

Clinical examination

- Weight 148 pounds, steady; height 63″.
- No significant clinical findings.

Laboratory investigations

- CMP: hypercalcemia: 10.8 mg/dL, otherwise no abnormality, eGFR >60 mL/min.
- Serum vitamin D: 35 ng/mL.
- Serum iPTH: 218 g/mL.

Multiple choice questions

1. ***In Mrs. TW's case, the laboratory findings are suggestive of:***
   A. Primary hyperparathyroidism.
   B. Secondary hyperparathyroidism.
   C. Osteoporosis.
   D. A and C.
   E. B and C.
   Correct answer: D
   Comment:
   The characteristic diagnostic features of Primary Hyperparathyroidism (PHPT) are hypercalcemia and an elevated or "inappropriately normal" serum parathyroid level. Normally an inverse relationship exists between serum calcium and parathyroid hormone levels.[1,2] In Mrs. TW's case, however, both the serum calcium and parathyroid hormone (PTH) levels are elevated. The likely diagnosis therefore is primary hyperparathyroidism (PHPT). As she also sustained a fragility fracture, she has osteoporosis regardless of her T-score. The final diagnosis therefore is osteoporosis and primary hyperparathyroidism.
   PHPT is a very common endocrine disorder and is the leading cause of hypercalcemia in outpatients. In the USA, its prevalence is estimated to be 0.86%.[3] Its epidemiology has changed as the introduction of multichannel serum auto-analyzers leads to the identification of several asymptomatic patients with the biochemical characteristic features of PHPT.[4–6] The proportion of patients presenting with the classical characteristic

features of nephrolithiasis and nephrocalcinosis, originally about two-thirds of the patient population, and osteitis fibrosa cystica (brown tumors and periosteal bone resorption of the long bones), originally about a third of the patient population, is shrinking. Primary hyperparathyroidism is now predominantly diagnosed in asymptomatic Black women, especially within the first 10years after the menopause.[7] It tends to have a worse prognosis in women than in men.[8,9] About 70%–80% of patients with primary hyperparathyroidism now present during the asymptomatic stage.[3]

A large descriptive epidemiological study performed on about 3.5 million enrollees in the Kaiser Permanente, Southern California, revealed that the incidence of PHPT (as diagnosed by hypercalcemia and elevated PTH or "inappropriately normal" PTH levels) fluctuated in women from 34 to 120 per 100,000 person-years (mean 66), and in men between 13 and 36 (mean 25). The incidence increased with age and the differences between the genders became more pronounced: 12–24 per 100,000 for both sexes under the age of 50years; 80 and 36 per 100,000 for women and men between the ages of 50 and 59years, respectively; and 196 and 95 for women and men aged 70–79years, respectively. The incidence of PHPT was higher among Black (92 women, 46 men) than White women (81 women, 29 men), Asians (52 women, 28 men), and Hispanics (49 women, 17 men). Of interest, the prevalence of PHPT tripled during the study period (1995–2010) increasing from 76 to 233 per 100,000 women and from 30 to 85 per 100,000 men.[10]

Patients with parathyroid cancer are usually much younger that those with PHPT: between the ages of 40 and 50years. Unlike PHPT which affects women more than men, parathyroid cancer affects both genders about equally. Their serum calcium and PTH levels are much higher than those seen in patients with PHPT. Nephrolithiasis, nephrocalcinosis, and bone diseases are more prominent in parathyroid cancer than in PHPT.[11]

Brown tumors are rare benign lesions developing during the remodeling process in advanced, long-lasting primary or secondary hyperparathyroidism. They are rarely seen nowadays as in most instances the diagnosis of hyperparathyroidism is made early during the increased remodeling process. They are sometimes misdiagnosed as nontreatable osteosarcomas. Characteristic diagnostic features of brown tumors include elevated serum parathyroid hormone and calcium levels. Bone imaging studies help exclude bone malignancy. Selective parathyroidectomy is the first-line therapy.[12]

Rarely, primary hyperparathyroidism is inherited as an autosomal dominant trait including multiple endocrine neoplasia type I (MEN1, MEN2, MEN4) and familial hypocalciuric hypercalcemia (FHH).[13]

2. ***Match the following:***
   (a) Hypercalcemia and elevated PTH level.
   (b) Hypercalcemia with suppressed PTH level.
   (c) Both.
   (d) Neither.

A. Primary hyperparathyroidism.
B. Secondary hyperparathyroidism.
C. Familial hypocalciuric hypercalcemia.
D. Lithium.
E. Thiazide diuretics.

Correct answers: A (a); B (b); C (a); D (a); E (c)

Comment:

In patients with hypoalbuminemia, the assayed serum calcium level should be first adjusted to the serum albumin level.[11,14] Directly assaying the ionized serum calcium level obviates the need to adjust the serum calcium level to the serum albumin level and is routinely done in several laboratories. In secondary hyperparathyroidism (SHPT), the serum calcium level is not elevated; instead, it is usually in the low normal range, but may also be low, depending on the efficacy of parathyroid hormone at maintaining the serum calcium within the normal range.

Several factors may contribute to hypercalcemia in patients on long-term thiazide therapy, including reduced renal calcium excretion, increased intestinal calcium absorption, metabolic alkalosis, and hemoconcentration. As the hypercalcemia is sometimes associated with elevated serum parathyroid hormone levels and as the hypercalcemia often persists after the discontinuation of the diuretic, it is possible that, in some patients, long-term thiazide therapy uncovers previously unknown hyperparathyrodism.[15,16]

Lithium induces hypercalcemia and elevated or nonsuppressed PTH levels by interfering with CaSRs. 10%–20% of patients on lithium develop hypercalcemia, a condition sometimes referred to as "lithium-associated hyperparathyroidism."[15,17–19] It is therefore recommended to assay the serum calcium levels at least annually in patients on lithium therapy. Other causes of hypercalcemia with suppressed PTH levels include sarcoidosis, malignancy-associated hypercalcemia, Addison's disease, vitamin D intoxication, and prolonged immobilization. The chloride/phosphate ratio is sometimes used to differentiate hypercalcemia due to PHPT from hypercalcemia due to other causes: a ratio greater than 33 is suggestive of PHPT.[20]

3. ***The main actions of parathyroid hormone include:***

A. Activation of osteoclastic bone resorption.
B. Increased renal calcium reabsorption from the distal convoluted tubules.
C. Stimulating the 1-alpha-hydroxylase enzyme in the kidneys.
D. A and B.
E. A, B, and C.

Correct answer: E

Comment:

The main function of PTH is to maintain the serum calcium level within a narrow range of normality. As soon as the calcium-sensing receptors (CaSRs) in the parathyroid chief cells detect any decrease in ionized serum calcium level they trigger the immediate release of PTH.[21]

PTH increases serum calcium level through three main mechanisms. First, activation of osteoclastic bone resorption, thus mobilizing calcium from bone matrix to the circulation; second, increasing renal calcium absorption in distal convoluted tubules, thus saving any calcium that would have otherwise been lost in the urine; and third, stimulation of 1-alpha hydroxylase enzyme in the kidneys to hydroxylate 25-hydroxy-vitamin D at the 1-position to yield 1,25 di-hydroxy-vitamin D, the most active vitamin D metabolite which increases intestinal calcium absorption.[11,21,22] When the serum calcium level normalizes, the CaSRs are no longer stimulated and the release of PTH is stemmed. Normally there exists an inverse relationship between serum calcium, especially ionized serum calcium, and the serum PTH level.[11]

- In **primary hyperparathyroidism (PHPT)**, the inverse relationship between serum calcium and PTH levels is not seen and both serum calcium and PTH levels are elevated because in these patients the production and release of PTH is autonomous and independent of the serum calcium level.
- In **normocalcemic hyperparathyroidism**, the serum calcium level is within the normal range, but the PTH is elevated in the absence of secondary causes of hyperparathyroidism. Normocalcemic hyperparathyroidism may be the precursor of PHPT.
- In **secondary hyperparathyroidism** (SHPT), the parathyroid glands try to maintain the serum calcium level within the range of normality by increasing the production and release of PTH stimulated by a low or decreasing serum calcium level. Therefore, in SHPT, the serum calcium is within or below the normal range, depending on the ability of the parathyroid glands to produce/release sufficient quantities of PTH to prevent hypocalcemia. The serum PTH is elevated.
- **Tertiary hyperparathyroidism** is characterized by an excessive/prolonged production of PTH after a long period of secondary hyperparathyroidism when the parathyroid glands were stimulated to produce/release larger quantities of PTH to prevent hypocalcemia from developing. In tertiary hyperparathyroidism, however, the excessive PTH production and release are no longer in response to any stimulus and the serum calcium level is elevated. Tertiary hyperparathyroidism is therefore the end result of prolonged SHPT. It is possible that the calcium-sensing receptors in the parathyroid glands have altered their set point and more PTH is produced/released even in the presence of hypercalcemia. Tertiary hyperparathyroidism is seen in patients with chronic kidney disease and postrenal transplant.[23]

4. ***Classical features of primary hyperparathyroidism include:***
   A. Osteitis fibrosa cystica.
   B. Increased bone turnover rate.
   C. Nephrolithiasis and nephrocalcinosis.
   D. A and C.
   E. A, B, and C.

   Correct answer: E

Comment:

The incidence of primary hyperparathyroidism increases with age in both sexes.[3] **Osteitis fibrosa cystica** refers to the radiological pathognomonic skeletal radiological features of primary hyperparathyroidism which include "salt-and-pepper" degranulation of the skull, subperiosteal resorption of the distal phalanges, tapering of the distal clavicle, bone cysts and brown tumors, often associated with skeletal deformities and fractures. Bone pain and swelling are often the presenting symptoms and usually affect the ribs, clavicles, pelvis, and mandible.[24] They sometimes are erroneously suspected of being bone metastases.[25]

The full spectrum of osteitis fibrosa cystica is rarely seen nowadays as in most instances the diagnosis of PHPT is made after finding an asymptomatic elevated serum calcium level which prompts the patient's investigation and diagnosis of PHPT, prior to its full-blown manifestation.

In Western countries, about 80% of patients with PHPT are diagnosed as a result of a blood profile done for some unrelated medical condition.[21,26]

Common skeletal manifestations include low BMD, low trabecular bone score (an indirect measure of trabecular microarchitecture and strength independent of BMD), and an increased fracture risk especially in cortical bones such as the distal 1/3 radius which are affected to a larger extent than the proximal femoral and lumbar vertebrae. This pattern of bone loss is different from that seen in postmenopausal women which tends to affect trabecular bone earlier and to a larger extent than cortical bone.[21,26]

Successful parathyroidectomy is associated with significant increases in BMD which tend to occur first and to a larger extent in the trabecular bones.[21,26] Similarly, bisphosphonates and estrogen increase BMD in patients who do not undergo surgery.[27] The administration of Cinacalcet, however, does not improve BMD although it reduces the serum calcium level.[26]

Levels of bone turnover markers are elevated in untreated patients with PHPT, and decrease rapidly, usually within hours after successful surgical parathyroidectomy.[28] This decrease is also seen, albeit less rapidly, in patients treated with estrogen, raloxifene, and bisphosphonates, but not cinacalcet. The decrease in levels of bone turnover markers is associated with an increase in BMD and a reduced fracture risk.[26]

Nephrocalcinosis and nephrolithiasis are characteristic features of PHPT because the kidneys have such a pivotal role in calcium metabolism regulating the concentration of serum calcium and phosphate and determining the whole body calcium and phosphate.[26] Factors regulating renal tubular calcium reabsorption include parathyroid hormone, calcium-sensing receptors, filtered sodium load, and tubular calcium transporters.[29] The reduction in glomerular filtration rate often seen in patients with PHPT is due to either complications of PHPT or comorbid conditions. Renal imaging for nephrocalcinosis and nephrolithiasis is recommended. Positive imaging is an indication for surgery. The risk of renal calculi formation should be assessed and above average fluid intake should be encouraged in patients who do not undergo surgery.[26]

A number of **nonspecific manifestations have been reported in patients with PHPT.**[30] Often patients are not aware of these and report dramatic improvements in their quality of life after successful parathyroidiectomy.[31–35] Psychiatric manifestations range from mild depression and anxiety to paranoid delusions, visual and auditory hallucinations. Patients often have shortened attention spans, impaired concentration, impaired memory, and impaired executive functions and complain of intellectual weariness.[36–38] Sleep and circadian rhythm disturbances are also reported.[39]

PHPT is also associated with an increased left ventricular mass; increased risk of coronary artery disease, hypertension, valvular and myocardial calcifications; and dysfunction of the cardiac microcirculation.[40] Arrhythmias and cardiac mortality in patients with PHPT are increased.[41] Abnormalities in the cerebral circulation have been reported.[42] Peptic ulcer disease and pancreatitis are also seen in primary hyperparathyroidism.[43]

Normocalcemic hyperparathyroidism is a variant of PHPT. Its diagnosis is established by finding a normal serum total calcium (adjusted for the albumin level) and ionized calcium in the presence of an elevated serum PTH level on at least three occasions over a period of 3–6 months, after causes of secondary hyperparathyroidism have been excluded. It has been postulated that NPHPT is the first phase of a biphasic disorder which eventually manifests itself at a later stage as hypercalcemic PHPT. NPHPT therefore is considered to be part of the diagnostic spectrum of PHPT.[15]

Common causes of elevated PTH and normal serum calcium levels include vitamin D insufficiency/deficiency; chronic renal diseases; hypercalciuria; gastrointestinal diseases (including gluten enteropathy) associated with calcium malabsorption; and a number of medications, including thiazides, bisphosphonates, denosumab, and lithium. These should be ruled out before making a diagnosis of normocalcemic PHPT.[15,44]

5. ***Match the following bone loss:***
   (a) Due to postmenopause estrogen deprivation.
   (b) Due to primary hyperparathyroidism.
   (c) Both.
   (d) Neither.
   A. Affects predominantly skeletal sites with high cortical bone content.
   B. Affects predominantly skeletal sites with high trabecular bone content.
   C. Increased fracture risk.
   D. Increased surface area of the distal radius.
   E. Reduced by bisphosphonates.

   Correct answers: A (b); B (a); C (c); D (b); E (c)

   Comment:

   Both estrogen deprivation and PHPT induce an increased rate of bone turnover, a reduced bone mass, and an increased fracture risk. However, whereas in postmenopausal women the rate of bone resorption is increased primarily through estrogen deficiency and an increased release of RANK-L which stimulates the formation/activation of osteoclasts, and affects initially the more vascular trabecular bone, such as the vertebrae, in PHPT the increased rate of bone turnover is triggered through the stimulation of receptors on the surface of osteoblasts and preosteoblasts down-regulating sclerostin leading to an increased differentiation, activity, and life span of osteoblasts and increased bone formation. A secondary effect is the increased release of RANK-L by osteoblasts, which activates osteoclastic bone resorption, thus increasing bone turnover.[45,46] PTH also decreases osteoprotegerin release further increasing osteoclastic bone-resorbing activity and hence rate of bone turnover. Initially hyperparathyroidism targets cortical more than trabecular bone, whereas estrogen deficiency targets trabecular more than cortical bone.[45,47]

6. ***Indications for parathyroid surgery include:***
   A. Hypercalcemia.
   B. Creatinine clearance below 60 mL/min.
   C. Asymptomatic patients with PHPT.
   D. A and C.
   E. A, B, and C.

Correct answer: E

Comments:

A solitary adenoma is the underlying etiology of primary hyperparathyroidism in 85%–90% of cases. Multiglandular hyperplasia affects about 15% of cases. Parathyroid carcinoma is very rare.[3,48] Parathyroid surgery should be considered in patients with PHPT especially in the following instances:

- Age under 50 years
- Serum calcium level more than 1.0 mg/dL (0.25 nmol/L) above the upper limit of the normal range, or
- Creatinine clearance less than 60 mL/min, 24-h urinary calcium exceeds 400 mg, presence of nephrolithiasis, nephrocalcinosis (X-ray, ultrasound, or CT), or
- DXA lowest T-score: −2.5 or lower at lumbar vertebrae, total hip, femoral neck, or distal 1/3 radius or
- Fragility fracture, including evidence of vertebral fracture by X-ray, CT, MRI, or VFA
- Medical surveillance is not possible.

Surgical parathyroidectomy is the only option that potentially cures PHPT.[8,49,50] The surgery is minimally invasive, usually performed under local anesthesia and conscious sedation. An index of successful surgery is the serum PTH level dropping by more than 50% into the normal range within 10 min of the surgical removal of the abnormal parathyroid gland(s). Cure rates exceed 98%.[11]

Several prospective studies have documented the positive effects of surgical parathyroidectomy in patients with primary hyperparathyroidism on BMD, fracture risk,

risk of developing renal calculi, and risk of renal impairment even in asymptomatic patients.[1,51–55]

Recommended monitoring of patients with PHPT who do not undergo surgery includes[48]:

- Annual serum calcium assay.
- Annual or every 2 years DXA (three sites), X-ray, or VFA if clinically indicated (height loss, back pain).
- Annual eGFR and serum creatinine.
- If renal calculi suspected: 24-h biochemical stone profile, renal imaging: X-ray, ultrasound, or CT.

7. ***Pharmacologic management of primary hyperparathyroidism includes:***
   A. Bisphosphonates.
   B. Calcium and vitamin D restriction.
   C. Cinacalcet.
   D. A and C.
   E. A, B, and C.

   Correct answer: D

   Comment:

   For patients with PHPT who refuse or cannot undergo surgery, oral bisphosphonates reduce serum calcium levels, increase BMD, reduce fracture risk, and improve survival, but to a lesser extent than surgical parathyroidectomy.[56] Calcium and vitamin D should not be restricted. Among patients with PHPT those who in addition have hypovitaminosis D tend to have higher rates of bone turnover, lower BMD, and an increased fracture risk.[57] Similarly, postsurgical parathyroidectomy, those patients who have low serum 25-hydroxy-vitamin D level tend to have smaller increases in BMD.[58] It is therefore recommended to assay the serum 25-hydroxy-vitamin D in all patients with PHPT and prescribe vitamin D supplementation to those with a serum level below 20 ng/mL.[2] Bisphosphonates, estrogen, and raloxifene are also useful in the management of patients who do not undergo surgical treatment as they induce an increase in BMD and reduce the fracture risk.[17,28,31]

   Cinacalcet, a calcimimetic, activates CaSR by increasing their affinity for ionized calcium. When administered in doses of 30–50 mg twice a day, the serum calcium normalizes in over two-thirds of patients and PTH levels decrease.[59] These changes, however, are associated with neither a significant increase in BMD nor with a reduced fracture risk.[31]

   It is important to ensure the patient has an adequate fluid intake to avoid volume contraction which may exacerbate the degree of hypercalcemia and may lead to a hypercalcemic crisis.[1]

8. ***Cinacalcet:***
   A. Decreases the production of PTH
   B. Increases the sensitivity of calcium receptors

C. Lowers the serum calcium
D. Is approved for the treatment of patients with primary and secondary hyperparathyroidism
E. All of the above

Correct answer: E

Comments:

Cinacalcet increases the sensitivity of calcium receptors to activation by extracellular calcium, thus decreasing the synthesis and secretion of PTH resulting in a lower serum calcium level. There is a paucity of research studies on Cinacalcet. One multicenter, international, phase 3 RCT enrolled 67 patients with moderate PHPT who could not undergo parathyroidectomy. For the first 6 months, patients were randomly allocated to either cinacalcet or placebo, and for the following 6 months, all subjects were receiving cinacalcet, starting at 30 mg twice a day. The dose (median) of cinacalcet titrated to maintain normocalcemia was 60.2mg/day. The serum calcium level normalized (<2.575 mmol/L) in 75.8% of patients receiving cinacalcet versus 0% in the placebo group. Similarly, PTH blood levels decreased by 23.8% versus 1.1% in the placebo group. The phosphate level increased from a mean of 0.665 to 0.885 mmol/L.[60]

A recent meta-regression study of 28 manuscripts reported that whereas the serum calcium levels normalized in 90% (CI 0.82–0.96) of the enrolled subjects, with a mean reduction of serum calcium levels of 0.412 mmol/L (CI 0.343–0.481 mmol/L), the serum PTH levels normalized in only 10% (CI 0.02–0.23) of the subjects. The main side effects reported included mild to moderate gastrointestinal symptoms (nausea or vomiting 23%) but only 3% hypocalcemia.[61]

9. ***Medical management of patients with primary hyperparathyroidism includes:***
A. Adequate calcium intake.
B. Adequate vitamin D intake.
C. Adequate hydration.
D. Hydrochlorothiazides.
E. A, B, and C.

Correct answer: E

Comments:

Optimum calcium intake should be maintained. Whereas calcium inhibits parathyroid proliferation, a low intake of calcium stimulates PTH production. Indeed, the 22-year-long Nurses' Health Study showed that the relative risk of PHPT was reduced in the group with the highest dietary calcium intake compared to the group with the lowest dietary calcium intake.[3]

Optimum vitamin D intake should also be maintained. Vitamin D insufficiency is more prevalent in patients with PHPT than in the general population, and an inverse relationship has been demonstrated between elevated PTH and low vitamin D levels. Vitamin D insufficiency also has been identified as an independent risk factor for postoperative hypocalcemia and the hungry bone syndrome.[3]

Adequate hydration should be maintained to avoid hypercalcemic crises. Hydrochlorothiazides also should be avoided because they stimulate calcium reabsorption in the distal renal tubule.

10. ***Familial hypocalciuric hypercalcemia (FHH):***
    A. Parathyroid hormone levels are always elevated.
    B. Parathyroidectomy is the treatment of choice.
    C. Hypermagnesemia is a characteristic feature.
    D. A, B, and C.
    E. A and B.

Correct answer: C

Comments:

Apart from primary hyperparathyroidism (PHPT), the main causes of hypercalcemia and elevated/high normal PTH level include familial hypocalciuric hypercalcemia (FHH), malignancy-associated hypercalcemia, lithium therapy, thiazide therapy, and tertiary hyperparathyroidism associated with chronic renal disease. In patients with primary hyperparathyroidism, the urinary calcium level is elevated and the serum phosphorus concentration is usually at the lower limits of normality.[12]

Familial Hypocalciuric Hypercalcemia (FHH), also known as Familial Benign Hypercalcemia, is a benign condition characterized by hypercalcemia, hypocalciuria (24-h urine calcium excretion less than 100 mg), normal to elevated levels of PTH, and hypermagnesemia. It is due to autosomal dominant loss-of-function mutations of the calcium-sensing receptors gene (CaSRs) in the parathyroid glands and kidneys. Apart from multiple myeloma, hypercalcemia associated with malignancy is a relatively rare and late finding in patients with malignancies who are rarely asymptomatic.[3,7]

In the parathyroid glands, CaSRs trigger the feedback inhibition of parathyroid hormone release in response to a rise in the serum calcium concentration. Loss-of-function mutations in CaSRs impair this feedback inhibition of parathyroid hormone secretion in response to a rise in the blood calcium concentration and lead to hypercalcemia with inappropriately normal or mildly elevated levels of parathyroid hormone. The degree of hypercalcemia depends on the degree to which the mutation affects the function of CaSRs.

In the kidneys, CaSRs are involved in the feedback inhibition of parathyroid-independent renal tubular calcium reabsorption. Loss-of-function mutations in CaSRs interfere with the feedback inhibition of calcium reabsorption in response to a rise in the serum calcium concentration. Calcium continues to be reabsorbed in the renal tubules resulting in hypercalcemia and hypocalciuria. The renal calcium/creatinine clearance ratio is usually less than 0.01 in patients with FHH, but higher in patients with PHPT.

Although usually asymptomatic, some patients with FHH may complain of generalized weakness, fatigue, difficulties concentrating, and polydipsia. Pancreatitis and chondrocalcinosis are rare complications. Often FHH does not require treatment and is accidentally discovered when the patient is having serum biochemical tests done for some unrelated condition. It should be differentiated from PHPT because whereas parathyroidectomy is usually the treatment of choice for primary hyperparathyroidism, parathyroidectomy in FHH is not indicated, and is inappropriate, because it does not affect the FHH-associated hypercalcemia. Genetic testing can assist in the diagnosis of FHH.[62–64]

Case summary

Diagnosis

- Primary hyperparathyroidism, osteoporosis.

Management recommendations

Further diagnostic tests

- Parathyroid scan to visualize parathyroid glands and identify any adenoma.

Treatment recommendations

1. Surgery is the preferred and the only curative option.
2. Medications: bisphosphonates, cinacalcet, vitamin D supplementation if needed.
3. Lifestyle changes: maintain healthy lifestyle, ensure adequate nutrition and hydration.

Follow-up recommendations

- Vary whether patient treated surgically or medically.

Key points

- Primary hyperparathyroidism is more common after the age of 40 years, in women than in men and in Blacks than in Whites.
- Most cases are asymptomatic and secondary to a benign adenoma.
- Diagnosis is established by hypercalcemia, elevated PTH, and no causes of secondary hyperparathyroidism.
- Surgical treatment is the preferred option.
- Medical treatment includes bisphosphonates and cinacalcet. If present, hypovitaminosis D should be corrected.

References

1. Khan AA, Hanley DA, Rizzoli R, et al. Primary hyperparathyroidism: review and recommendations on evaluation, diagnosis and management. A Canadian and International consensus. *Osteoporos Int.* 2017;28 (1):1–19.
2. Eastell R, Arnold A, Brandi ML, et al. Diagnosis and management of asymptomatic primary hyperparathyroidism. *J Clin Endocrinol Metab.* 2009;94(2):340–350.
3. Dandurand K, Ali DS, Aliya K. Primary hyperparathyroidism: a narrative review of diagnosis and medical management. *J Clin Med.* 2021;10(8):1604.
4. Clarke BL. Epidemiology of primary hyperparathyroidism. *J Clin Densitometry.* 2013;16(10):8–13.
5. Melton III LJ. The epidemiology of primary hyperparathyroidism in North America. *J Bone Miner Res.* 2002;17 (Suppl. 2):12–17.
6. Wermers RA, Khosla S, Atkinson EJ, et al. Incidence of primary hyperparathyroidism in Rochester, Minnesota, 1993-2001: an update on the changing etiology of the disease. *J Bone Miner Res.* 2006;21:171–177.
7. Silverberg SJ, Walker MD, Bilezikian JP. Asymptomatic hyperparathyroidism. *J Clin Densitom.* 2013;16 (1):14–21.
8. Dadon T, Tsvetov G, Levi S, Gorshtein A, Slutzky-Shraga I, Hirsch D. Gender differences in the presentation, course and outcomes of primary hyperparathyroidism. *Maturitas.* 2021;145:12–17. https://doi.org/10.1016/j.maturitas.2020.11.007. Mar. Epub 2020 December 14. PMID: 33541557.
9. Cormier C, Koumakis E. Bone and primary hyperparathyroidism. *Joint Bone Spine.* 2022;89(1):105129. https://doi.org/10.1016/j.jbspin.2021.105129. Epub 2021 January 20. PMID: 33484857.
10. Yeh M, Ituarte PHG, Zhou HC, et al. Incidence and prevalence of primary hyperparathyroidism in a racially mixed population. *J Clin Endocrinol Metab.* 2013;98(3):1122–1129.
11. Bilezekian JP, Bandeira L, Khan A, Cusano NE. Hyperparathyroidism. *Lancet.* 2018;391:168–178.
12. Gallo D, Rosetti S, Marcon I, et al. When primary hyperparathyroidism comes as good news. *Endocrinol Diabetes Metab Case Rep.* 2020;2020:20-0046. https://doi.org/10.1530/EDM-20-0046. PMID: 32554826. PMCID: PMC7354736. Epub ahead of print.
13. Giusti F, Cavalli L, Cavalli T, Brandi ML. Hereditary hyperparathyroidism syndromes. *J Clin Densitom.* 2013;16(1):69–74.
14. Bilzekian JP, Khan AA, Potts Jr JT. Guidelines for the management of asymptomatic primary hyperparathyroidism: summary statement from the Third International Workshop. *J Clin Endocrinol Metab.* 2009;94(2):335–339.
15. Eastell R, Brandi ML, Costa AG, et al. Diagnosis of asymptomatic primary hyperparathytroidism: proceedings of the fourth international workshop. *J Clin Endocrinol Metab.* 2014;99(10):3570–3579.

16. Wermers RA, Kearns AE, Jenkins GD, Melton LJ. Incidence and clinical Spectrum of thiazide-associated hypercalcemia. *Am J Med.* 2007;120(10):911–915.
17. Khairallah W, Fawaz A, Brown EM, et al. Hypercalcemia and diabetes insipidus in a patient previously treated with lithium. *Nat Clin Pract Nephrol.* 2007;3:397–404.
18. Szalat A, Mazeh H, Freund HR. Lithium-associated hyperparathyroidism: report of four cases and review of the literature. *Eur J Endocrinol.* 2009;160:317–323.
19. McKnight R, Adida M, Budge K. Lithium toxicity: a systematic review and meta-analysis. *Lancet.* 2012;379:721–728.
20. Boughey JC, Ewart CJ, Yost MJ, et al. Chloride/phosphate ratio in primary hyperparathyroidism. *Am Surg.* 2004;70(1):25–28.
21. Makras P, Anastasilakis AD. Bone disease in primary hyperparathyroidism. *Metabolism.* 2018;80:57–65.
22. Khan A. Medical management of primary hyperparathyroidism. *J Clin Densitom.* 2013;16(1):60–63.
23. Jamal SA, Miller PD. Secondary and tertiary hyperparathyroidism. *J Clin Densitom.* 2013;16(1):64–68.
24. Lewiecki EM, Miller PD. Skeletal effects of primary hyperparathyroidism: bone mineral density and fracture risk. *J Clin Densitom.* 2013;16(1):28–32.
25. Meydan N, Barutca S, Guney E, et al. Brown tumors mimicking bone metastases. *J Natl Med Assoc.* 2006;98 (6):950–953.
26. Silverberg SJ, Bilezikian JP. Evaluation and management of primary hyperparathyroidism. *J Clin Endocrinol Metab.* 1996;81(6):2036–2040.
27. Sankaran S, Gamble G, Bolland M, et al. Skeletal effects of interventions in mild primary hyperparathyroidism: a meta-analysis. *J Clin Endocrinol Mtab.* 2010;95:1653–1662.
28. Costa AG, Bilezikian JP. Bone turover markers in primary hyperparathyroidism. *J Clin Densitom.* 2013;16 (1):22–27.
29. Peacock M. Primary hyperparathyroidism and the kidney: biochemical and clinical spectrum. *J Bone Miner Res.* 2002;17(Suppl. 2):N87–N94.
30. Walker MD, Rubin M, Silverberg SJ. Nontraditional manifestations of primary hyperparathyroidism. *J Clin Densitim.* 2013;16(1):40–47.
31. Silverberg SJ, Clarke BL, Peacock M, et al. Current issues in the presentation of asymptomatic primary hyperparathyroidism: proceedings of the fourth international workshop. *J Clin Endocrinol Metab.* 2014;99 (10):3580–3594.
32. Sheldon DG, Lee FT, Neil NJ, Ryan Jr JA. Surgical treatment of hyperparathyroidism improves health-related quality of life. *Arch Surg.* 2002;137(9):1022–1026.
33. Mittendorf EA, Wefel JS, Meyers CA, et al. Imrovement in sleep disturbance and neurocognitive function after parathyroidectomy in patients with primary hyperparathyroidism. *Endocr Pract.* 2007;13(4):338–344.
34. Chiang CY, Andrews DG, Anderson D, et al. A controlled prospective study of neuropsychological outcomes post parathyroidectomy in primary hyperparathyroid patients. *Clin Endocrinol (Oxf).* 2005;62(1):99–104.
35. Roman SA, Sosa JA, Mayes L, et al. Parathyroidectomy improves neurocognitivedeficits in patients with primary hyperparathyroidism. *Surgery.* 2005;138(6):1121–1129.
36. Okamoto T, Kamo T, Obara T. Outcome study of psychological distress and nonspecific symtoms in patients with mild primary hyperparathyroidism. *Arch Surg.* 2002;137(7):1022–1028.
37. Coker LH, Rorie K, Cantley L, et al. Primary hyperparathyroidism, cognition and health-related quality of life. *Ann Surg.* 2005;242(5):642–650.
38. Roman S, Sosa JA. Psychiatric and cognitive aspects of primary hyperparathyroidism. *Curr Opin Oncol.* 2007;19(1):1–5.
39. Walker RP, Paloyan E, Gopalsami C. Symptoms in patients with primary hyperparathyroidism: muscle weakness or sleepiness. *Endocr Pract.* 2004;10(5):404–408.
40. Marini C, Giusti M, Armonino R, et al. Reduced coronary flow reserve in patiuents with primary hyperparathyroidism: a study by G-SPECT myocardial perfusion imaging. *Eur J Nucl Med Mol Imaging.* 2010;37(12):2256–2263.
41. Curine M, Letizia C, Amato S, et al. Increased risk of cardiac death in primary hyperparathyroidism. *Int J Cardiol.* 2007;121(2):200–202.

42. Cermik TF, Kaya M, Ugur-Altun B, et al. Regional cerebral blood flow abnormalities in patients with primary hyperparathyroidism. *Neuroradiology*. 2007;49(4):379–385.
43. Abboud B, Daher R, Boujaoude J. Digestive manifestations of parathyroid disorders. *World J Gastroenterol*. 2011;17:4063–4066.
44. Cusano NE, Siverberg SJ, Bilezikian JP. Normocalcemic primary hyperparathyroidism. *J Clin Densitom*. 2013;16(1):33–39.
45. Fu Q, Jilka RL, Manolagas SC, O'Bren CA. Parathyroid hormone stimulates receptor activator of NFkappaB ligand and inhibits osteoproteregin expression via protein kinase A activation of CAMP-response element-binding protein. *J Biol Chem*. 2002;277(50):48868–48875.
46. Bellido T, Ali AA, Gubrij I, et al. Chronic elevation of parathyroid hormone in mice reduces expression of sclerostin by osteocytes. *Endocrinology*. 2005;146(11):4577–4583.
47. Dempster DW, Muller R, Zhou H, et al. Preserved three-dimensional cancellous bone structure in mild primary hyperparathyroidism. *Bone*. 2007;41(1):19–24.
48. Bilezekian JP, Brandi ML, Eastell R, et al. Guidelines for the management of asymptomatic primary hyperparathyroidism: summary statement from the fourth international workshop. *J Clin Endocrinol Metab*. 2014;99(10):3561–3569.
49. Udelsman R, et al. Surgery for asymptomatic primary hyperparathyroidism: proceedings of the third international workshop. *J Clin Endocrinol Metab*. 2009;94(2):366–372.
50. Udelsman B, Udelsman R. Surgery in primary hyperparathyroidism: extensive personal experience. *J Clin Densitom*. 2013;16(1):54–59.
51. Ambrogini E, Cetani F, Cianferotti L, et al. Surgery or surveillance for mild asymptomatic primary hyperparathyroidism: a prospective, randomized clinical trial. *J Clin Endocrinol Metab*. 2007;92:3114–3121.
52. Bollerslev J, Jansson S, Mollerup CL, et al. Medical observation, compared with parathyroidectomy, for asymptomatic primary hyperparathyroidism: a prospective, randomized clinical trial. *J Clin Endocrinol Metab*. 2007;92:1687–1692.
53. Rao DS, Phillips ER, Divines GW, Talpos GB. Randomized controlled clinical trial of surgery versus no surgery in patients with mild asymptomatic primary hyperparathyroidism. *J Clin Endocrinol Metab*. 2004;89:5415–5422.
54. Rubin MR, Bilezikian JP, McMahon DJ, et al. The natural history of primary hyperparathyroidism with or without parathyroid surgery after 15 years. *J Clin Endocrinol Metab*. 2008;93:3462–3470.
55. Lundstam K, Heck A, Mollerup C, et al. Effects of parathyroidectomy versus observation on the development of vertebral fractures in mild primary hyperparathyroidism. *J Clin Endocrinol Metab*. 2015;100:1359–1367.
56. Fang WL, Tseng LM, Chen SY, et al. The management of high-risk patients with primary hyperparathyroidism: minimally invasive parathyroidectomy vs medical treatment. *Clin Emdocrinol*. 2008;68:520–528.
57. Inoue Y, Kaji H, Hisa I, et al. Vitamin D status affects osteopenia in postmenopausal patients with hyperparathyroidism. *Endocr J*. 2008;55:57–65.
58. Pradeep PV, Mishra A, Agarwal G, et al. Long-term outcome after parathyroidectomy in patients with advanced primary hyperparathyroidism and associated vitamin D deficiency. *World J Surg*. 2008;32(5):829–835.
59. Peacock M, Bilzekian JP, Bolognese MA, et al. Cinacalcet hydrochloride reduces hypercalcemia in primary hyperparathyroidism across a wide spectrum of disease severity. *J Clin Endocrinol Metab*. 2011;96:8–19.
60. Khan A, Bilezikian J, Bone H, et al. Cinacalcet normalizes serum calcium in a double-blind randomized, placebo-controlled study in patients with primary hypoparathyroidism with contraindications to surgery. *Eur J Endocrinol*. 2015;172:527–535.
61. Ng CH, Chin YH, Tan MHQ, et al. Cinacalcet and primary hyperparathyroidism: systematic review and meta regression. *Endocr Connect*. 2020;9:724–735.
62. Stokes VJ, Nielsen MF, Hannan FM, Thakker RV. Hypercalcemic disorders in children. *J Bone Miner Res*. 2017;32(11):2157–2170.
63. Christensen SE, Nissen PH, Vestergaard P, Mosekilde L. Familial hypocalciuric hypercalcaemia: a review. *Curr Opin Endocrinol Diabetes Obes*. 2011;18(6):359–370.
64. Dowthwaite SA, Young JE, Pasternak JD, Young J. Surgical management of primary hyperparathyroidism. *J Clin Densitom*. 2013;16(1):48–53.

SECTION 4

Diet, calcium, magnesium, vitamin D, and lifestyle changes

CHAPTER 29

Calcium and vitamin D disorders. Part I: Mild hypocalcemia☆

Learning objectives

- Symptoms of mild hypocalcemia.
- Diagnosis of hypocalcemia, appropriate laboratory studies.
- Management of mild hypocalcemia.

The case study

Reason for seeking medical help

About 3weeks ago, Mrs. RL, a 52-year-old Caucasian woman, had a comprehensive metabolic profile done as part of her annual medical check which revealed a marginally low serum calcium level: 8.3mg/dL (normal range 8.5–10.2). She is essentially asymptomatic and is referred to the bone clinic to manage her marginally low serum calcium level.

Past medical/surgical history

- Fractured left radius roller skating at age 12.
- Hysterectomy at age 42years, hormonal replacement therapy for 3years.
- Basal cell carcinoma surgically removed about 3 years ago.
- Seasonal allergies.
- She is unable to tolerate dairy products and has avoided them since she realized her possible intolerance, when she was in her mid-twenties. A diagnosis of possible lactose intolerance was made.

☆ RL, 62-year-old Caucasian woman, with osteopenia, hypocalcemia.

Diagnosis and Treatment of Osteoporosis. https://doi.org/10.1016/B978-0-323-99550-4.00025-3
Copyright © 2024 Elsevier Inc. All rights are reserved, including those for text and data mining, AI training, and similar technologies.

Personal habits

- Active lifestyle, walking about 3 miles, 4 days a week in her neighborhood with a walking group, bikes a local trail about 15 miles, once a week with a cycling club.
- Working full time as a nurse manager in the ER.
- Minimal sun exposure due to history of carcinoma, wears a wide-brim hat and UV protectant, long sleeve shirt, and sunscreen when outdoors.
- Avoids milk and dairy products because of her fear of lactose intolerance.
- Four cans of Diet Pepsi daily.
- Six cups of coffee daily.
- Does not smoke cigarettes.
- One glass of wine twice a week, no binge drinking.

Medication

- Probiotics.
- Fish oil.
- Calcium chew, 600 mg daily, when she remembers it: approximately once a week.
- Zyrtec prn for allergies.

Family history

- Mother had kyphosis, no fractures, deceased about 10 years ago.

Clinical examination.

- Weight: 154 lbs.
- No significant clinical findings.

DXA scan

- The BMD of both hips, upper 4 lumbar vertebrae, and distal nondominant radius are within the normal limits.

Laboratory investigations

- Hypocalcemia, serum calcium: 8.3, after adjusting for serum albumin.
- Comprehensive metabolic profile: within normal limits.
- Serum 25-hydroxy-vitamin D: 32 ng/mL.

Multiple choice questions

1. ***Factors contributing to RL's low serum calcium level include:***
   A. Lactose intolerance.
   B. Malabsorption.
   C. Low calcium intake.
   D. Excessive caffeine and sodium intake.
   E. Any of the above-mentioned possibilities.
   Correct answer: E
   Comment:
   RL has been avoiding dairy products since her late twenties. The National Osteoporosis Foundation recommends 1200 mg of calcium daily for women over 50 years of age.[1] She is taking 600 mg calcium chew when she remembers to take it, and probably is not getting enough calcium. In addition, she is having an excessive amount of caffeine and sodium daily. Both increase the amount of calcium lost in the urine and induce a negative calcium balance. Her serum 25-hydroxy-vitamin D level, however, is 32ng/mL, within the normal range, and therefore not a contributing factor to her low calcium level.
2. ***Laboratory studies recommended for RL include:***
   A. 24-h urinary calcium.
   B. 24-h urinary sodium.
   C. Ionized serum calcium.
   D. IPTH.
   E. All of the above.
   Correct answer: E
   Comment:
   Assaying the 24-h urinary calcium and sodium will show if RL is losing an excessive amount of calcium via urine and this may be the etiology of her low serum calcium level. If RL is losing calcium through her urine, hydrochlorothiazide is a therapeutic management option to help her kidneys retain calcium and ultimately increase her serum calcium level.[2]
   The serum iPTH level is expected to be elevated to compensate for the low serum calcium level. A low, or low normal ionized serum calcium level is suggestive of hypoparathyroidism.
3. ***The alternative dietary sources of calcium that RL can consume if she has lactose intolerance include:***
   A. Soy milk, almond milk, oat milk, coconut milk.
   B. Orange juice (fortified with calcium).
   C. Broccoli, kale, spinach.
   D. Bread (fortified with calcium).
   E. Any of the above.
   Correct answer: E

Comment:

All of the items listed are options for lactose-intolerant patients. There are multiple other foods that can be utilized as well including almonds and sweet potatoes. Patient education is important to ensure an adequate daily calcium intake. Several foods are fortified with calcium. For instance, orange juice fortified with calcium has a similar calcium content as milk.[3]

4. ***Chronic calcium deficiency can cause:***
   A. Osteoporosis.
   B. Rickets.
   C. Osteomalacia.
   D. Secondary hyperparathyroidism.
   E. All of the above.

   Correct answer: E

   Comment:

   Low calcium intake can lead to osteoporosis by decreasing bone mineral density. Calcium deficiency in children can lead to rickets.[4] Osteomalacia is the softening of bones in adults, resulting from hypocalcemia and hypovitaminosis D.[4]

   Hypocalcemia stimulates the calcium-sensing cells in the parathyroid glands to release parathyroid hormone which stimulates bone-resorbing cells to increase the serum calcium to the normal ranges, leading to secondary hyperparathyroidism, which is characterized by an elevated parathyroid hormone level and a low or low normal serum calcium level. In primary hyperparathyroidism, both the serum calcium level and the serum parathyroid hormone level are increased.

5. ***Symptoms of hypocalcemia include:***
   A. Neuromuscular irritability.
   B. Renal calcification.
   C. Depression.
   D. Seizures.
   E. All of the above.

   Correct answer: E

   Comment:

   Hypocalcemia may manifest itself through a wide variety of symptoms but is usually asymptomatic especially in mild cases, as with RL. Symptoms range from neuromuscular symptoms, such as numbness and tingling of the hands and feet, to more severe ones associated with depression, cataracts, and seizures.[4]

6. ***RL's 24-h urine calcium and sodium comes back:***
   - 24-h calcium: 200 mEq/L normal range 100–300 mEq/L.
   - 24-h sodium: 150 mEq/L normal range 40–220 mEq/L.

Given the above results, the best course of action is:

A. Start a low-dose hydrochlorothiazide
B. Increase daily dietary calcium intake
C. Add 1200-mg calcium supplement
D. A and C
E. A and B

Correct answer: B

Comment:

The 24-h urinary calcium and sodium are within normal limits, meaning RL is not losing an excessive amount of calcium through her urine. She therefore probably is not ingesting enough calcium. Focusing on calcium-rich foods is the best option for RL at this stage. HCTZ can be considered if RL had hypercalciuria. Hydrochlorothiazide reduces the renal calcium excretion and has shown to reduce the fracture risk by reducing calcium lost via urinary output, and increasing the BMD.[5]

7. ***The optimal initial treatment for RL's low calcium level is:***

A. Calcium citrate tablets 1200 mg daily.
B. Calcium carbonate tablets 1200 mg daily.
C. Increase dietary calcium intake 1200 mg.
D. Reduce sodium and caffeine intake.
E. C and D.

Correct answer: E

Comment:

Ideally RL should attempt to obtain calcium through dietary sources. If she is unable to do that, then she needs a calcium supplement. Calcium citrate is more easily absorbed than calcium carbonate, especially in older people who may have a low gastric acidity: reduced gastric acidity may interfere with the gastric absorption of calcium. In RL's case, she is not taking any PPIs or H2 blockers that decrease the amount of acidity in the stomach, so she can take either supplement if needed. Also, it is important to emphasize the upper limit of calcium intake is 2000 mg/day.

8. ***RL has increased her daily dietary calcium intake to about 1500 mg and has reduced her caffeine and sodium intake. Recheck of her calcium level is 9.0. The plan of action is:***

A. Continue with 1200 mg of dietary calcium.
B. Stop efforts to increase oral calcium supplementation.
C. Repeat her DXA scan in 2 years.
D. B and C.
E. A, C, and D.

Correct answer: E

Comment:

RL's dietary calcium has improved. She now needs to maintain her present increased dietary calcium intake, which can potentially increase the BMD.[6] At present, therefore, she does not need any medication. She nevertheless needs to maintain her improved diet and increased calcium intake. Her DXA scan should be repeated in 2 years to determine if she had any changes in BMD and whether any modification or pharmacologic therapy is needed.

9. ***Factor(s) that can interfere with dietary calcium include:***
   A. Caffeine intake.
   B. Vitamin D level.
   C. Malabsorption.
   D. Sodium intake.
   E. All of the above.

   Correct answer: E

   Comment:

   Caffeine reduces the renal reabsorption of calcium, thus increasing the urinary calcium loss and decreasing the bioavailability of oral calcium.[4] Caffeine also increases the urinary excretion of magnesium, sodium, and chloride.

10. ***Medications that interact with calcium include:***
   A. Levothyroxine.
   B. Quinolones.
   C. Beta blockers.
   D. Insulin.
   E. A and B.

   Correct answer: E

   Comment:

   Levothyroxine should not be taken within 4h of a calcium supplement. Quinolones need a two-hour window before or after taking a calcium supplement.[4] RL is not currently taking either medication, but it is important to keep this in mind should she be prescribed any of these tablets.

Key points

- Hypocalcemia is most of the time silent, but can also present with a broad range of symptoms including depression, seizure, and neuromuscular complaints.
- Laboratory studies for a low calcium level include 24-h urinary calcium and sodium to determine if calcium is being lost through the urine.
- First-line treatment for hypocalcemia is dietary calcium intake based on age-related requirements.

References

1. National Osteoporosis Foundation; 2022. https://www.bonehealthandosteoporosis.org/healthy-bones-guide-calcium-bones/.
2. Cheng L, Zhang K, Zhang Z. Effectiveness of thiazides on serum and urinary calcium levels and bone mineral density in patients with osteoporosis: a systematic review and meta-analysis. *Drug Des Devel Ther.* 2018;12:3929–3935. Published 2018 November 14 https://doi.org/10.2147/DDDT.S179568.
3. Hodges JK, Cao S, Cladis DP, Weaver CM. Lactose intolerance and bone health: the challenge of ensuring adequate calcium intake. *Nutrients.* 2019;11(4):718. Published 2019 March 28 https://doi.org/10.3390/nu11040718.
4. National Institutes of Health. Calcium; 2021. https://ods.od.nih.gov/factsheets/Calcium-HealthProfessional/.
5. Kang KY, Kang Y, Kim M, et al. The effects of antihypertensive drugs on bone mineral density in ovariectomized mice. *J Korean Med Sci.* 2013;28(8):1139–1144. https://doi.org/10.3346/jkms.2013.28.8.1139.
6. Yao X, Hu J, Kong X, Zhu Z. Association between dietary calcium intake and bone mineral density in older adults. *Ecol Food Nutr.* 2021;60(1):89–100. https://doi.org/10.1080/03670244.2020.1801432.

Calcium and vitamin D disorders: Part II: Hypovitaminosis D

Learning objectives

- Factors modulating vitamin D metabolism.
- The diagnosis and management of hypovitaminosis D.

The case study

Reason for seeking medical help

- PDH, a 56-year-old Caucasian woman, is referred because about a year ago she was found to have hypovitaminosis D: serum 25-hydroxy-vitamin D: 16 ng/mL and osteopenia: T-score −1.1 at the upper 4 lumbar vertebrae. She received 2 courses of 3-month ergocalciferol supplements (50,000 IU once a week), 3 months of cholecalciferol 2000 units daily, and another 3 months of cholecalciferol 5000 units with little change in her serum vitamin D level: 15, 17, 17, and 16 ng/mL at 3, 6, 9, and 12 months, respectively. She was adherent to the prescribed medication. About 3 weeks ago she tried sublingual vitamin D tablets but could not tolerate them: they caused severe oral irritation.

Past medical and surgical history

- No relevant medical history.
- Natural menopause about 2 years ago, no HRT.
- Several allergies.

Personal habits

- Physically active lifestyle: night nurse on ICU.
- Avoids outdoor activities because of allergies.
- Avoids milk and dairy products, thinks she may be lactose intolerant.

Diagnosis and Treatment of Osteoporosis. https://doi.org/10.1016/B978-0-323-99550-4.00017-4
Copyright © 2024 Elsevier Inc. All rights are reserved, including those for text and data mining, AI training, and similar technologies.

- No cigarette smoking.
- No excessive sodium, caffeine, or alcohol intake.

Medications

- Calcium carbonate 1200 mg daily.
- Multivitamin tablet daily.
- Cholecalciferol, 2000 units daily with breakfast.

Family history

- Negative for osteoporosis, malabsorption, and lactose intolerance.

Clinical examination

- Weight 98 pounds, height 62″. She always had a low body weight.
- No significant clinical findings.

Laboratory result(s)

- Comprehensive metabolic profile: no abnormality except from marginally elevated alkaline phosphatase: 130 UL.
- Thyroid stimulation hormone (TSH), sedimentation rate: within normal limits.
- Serum 25-hydroxy-vitamin D/16 ng/mL, parathyroid hormone (PTH) 112 pg/mL, and calcium 8.9 mg/dL.

Multiple choice questions

1. ***In PDH's case, the following tests are indicated:***
   A. Tissue transglutaminase.
   B. Serum 1,25-hydroxy-vitamin D.
   C. 24-h urinary calcium and sodium excretion.
   D. A and B.
   E. A and C.
   Correct answer: A
   Comment:
   PDH's serum 25-hydroxy-vitamin D level has essentially remained unchanged for the past year even though she has been on several courses of different vitamin D supplements. Given her low body weight, she may have malabsorption which may be the reason for her nonresponse to orally administered vitamin D and her low body weight. Assaying the

serum tissue transglutaminase level is the next step. If positive, a duodenal biopsy may be indicated. Patients with gluten sensitivity respond well to gluten-free diets.

In PDH's case, at this stage, it is not necessary to assay the 24-h urine sodium and calcium excretion. The pressing issue is to identify the reason for her not responding to orally administered vitamin D. Besides, her vitamin D deficiency and associated secondary hyperparathyroidism will increase the tubular calcium resorption and affect the urine calcium excretion.

2. ***Hypovitaminosis D may present with:***
   A. Proximal muscle weakness.
   B. Repeated falls.
   C. Stress fractures.
   D. A and B.
   E. A, B, and C.

   Correct answer: E

   Comment:

   Muscle weakness, especially proximal muscle weakness, is a cardinal clinical feature of hypovitaminosis D.[1] In late stages the myopathy is such that patients have a waddling gait. Several studies also documented decreased reaction time, impaired balance, and an increased risk of falls especially in older people with low serum vitamin D levels. Conversely, vitamin D supplementation was associated with improvements in muscle strength, walking distance, and a decrease in general discomfort.[2]

   The positive effects of vitamin D supplementation on falls and fracture risk have been reported by several investigators and a meta-analysis of 11 randomized clinical trials concluded that hip fractures and nonvertebral fractures are reduced by 30% and 14%, respectively, when vitamin D is administered in mean doses of 800 IU/day (range 792–2000).[3] Another meta-analysis concluded that the more pronounced benefits were observed at mean doses of vitamin D between 700 and 1000 IU daily to maintain serum vitamin D levels between 30 and 44 ng/mL.[4] Stress fractures occur more frequently in subjects with serum vitamin D levels below 30 ng/mL than in those with higher levels.[2]

3. ***The diagnosis of hypovitaminosis D is confirmed by finding:***
   A. Low serum 25-OHD.
   B. Low serum 1,25-OHD.
   C. Elevated serum iPTH level.
   D. A and B.
   E. A, B, and C.

   Correct answer: A.

   Comment:

   Low serum 25-OH vitamin D is the gold standard to diagnose vitamin D deficiency. Unfortunately, there is no uniform assay methodology and no agreement as to what the "normal" serum 25-OHD level is. The guidelines of the Institute of Medicine (IOM) consider a serum level of 20ng/mL as "sufficient."[5] The US Endocrine Society guidelines state this level should be 30ng/mL. The US Endocrine Society also recommends that "deficiency" be defined as 20ng/mL or less, "insufficiency" at levels between 20 and 29 ng/mL, and "sufficiency" at levels 30ng/mL or higher.[6]

It is also suggested that a level between 40 and 60ng/mL is ideal and that levels up to 100ng/mL are "safe." Furthermore, whereas the IOM guidelines are that the upper limit of vitamin D intake should not exceed 4000IU, the Endocrine Society considers the upper limit to be 10,000IU daily.[6] Patients with low 25-OHD often have secondary hyperparathyroidism; the serum calcium level, however, remains within the normal range until very late cases when secondary hyperparathyroidism is no longer able to compensate for the low vitamin D level.

4. ***Comparing ergocalciferol (D2) to cholecalciferol (D3), the following is/are true:***
   A. D2 induces larger initial increases in serum 25-hydroxy-vitamin D (25-OHD) levels.
   B. D3-induced increases in 25-OHD last longer than those induced by D2.
   C. Peak serum 25-OHD concentration is reached 12h after oral administration.
   D. A and B.
   E. A, B, and C.

   Correct answer: B

   Comment:

   The relative potencies of ergocalciferol (D_2) and cholecalciferol (D_3) were evaluated by administering a single 50,000IU dose of each compound to a group of healthy male volunteers. Over the first 3days both vitamin D preparations induced similar increases in the serum vitamin D level. Subsequently, however, the increase in vitamin D level induced by D3 continued to rise for the following 14days, whereas the increases induced by D2 rapidly fell and by day 14 were not different from baseline values. The 28-day area under the curve postoral administration was 60.2ng/dL and 204.7ng/dL for D2 and D3, respectively ($P < .002$). The relative potency D3:D2 was 9.5:1.[7] For each 100IU vitamin D ingested, the serum 25-hydroxy-vitamin D level is expected to increase by 0.6–1.0ng/mL.[8]

5. ***Vitamin D deficiency leads to bone demineralization by affecting:***
   A. Calcium absorption through the intestinal tract.
   B. Rate of bone resorption.
   C. Urinary calcium excretion.
   D. A and B.
   E. A, B, and C.

   Correct answer: E

   Comment:

   The ionized serum calcium level which is essential for most cellular functions is maintained within a narrow range of normality through a finely balanced and acutely responsive calcium/parathyroid hormone/vitamin D axis. Low serum vitamin D levels lead to impaired absorption of calcium from the duodenum and trigger a negative calcium balance which initially is swiftly counteracted by an increased parathyroid hormone secretion, which increases renal calcium resorption and rapidly mobilizes and activates osteoclasts to increase bone resorption and transfer calcium from bones to the circulation.

6. ***Skin production of vitamin D:***
   A. Ordinary glass blocks UV-B.
   B. Is not affected by sunscreen lotions.
   C. May reach toxic levels if exposure is too intense.
   D. A and B.
   E. A, B, and C.

   Correct answer: A

   Comment:

   UV-B rays do not sufficiently penetrate glass and therefore not enough vitamin D may be produced if sun exposure is through glass.[9] Vitamin D can be ingested or produced in the skin through the action of UV light (UV-B wavelength: 290–315 nm) on 7-dehydrocholesterol. Several factors affect the rate at which vitamin D is produced in the skin, including geographical latitude, ozone levels, season, time of day, clear or cloudy sky, air pollution, clothes worn, skin pigmentation, and use of sunscreen products. A properly applied sunscreen with a sun-protecting factor of 15 blocks almost completely the production of vitamin D in the skin.[2] Vitamin D synthesis occurs mostly between 10:00am and 3:00pm.[9] Five to 15 min of unprotected exposure to sunshine during this time period, when UV-B rays are available from the sun, is adequate to provide enough vitamin D for 1 day.[10] Excessive sun exposure does not lead to high serum vitamin D levels because of its rapid photodegradation into biologically inactive metabolites.[9] Relatively few foods naturally contain vitamin D and include egg yolk, fish oil, and fatty fish such as mackerel, salmon, and herring. Several foods, however, are fortified with vitamin D.

7. ***Steps in the formation and activation of vitamin D include:***
   A. Binding to vitamin D binding protein (DBP).
   B. Hepatic hydroxylation to 25-hydroxy-vitamin D.
   C. Renal hydroxylation to 1,25-di-hydroxy-vitamin D.
   D. B and C.
   E. A, B, and C.

   Correct answer: E

   Comment:

   Whether absorbed through the intestinal tract or formed in the skin, once vitamin D reaches the circulation it is bound to vitamin D Binding Protein (DBP). In the liver it is hydroxylated to become 25-hydroxy-vitamin D (25-OHD) and has a half-life of 2–3 weeks. In the kidneys, under the influence of parathyroid hormone, it is further hydroxylated either by 1α-hydroxylase enzyme to 1,25-di-hydroxy-vitamin D: ($1,25(OH)_2D$): the most active metabolite or by other enzymes to form fewer active metabolites.

$1,25(OH)_2D$ also can be produced for local use by some cells. When it reaches the target cells $1,25(OH)_2D$ diffuses through the cell and nuclear membranes, binds to intranuclear vitamin D receptors (VDR), acts as a transcription factor, and modifies the expression of a number of genes associated with metabolic pathways. $1,25(OH)_2D$ also binds to Membrane-Associated Rapid Response Steroid-binding (MARRS) vitamin D receptors located in plasma membrane caveolae to regulate cytosolic calcium concentration and affect the activity of a number of enzymes.[10] Vitamin D receptors have been identified in a number of tissues, including parathyroid glands, brain, pancreas, stomach, ovaries, and testicles.

8. ***Low serum vitamin D levels are associated with increased risks of:***
   A. Depression.
   B. Dementia.
   C. Overall mortality.
   D. A and C.
   E. A, B, and C.

   Correct answer: E.

   Comment:

   Vitamin D regulates cellular calcium homeostasis and has neuroprotective functions. Vitamin D receptors are found in the brain and regulate several cellular functions including the production and release of neurotrophic factors such as nerve growth factor and the synthesis of neurotransmitters, including acetylcholine, GABA, and catecholamines.[11]

   There is evidence to show an increased risk of neuropsychological diseases in patients with low vitamin D levels[12]: specifically depression,[11,13] dementia, including Alzheimer's disease, epilepsy, multiple sclerosis, and schizophrenia.[14] It is, however, still not clear whether this is a causal or associative relationship. Several studies have documented an increased overall mortality with lower serum vitamin D levels.[9]

9. ***Patients with low serum vitamin D levels are more at risk of:***
   A. Prostate cancer.
   B. Colon cancer.
   C. Breast cancer.
   D. A and B.
   E. A, B, and C.

   Correct answer: E

   Comment:

   A number of studies have shown that patients with low serum vitamin D levels are more at risk of developing cancer and that higher levels of serum vitamin D levels may exert a protective effect against some types of cancer including prostate, breast, and colorectal. Other studies did not identify this tendency, and definite proof of a causative relationship is lacking.[9]

   A meta-analysis concluded that for each 4ng/mL increase in the serum vitamin D level, the risk of colorectal cancer was reduced by 6%.[15] Several other studies have documented negative effects of low serum vitamin D levels on different types of cancer incidence and mortality.[9] There is also mounting evidence that the relationship between serum vitamin D levels and cancer incidence may be U-shaped or J-shaped, with those at the lowest and highest levels having a higher risk than those at midrange levels.[9] A large study on 247,574 individuals suggested a J-shaped or U-shaped relationship between overall mortality and serum vitamin D levels, with the lowest mortality at levels between 20 and 24ng/mL.[16]

10. ***Patients with low serum vitamin D levels are more at risk of:***
    A. Chronic kidney disease.
    B. Diabetes mellitus, type 2.
    C. Autoimmune diseases.
    D. A and B.
    E. A, B, and C.

    Correct answer: E

    Comment:

    Vitamin D deficiency is prevalent among patients with chronic kidney diseases and accelerates its progression.[16] A 5-year prospective on 6180 adults documented that patients with serum vitamin D levels less than 15ng/mL at baseline had a higher incidence of albuminuria and low eGFR.[17] Observational studies have shown an association between serum 25-OHD levels below 30ng/mL, hypertension, and the metabolic syndrome.[18,19] Several observational studies also documented an association between serum 25-OHD levels and type 2 diabetes mellitus, autoimmune diseases, and respiratory tract diseases.[9] It is nevertheless still debatable whether these associations are true causative ones or merely associations due to some other common factor(s).

Key points

- There is no consensus as to what constitutes hypovitaminosis D. The Institute of Medicine defines it as a level below 20ng/mL, whereas the US Endocrine Society defines it as below 30ng/mL.
- Assaying the serum 25-hydroxy-vitamin D levels determines the patient's vitamin D status.
- Apart from its deleterious effect on bones, vitamin D deficiency may be associated with a number of disease states, including hypertension, diabetes mellitus, cancer, autoimmune dysfunction, depression, cognitive impairment, and Alzheimer's disease.
- Ergocalciferol and cholecalciferol are useful to treat hypovitaminosis D. Given the present evidence, cholecalciferol appears to be superior to ergocalciferol.

References

1. Holick MF. Vitamin D deficiency. *N Engl J Med.* 2007;357(3):266–281.
2. Ogan D, Pritchett K. Vitamin D, and the athlete: risks, recommendations, and benefits. *Nutrients.* 2013;5:1856–1868.
3. Bischoff-Ferrari HA, Willett WC, Orav EJ, et al. A pooled analysis of vitamin D dose requirements for fracture prevention. *N Engl J Med.* 2012;367(1):40–49.

4. Pramyothin P, Holick MF. Vitamin D supplementation: guidelines and evidence for subclinical deficiency. *Curr Opin Gastroenterol.* 2012;28(2):139–150.
5. Ross AC, Manson JE, Abrams SA, et al. The 2011 report on dietary reference intakes for calcium and vitamin D from the Institute of Medicine: what clinicians need to know. *J Clin Endocrinol Metab.* 2011;96(1):53–58.
6. Holick MF, Binkley NC, Bischoff-Ferrari HA, et al. Evaluation, treatment, and prevention of vitamin D deficiency: an Endocrine Society clinical practice guideline. *J Clin Endocrinol Metab.* 2011;96(7):1911–1930.
7. Armas LA, Hollis BW, Heaney RP. Vitamin D2 is much less effective than vitamin D3 in humans. *J Clin Endocrinol Metab.* 2004;89:5387–5391.
8. Heaney RP, Davies KM, Chen TC, et al. Human serum 25-hydroxycholecalciferol response to extended oral dosing with cholecaciferol. *Am J Clin Nutr.* 2003;77(1):201–210.
9. Hossein-Nezhad A, Holick MF. Vitamin D and health: a global perspective. *Mayo Clin Proc.* 2013;88 (7):720–755.
10. Holick MF. The vitamin D epidemic and its health consequences. *J Nutr.* 2005;135:2739S–2748S.
11. Harms LR, Burne TH, Eyles DW, McGrath JJ. Vitamin D and the brain. *Best Pract Res Clin Endocrinol Metab.* 2011;25:657–669.
12. (a) Wozosek M, Lukasszkiiewicz J, Wrzosek M, et al. *Pharmacol Rep.* 2013;65:271–278. (b) Lapid MI, Cha SS, Takahashi PY. Vitamin D and depression in geriatric primary care patients. *Clin Interv Aging.* 2013;8:509–514.
13. Jamilian H, Bagherzadeh K, Nazeri Z, Hassanijirdehi M, Vitamin D. Parathyroid hormone, serum calcium and phosphorus in patients with schizophrenia and major depression. *Int J Psychiatry Clin Pract.* 2013;17:30–34.
14. Dursun E, Gezen-Ak D, Yilmazer S. A novel perspective for Alzheimer's disease: vitamin D receptor suppression by amyloid-B and preventing the amyloid-B induced alterations by vitamin D in cortical neurons. *J Alzheimers Dis.* 2011;23:207–219.
15. Chung M, Lee J, Terasawa T, et al. Vitamin D with or without calcium supplementation for prevention of cancer and fractures: an updated meta-analysis for the US preventive services task force. *Ann Intern Med.* 2011;155 (12):827–838.
16. Li YC. Vitamin D in chronic kidney disease. *Contrib Nephrol.* 2013;180:98–109.
17. Damasiewicz MJ, Magliano DJ, Daly RM, et al. Serum 25-hydroxyvitamin D deficiency and the 5-year incidence of CKD. *Am J Kidney Dis.* 2013;62(1):58–66.
18. Anderson JL, May HT, Horne BD, et al. Relation of vitamin D deficiency to cardiovascular risk factors, disease status and incident events in a general healthcare population. *Am J Cardiol.* 2010;106(7):963–968.
19. Durup D, Jorgensen HL, Christensen J, et al. A reverse J-shaped association of all-cause mortality with serum 25-hydroxyvitamin D in general practice. *J Clin Endocrinol Metab.* 2012;97(8):2644–2652.

Calcium and vitamin D disorders: Part III: From hypovitaminosis to hypervitaminosis D[☆]

Learning objectives

- Signs and symptoms of hypervitaminosis D.
- The management of hypervitaminosis D.
- Diseases that increase the risk of hypovitaminosis D and hypervitaminosis D.

The case study

Reasons for seeking medical help

- About 3 years ago MH was diagnosed with osteoporosis as evidenced by the lowest T-score −2.5 in her upper 4 lumbar vertebrae.
- At that time, she was found to also have a marginally elevated serum alkaline phosphatase (bone isoenzyme) and hypovitaminosis D (25-hydroxy): 14 ng/mL. Her only complaint was easy fatigue and generalized weakness at times. Other common diseases, including psychological and psychiatric ones, had been ruled out, and her symptoms were attributed to vitamin D deficiency.
- She was prescribed ergocalciferol 50,000 units daily for only 3 months and was instructed to take over-the-counter vitamin D3 (cholecalciferol) 2000 units tablets once a day. She was scheduled for a follow-up clinic visit 3 months later with repeat assay of her serum vitamin D level at that time.
- MH, however, showed up for neither her laboratory work-up nor follow-up appointment. She did not think she needed medical care. The medical office was unable to reach her.

☆ MH, 57-year-old Caucasian woman, initially with hypovitaminosis D, now with vitamin D toxicity.

Diagnosis and Treatment of Osteoporosis. https://doi.org/10.1016/B978-0-323-99550-4.00024-1
Copyright © 2024 Elsevier Inc. All rights are reserved, including those for text and data mining, AI training, and similar technologies.

- She continued to take OTC vitamin D3, 2000 units once a day, but then increased it to 2000 units twice a day since her last clinic visit about 2 years ago. She also increased her sun exposure in addition to ultraviolet light.
- Her generalized muscle weakness improved, and she had bouts of "increased energy." This was nevertheless short-lived.
- She now returns to the clinic, about 2 years after her initial encounter, because she was experiencing abdominal pain, polyuria, nausea, and occasional vomiting. She also developed at least three renal calculi which she passed spontaneously. In addition, she also experienced bouts of confusion.

Past medical and surgical history

- Natural menopause age 47 years, 1 year of HRT, then discontinued it.
- Essentially healthy until this present episode.

Lifestyle

- Sedentary lifestyle: works as a receptionist 5 days a week. She walks with her husband on Saturday mornings for about 45 min.
- Suspected to have lactose intolerance.
- History of cigarette smoking half a pack a day for about 4 years in her 20s.
- Caffeine intake three cups of coffee daily.
- Alcohol consumption, occasionally, about once a month.
- No excessive sodium intake.

Medication(s)

- Vitamin D3 2000 units bid. Frequently, at least 3 times a week, she would double the vitamin D dose when she felt tired and weak and in need of "that bout of extra energy." She also purchased an "ultraviolet lantern" to stimulate the cutaneous production of vitamin D. She uses it daily, sometimes twice a day during weekends.
- Calcium carbonate tablets, on average 4 a day.
- Multiple vitamin and mineral supplements, purchased over the counter, 3–4 tablets a day.

Family history

- Unknown; she was adopted soon after birth.

Clinical examination

- Weight: 152 lbs., height: 63″.
- Clinical examination does not reveal any significant finding.

Laboratory result(s)

- Serum 25-OH vitamin D: 124 ng/mL.
- Comprehensive metabolic profile: no abnormal findings.

Multiple choice questions

1. ***Factors that initially may have contributed to MH's vitamin D deficiency include:***
   A. Lactose intolerance.
   B. Limited sun exposure.
   C. Ethnicity.
   D. Low daily calcium and vitamin D intake.
   E. All of the above
   Correct answer: E
   Comment:
   Patients who are lactose intolerant and do not use alternative sources of dietary calcium and vitamin D are at risk of developing vitamin D deficiency: hypovitaminosis D. Limited sun exposure from staying indoors can also increase the risk of vitamin D deficiency. Similarly, an increase in melanin pigments in the skin, as with African Americans, can decrease the cutaneous vitamin D production from sunlight further increasing the risk of vitamin D deficiency.[1] A decreased vitamin D level increases the risk of diabetes mellitus and insulin resistance.[2]
2. ***At this stage the following laboratory tests are indicated for Ms. MH:***
   A. Vitamin D (25-hydroxy).
   B. CMP and ionized serum calcium level.
   C. HGB A1C.
   D. A and B.
   E. A, B, and C.
   Correct answer: E
   Comment:
   MH initially was prescribed 3 months of vitamin D2 (ergocalciferol) 50,000 units once a week in addition to vitamin D3 (cholecalciferol) obtained over the counter. After 3 months, she continued taking vitamin D3, 2000 units BID, and often increased the dose, especially as she felt that the vitamin D supplements increased her "level of energy." She also increased the amount of exposure to sun and ultraviolet rays. At this point, she needs her serum vitamin D level assayed to fine-tune the treatment regimen and tailor it to her individual circumstances.

   A comprehensive metabolic profile is justified to identify the underlying cause of her renal calculi and whether she has sustained any renal impairment. Ionized serum calcium assay is also relevant. As excessive vitamin D intake increases the risk of hyperglycemia and diabetes mellitus, an assay of serum HGB A1C is therefore also justified.

3. ***Vitamin D toxicity presents with these symptoms:***
   A. Nausea/vomiting.
   B. Muscle weakness.
   C. Hypercalcemia.
   D. Decreased appetite.
   E. All of the above.

   Correct answer: E

   Comment:

   Excessive amounts of vitamin D can increase calcium absorption causing renal calculi, polyuria, polydipsia, nausea and vomiting, muscle weakness, dehydration, and decreased appetite.[3] MH specifically complained of muscle weakness. Other manifestations of vitamin D toxicity include confusion, apathy, and abdominal pain.[3]

4. ***MH's laboratory tests reveal:***

   Serum vitamin D (25-hydroxy-vitamin D) hypervitaminosis D: 145 ng/mL.
   Comprehensive metabolic profile: within normal limits, except for marginal hypercalcemia (serum calcium 10.5 mg/dL: normal range 8.6–10.3 mg/dL).
   HGB A1C 6.5%, within normal range.
   At this stage the treatment plan for Ms. MH is:
   A. Discontinue calcium supplementation.
   B. Discontinue vitamin D3 and any type of vitamin D supplementation, including vitamin D2.
   C. Recheck serum vitamin D level in 3 months.
   D. A and B.
   E. A, B, and C.

   Correct answer: E

   Comment:

   Vitamin D intoxication can occur with serum concentrations above 80 ng/mL. However, concentrations are much greater with symptomatic hypervitaminosis D.[4] MH developed several renal calculi and experienced vitamin D toxicity symptoms (muscle weakness and nausea). If she continues with vitamin D supplementation, even at a lower dose, her vitamin D level will continue to rise. The best course of action is to stop her supplementation and recheck her level in 3 months.

5. ***Additional laboratory studies include:***
   A. Serum parathyroid hormone (PTH).
   B. Ionized serum calcium.
   C. 24-h urinary calcium.
   D. A and B.
   E. All of the above.

   Correct answer: E

Comment:

All of the above tests are needed to monitor MH's condition. PTH blood levels will decrease as calcium levels increase due to hypervitaminosis D. To counteract the increase in calcium, the kidneys will increase urinary calcium excretion to try maintaining homeostasis. This, however, increases the risk of renal calculi.

6. ***If MH continues with her vitamin D supplementation, the following may occur:***

   A. Renal calculi.
   B. Hypercalciuria.
   C. Decreased PTH.
   D. A and B.
   E. All of the above.

   Correct answer: E

   Comment:

   As vitamin D levels increase to 150 ng/mL, calcium levels tend to increase causing a decrease in PTH to compensate for the increased calcium level, as well as an increase in calcium excreted through the urine. The patient then becomes at an increased risk of developing renal calculi.[3]

7. ***Three months later: MH returns. Her serum vitamin D (25-hydroxy) level is now 98 ng/mL. She no longer has muscle weakness or nausea. The treatment plan should include:***

   A. No vitamin D supplementation.
   B. Start treatment for her osteoporosis.
   C. Start 1000 unit vitamin D3 (cholecalciferol) daily.
   D. A and B.
   E. B and C.

   Correct answer: D

   Comment:

   MH now has a vitamin D level within the normal range. At this stage, therefore she does not need any supplementation. She nevertheless would benefit from a yearly vitamin D level assay to detect early mild hypervitaminosis D while she is still in the asymptomatic phase.

   With a low vitamin D level, MH may experience generalized bone pain when she starts treatment for osteoporosis, so it is important to ensure that she has a normal serum vitamin D level prior to initiating treatment for osteoporosis.

8. ***Hypervitaminosis D typically occurs from:***

   A. Increased exposure to the sun.
   B. Diet consisting of foods with high vitamin D content.
   C. Exogenous sources of vitamin D as over-the-counter supplements.
   D. A and B.
   E. A, B, and C.

   Correct answer: C

Comment:

Typically, patients take mega doses of exogenous vitamin D, readily available as supplements, obtained over the counter, with no medical prescription required, and taken each day may lead to vitamin D toxicity. Whereas the body is able to regulate the amount of vitamin D absorbed from food sources, it is sometimes not able to maintain a normal vitamin D level from large doses of vitamin D intake.[3]

9. ***Patients at a greater risk to develop hypervitaminosis D include:***
   A. Patients with hypocalcemic disorders, such as hypoparathyroidism, osteomalacia.
   B. Patients with lymphomas.
   C. Patients with Williams-Beuren syndrome.
   D. Patients with tuberculosis.
   E. All of the above.

   Correct answer: E

   Comment:

   Hypersensitivity to vitamin D occurs in patients with lymphomas and granuloma disorders, such as tuberculosis and giant cell polymyositis. PTH levels are suppressed in these cases.[3] In tuberculosis, elevated serum levels of vitamin D are due to macrophages increasing extrarenal synthesis of 1, 25(OH)2D. The pathophysiology of how patients with Williams-Beuren syndrome develop hypervitaminosis D is still obscure.[3]

10. ***The earliest renal sign of vitamin D toxicity is:***
    A. Hypercalciuria.
    B. Polyuria.
    C. Dehydration.
    D. Renal calculi.
    E. All of the above are early signs.

    Correct answer: A

    Comment:

    Hypercalciuria, polyuria, dehydration, and renal calculi are signs of hypervitaminosis D. Hypercalciuria occurs first. Gastrointestinal symptoms, such as nausea/vomiting, constipation, as well as neuropsychiatric symptoms can also occur.[3] It is important to emphasize to patients the need for regular follow-ups.

Key points

- Hypervitaminosis D mainly occurs from exogenous sources, making it preventable in most cases.
- Signs and symptoms of hypervitaminosis D include nausea/vomiting, muscle weakness, dehydration, polyuria, hypercalcemia, and renal calculi.
- The main treatment for hypervitaminosis D is to discontinue vitamin D supplementation and decrease dietary calcium intake. Further treatment is dependent on the patient's symptoms.
- Several diseases can increase the patient's risk of developing vitamin D toxicity. These include tuberculosis, osteomalacia, hypoparathyroidism, Williams-Beuren syndrome, and lymphomas.

References

1. Jin J. Screening for vitamin D deficiency in adults. *JAMA*. 2021;325(14):1436–1442.
2. Berridge M. Vitamin D deficiency and diabetes. *Biochem J*. 2017;474:1321–1332.
3. Marcinowska-Suchowierska E, Kupisz-Urbanska M, Lukaszkiewicz J, et al. Vitamin D toxicity—a clinical perspective. *Front Endocrinol*. 2018;9.
4. Tebben P, Singh R, Kumar R. Vitamin D-mediated hypercalemia: mechanisms, diagnosis, and treatment. *Endocr Rev*. 2016;37(5):521–554.

Magnesium[☆]

Learning objectives

- Signs and symptoms of magnesium deficiency.
- Identifying individuals at risk of magnesium deficiency.
- Impact of magnesium deficiency.

The case study

Reason for seeking medical help

Mrs. JL is experiencing nausea and vomiting for the past 3 days, as well as intermittent muscle cramps. She is known to have osteoporosis as evidenced by a T-score of −2.5 in her left femoral neck and has been on alendronate for about 2 years.

Past medical/surgical history

- Surgical menopause age 48; 3 years of HRT.
- Fractured right radius as a child skateboarding.

Personal habits

- Physically active: walks her two dogs daily.
- Babysits her 4-year-old grandson 3 days a week.
- No cigarette smoking.
- Drinks one cup of coffee daily, and two glasses of sweet tea.
- Drinks two glasses of almond milk, one cup of yogurt daily.

☆ JL, 80-year-old White woman, with magnesium deficiency.

Diagnosis and Treatment of Osteoporosis. https://doi.org/10.1016/B978-0-323-99550-4.00021-6
Copyright © 2024 Elsevier Inc. All rights are reserved, including those for text and data mining, AI training, and similar technologies.

Medication

- Alendronate 70 mg weekly.
- Multivitamin daily.
- Fish oil.
- Vitamin D3 1000 units daily.

Family history

- Negative for osteoporosis.

Clinical examination

- Weight: 118 lbs, height 66″.

Laboratory investigations

- Serum 25-hydroxy-vitamin D: 30 ng/mL.
- Calcium 8.9 mg/dL.
- Magnesium: 0.65 mmol/L.
- Comprehensive metabolic profile: within normal limits.

Multiple choice questions

1. ***Magnesium homeostasis:***
   A. A cause-and-effect relationship between dietary magnesium intake and osteoporosis has not been established.
   B. A tight control of magnesium homeostasis is essential for bone health.
   C. Lower blood levels of magnesium are associated with osteoporosis.
   D. B and C.
   E. All of the above.

   Correct answer: D

   Comment:

   Several studies have shown that about a third of patients with osteoporosis have hypomagnesaemia, and that about 20% of patients with osteoporosis constantly consume diets low in magnesium.[1] Total magnesium in an adult body ranges from 20 to 28 g: approximately 60% in bones, 39% in intracellular compartments, and about 1% in extracellular fluids.

   A cause/effect relationship between dietary magnesium intake and osteoporosis has been established.[1] Magnesium is found in many foods in varying concentrations. Its concentration in leafy vegetables is 30–60 mg/100 g. Larger quantities are present in legumes (80–170mg/100g), nuts (130–264mg/100), and whole grain in wheat bran (up to 550 mg/100 g).

As much as 80% of the magnesium in food is removed during refining treatments; for instance, white bread contains only 15mg/100g. Coffee contains about 80mg/100g. Dried fruit, potatoes, meat, fish, and milk are less rich in magnesium. The magnesium content of bottled water varies between 1 and 109 mg/mL, with an average of 15 mg/mL.[1]

The bioavailability of magnesium also varies according to other specific components of the diet such as phytates, calcium, phosphorus, and long-chain fatty acids which may reduce magnesium gastrointestinal absorption. Cooking, also, may reduce the bioavailability of magnesium.

Magnesium can be taken orally as citrate, carbonate, or oxide, in doses between 250 and 1800 mg daily. An increase in bone mineral density and a reduction in fracture risk have been recorded in individuals taking magnesium supplements.[1]

2. ***The effects of magnesium deficiency include:***
   A. Increased bone fragility.
   B. Impaired vitamin D synthesis and activation.
   C. Impaired neurotransmission.
   D. All of the above.
   E. None of the above.

Correct answer: D

Comment:

Magnesium contributes to a number of body functions, including a direct effect on bone fragility, vitamin D synthesis, electrolyte balance, neurotransmission, and muscle contraction, including heart muscles, cell division, protein synthesis, and maintenance of bones and teeth. Magnesium is also an essential cofactor for vitamin D synthesis and activation which in turn may increase intestinal magnesium absorption.

An important issue to consider is that routinely measured serum magnesium levels do not always accurately reflect the total body magnesium status, so a patient with a "normal serum magnesium" level may in fact have magnesium deficiency.

3. ***Symptoms of magnesium deficiency include:***
   A. Nausea/vomiting.
   B. Fatigue.
   C. Seizures.
   D. Muscle cramps.
   E. All of the above.

Correct answer: E

Comment:

The first signs of hypomagnesemia are nausea, vomiting, and fatigue.[2] JL presents with nausea and vomiting. As the deficiency progresses, numbness, muscle cramps, and seizure occur and eventually, abnormal heart rhythms can develop.[2]

4. ***Individuals at risk of magnesium deficiency include those with:***
   A. Crohn's disease.
   B. Type II diabetes mellitus.
   C. Alcoholic dependency.
   D. Older adults.
   E. All of the above.

   Correct answer: E

   Comment:

   Celiac and Crohn's disease can lead to a decrease in magnesium levels due to malabsorption and diarrhea.[2] Diabetes mellitus can cause an increase in urinary excretion of magnesium. Alcohol dependence and hypomagnesemia can develop as a result of the combination of gastrointestinal issues, such as diarrhea and overall poor nutritional status.[2] In the case of older adults, they tend to consume less foods that contain magnesium and have a decreased ability to absorb the magnesium they consume.[2] In JL's case, her main risk factor is her age, as she does not have Crohn's disease, type II diabetes, or alcohol dependency.

5. ***The best course of action with JL is to:***
   A. Supplement magnesium.
   B. Increase her dietary intake of magnesium.
   C. Supplement magnesium and potassium.
   D. Supplement magnesium, potassium, and calcium.
   E. A and B.

   Correct answer: E

   Comment:

   JL should be educated about food sources that contain magnesium and her Recommended Daily Allowance (RDA) of magnesium. If she is already eating a diet rich in these foods, she may have a decreased ability to absorb magnesium and would benefit from magnesium supplementation.

6. ***JL is on a bisphosphonate. Important teaching regarding magnesium supplementation include:***
   A. Taking the bisphosphonate with the magnesium supplement at the same time to increase the absorption of both.
   B. Taking the magnesium supplement at least 2h after her bisphosphonate.
   C. Taking the magnesium supplement 30min after her bisphosphonate.
   D. Stopping the bisphosphonate and prescribe zoledronic acid instead.
   E. Taking the magnesium supplement 30min before the bisphosphonate.

   Correct answer: B

   Comment:

   The intake of magnesium supplement should be separated from the bisphosphonate by at least 2h to prevent a decrease in the amount of bisphosphonate absorbed.[2] The bisphosphonate should be taken first while fasting.

7. ***Foods that contain magnesium include:***
   A. Pumpkin seeds.
   B. Peanut butter.
   C. Avocado.
   D. Yogurt.
   E. All of the above.

   Correct answer: E

   Comment:

   Magnesium is found in a wide variety of foods. Pumpkin and chia seeds have the largest amount per serving. Magnesium can be found in meat; vegetables such as spinach, broccoli; fruits; and various nuts.[2] The recommended daily allowance of magnesium is 320 mg for women older than 51 years old, as is JL's case.[2]

8. ***Magnesium deficiency can result in:***
   A. Osteoporosis.
   B. Sarcopenia.
   C. Cardiovascular disease.
   D. Kidney disease.
   E. A, B, and C.

   Correct answer: E

   Comment:

   Magnesium deficiency is intertwined with all three diseases: osteoporosis, sarcopenia, and cardiovascular diseases.[3–6] Sarcopenia is the loss of muscle mass and function. Magnesium is involved in muscle contractions as well as bone formation.[2] Magnesium supplementation can decrease blood pressure which is a risk factor for patients with cardiovascular diseases.[2]

   Magnesium levels can be measured in a variety of ways. With only about 1% of magnesium residing in serum levels, sometimes a magnesium tolerance test is used to assess magnesium status.[2] This involves infusing magnesium and then measuring urinary output and is far more invasive. Magnesium status should be evaluated clinically as well as by laboratory studies.[2–4] In JL's case, she exhibits both clinical symptoms and has a low magnesium level.

9. ***Magnesium is closely linked with:***
   A. Calcium.
   B. Vitamin D.
   C. PTH.
   D. A and B.
   E. All of the above.

   Correct answer: E

   Comment:

   Magnesium is needed for calcium and vitamin D metabolism.[1–6] Calcium levels are decreased with insufficient magnesium intake.[2–6] When magnesium levels decrease, the body tries to compensate by increasing PTH levels to maintain homeostasis.[1–6]

10. ***Magnesium deficiency can lead to osteoporosis by:***
    A. Increasing bone turnover.
    B. Affecting calcium, PTH, and vitamin D.
    C. Inducing inflammation and bone remodeling.
    D. Inducing endothelial dysfunction.
    E. All of the above.

    Correct answer: E

    Comment:

    Magnesium affects the body's homeostasis by all of the processes mentioned before and can lead to bone mineral density loss if not corrected.[6] Serum levels of magnesium are not an accurate picture of a person's magnesium status as they consider neither intracellular magnesium nor magnesium in the bones.[2]

    Other methods of measuring magnesium include ionized magnesium, magnesium tolerance test, and measuring magnesium levels in the saliva and urine.

Key points

- Magnesium plays an essential role in bone health.
- Magnesium deficiency causes a variety of symptoms, including nausea, vomiting, fatigue, muscle cramps, and seizures.
- Diseases due to malabsorption or gastrointestinal issues can cause magnesium deficiency, such as celiac disease or Crohn's disease.
- Older individuals are more likely to develop magnesium deficiency as they tend to consume less magnesium-rich foods.
- Complications from magnesium deficiency include osteoporosis, cardiovascular, and kidney diseases.

References

1. Rondanelli M, Faliva AM, Tartara A, et al. An update on magnesium and bone health. *Biometals.* 2021;34:715–736.
2. National Institutes of Health. *Magnesium.* 2021.
3. Pickering ME. Cross-talks between the cardiovascular disease-sarcopenia-osteoporosis triad and magnesium in humans. *Int J Mol Sci.* 2021;22(16):9102. Published 2021 August 23 https://doi.org/10.3390/ijms22169102.
4. Mederle OA, Balas M, Ioanoviciu SD, Gurban CV, Tudor A, Borza C. Correlations between bone turnover markers, serum magnesium and bone mass density in postmenopausal osteoporosis. *Clin Interv Aging.* 2018;13:1383–1389. Published 2018 August 3 https://doi.org/10.2147/CIA.S170111.
5. Erem S, Atfi A, Razzaque MS. Anabolic effects of vitamin D and magnesium in aging bone. *J Steroid Biochem Mol Biol.* 2019;193:105400. https://doi.org/10.1016/j.jsbmb.2019.105400.
6. Chang J, Yu D, Ji J, Wang N, Yu S, Yu B. The association between the concentration of serum magnesium and postmenopausal osteoporosis. *Front Med (Lausanne).* 2020;7:381. Published 2020 Aug 4 https://doi.org/10.3389/fmed.2020.00381.

CHAPTER 33

Physical exercise and bone health☆

Learning objectives

- Identify physical exercises that should be incorporated in the management of osteoporosis.
- Identify physical exercises that should be avoided in patients with osteoporosis.
- Recognize when to refer a patient for physical therapy.

The case study

Reasons for seeking medical help

- JC, a 68-year-old Asian woman, was recently diagnosed with osteoporosis as evidenced by a T-score of −2.5 in her upper four lumbar vertebrae. Her VFA does not show any fractures. She is now taking alendronate 70 mg weekly as directed and is not experiencing adverse effects. She would like to exercise, but is unsure which physical exercises are appropriate for her.
- She is also concerned that her balance has deteriorated since she stopped doing yoga after her hip surgery for osteoarthritis. She currently lives alone and would like to stay as independent as possible.

Past surgical and medical history

- Right hip replacement due to osteoarthritis at age 62 years. Good results except for occasional bouts of unsteadiness, occurring with no definite precipitating factors. She, however, experienced three near-falls during the past 2 weeks. She saw her primary care provider who recommended she continue walking and use a walking aid if necessary. She is reluctant to follow that advice and is seeking help.
- Natural menopause at age 52 years, received hormonal replacement therapy for about 6 months then discontinued it because of fear of adverse effects.

☆ JC, a 68-year-old Asian woman, with osteoporosis.

Diagnosis and Treatment of Osteoporosis. https://doi.org/10.1016/B978-0-323-99550-4.00003-4
Copyright © 2024 Elsevier Inc. All rights are reserved, including those for text and data mining, AI training, and similar technologies.

Lifestyle

- Gardens regularly, weather permitting.
- Took yoga classes for about 4 months prior to her hip replacement surgery. She enjoyed these exercises and is happy to continue, but is concerned they may not be appropriate for her, especially since she experienced bouts of unsteadiness.
- Walks daily, about 45 min.
- No cigarette smoking.
- No excessive sodium, caffeine, or alcohol intake.

Medication(s)

- Multivitamin daily.
- Vitamin D3 1000 units daily.
- Calcium 1200 mg daily.

Family history

- Negative for osteoporosis.

Clinical examination

- Weight 100 lbs., height 62″.
- Mild kyphosis.
- No significant clinical findings.

Laboratory results

- Comprehensive Metabolic Profile (CMP): All results within normal limits.
- Serum 25-hydroxy-vitamin D: 42 ng/mL.

Multiple choice questions

1. ***Exercises to incorporate in a program for osteoporosis include:***
   A. Planks.
   B. Pelvic bridges.
   C. Wall angels.
   D. Reverse sit-ups.
   E. All of the above.
   Correct answer: E

Comment:

Ideally, a physical exercise program should be developed, individualized, and tailored to meet JC's specific personal needs, capabilities, and circumstances. Ideally this should be done in conjunction with a physical therapist or an occupational therapist experienced with the needs and problems of patients with osteoporosis who have undergone hip replacement surgery.

Trunk flexion exercises such as sit-ups may increase pressure on the vertebral column. Plank exercises are preferable for patients with osteoporosis. Planks strengthen the rectus abdominis. Pelvic bridges strengthen the gluteal muscles and pelvic floor, as well as hip flexors.

Supine poses are a good choice for patients with kyphosis and balance issues because they do not increase the pressure on the thoracic vertebrae and do not increase the risk of falling. They also tend to isolate the hip flexors, which help in stabilization of the core and spine. Wall angels are beneficial to improve posture and strengthen back extensor muscles.

In JC's case, she has mild kyphosis which can potentially be improved by performing these exercises. In addition, many exercises can be performed from a seated position. This is especially helpful if the patient has difficulty standing and/or walking due to arthritic pain. These exercises include ankle plantar flexion and dorsiflexion, knee flexion and extension, hip flexion, extension, abduction, adduction, shoulder, and elbow flexion. It is also useful to use rubber balls, a small one to exercise the muscles of the hand and a larger one for hips, knees, and ankles. Many of these exercises can be performed while the patient is sitting down.

2. ***Balance exercises appropriate for fall prevention in patients with osteoporosis include:***
   A. Tai Chi.
   B. Sit to standing exercises.
   C. Yoga.
   D. Whole body vibration machines.
   E. A, B, and C.

   Correct answer: E

   Comment:

   Tai Chi performed regularly improves balance, coordination, muscle strength, and helps fall prevention.[1] Tai Chi also improves bone mineral density in the lumbar vertebrae.[1] Sitting to standing exercises target core muscles which aid in balance. Yoga also helps with balance and proprioception. Results of research concerning whole body vibration machines and balance in older individuals are inconclusive at present.[2]

3. ***A physical exercise program for osteoporosis should be:***
   A. Individualized.
   B. Ideally supervised by a licensed health care professional with expertise managing patients with osteoporosis.
   C. Easily accessible.

D. In a gym setting.
E. A, B, and C.

Correct answer: E

Comment:

Physical exercise programs should be, at least initially, supervised by a licensed health care professional. Programs should be tailored to the individual needs, regarding cardiovascular health, strength, balance, accessibility, and cognitive functions. It does not need to be in a gym setting. It should be developed for the patient to perform in his or her home, preferably with minimal equipment to keep it cost efficient and more accessible.

4. ***Exercises to avoid by patients with a diagnosis of osteoporosis include:***

A. Sit-ups.
B. Deep spinal twists.
C. Forward bends.
D. Rounding of the back.
E. All of the above.

Correct answer: E

Comment:

JC should avoid exercises that involve rounding of the spine, such as sit-ups, cat/cow in yoga, forward bends with a rounded back, and weighted movements at the end range of flexion.[3] These exercises may increase the risk of sustaining a vertebral compression fracture. In addition, deep twisting motions can cause compression fractures. It is also important for JC to remember to use a hip hinge when picking up objects from the floor, as this decreases the pressure on her back and is proper lifting form.

5. ***Aerobic exercise benefits other disease processes including:***

A. Diabetes mellitus.
B. Cardiovascular diseases.
C. Sarcopenia.
D. Neurodegeneration.
E. All of the above.

Correct answer: E

Comment:

Physical exercise is an effective method of improving glycemic control in patients with type II diabetes mellitus.[4] Aerobic exercises can help decrease muscle wasting that occurs with sarcopenia.[5] Aerobic exercises help decrease neurodegeneration, increase neuron formation and mitochondrial biogenesis, and modulate amyloid-degrading enzymes.[6]

6. ***Peak bone mass occurs in the following groups:***

A. Teenage years.
B. 20s–30s.
C. 40s.

D. At the beginning of the menopause.
E. After the menopause.

Correct answer: B

Comment:

Peak bone mass is not reached at the same time in all the skeleton. In most bones, however, it is reached in the 20s–30s. Physical activity has the greatest impact on adolescents as they still develop their bone mass to reach the highest genetically determined level.[7]

7. ***JC comes back to the office to follow-up on her osteoporosis regarding exercises. She has heard that free weights will help her but has never lifted weights. The following is recommended:***

A. Buy a light set of free weights for at-home use.
B. Work with a personal trainer for an appropriate plan and for guidance on correct form.
C. Work with a personal trainer but encourage weight machine use.
D. Do not lift free weights.
E. Use a mix of free weights and machines at a gym.

Correct answer: B

Comment:

JC has mild kyphosis and no history of lifting weights. Given this, and her eagerness to develop an exercise programs tailored to her own individual needs, a good recommendation is for her to seek help from a personal qualified trainer who would ensure she has correct lifting form and to help create a workout plan individualized to meet her own needs.

As a general rule, a combination of resistive and aerobic exercises will be helpful. It is also important for JC to fully understand that experiencing pain while performing a physical exercise is an important sign that the intensity of that particular exercise at that particular time is being exceeded and is an important warning signal to stop performing this exercise. She may try again a few days later.

8. ***In addition, JC would like help for her mild kyphosis. Recommendations include:***

A. Refer to physical therapy for individualized exercises.
B. Advise JC to "stand up straight" and work on standing straight multiple times throughout the day.
C. Discuss a few exercises and provide an educational handout.
D. Consider kyphoplasty.
E. A and C.

Correct answer: E

Comment:

Having a reliable reference to give patients as well as a few basic exercises for them to do is a great first step in improving the patients' posture and overall wellness. Referring to physical therapy is another option and can help patients with more in-depth care as well as developing an individualized plan. Given the low magnitude of the pain JC is experiencing, there is no need to consider kyphoplasty.

9. ***JC returns 6 months later for a follow-up visit. She is feeling well, but is asking whether a whole body vibration machine would speed up her progress. The best response is:***
   A. The results of the research are conflicting.
   B. It is highly recommended.
   C. Resistance exercises are a more appropriate option.
   D. A combination of weight-bearing and resistance exercises are more appropriate options.
   E. A and D.

   Correct answer: E

   Comment:

   Kyphosis can be improved by exercises that target paravertebral muscles.[8] Research regarding whole body vibration machines is at present inconclusive. Most published studies have a small sample size. There also is little consistency on the minimum amount used to show an improvement in bone density. Both weight-bearing exercise and resistance exercises are recommended to help increase bone density in patients with a diagnosis of osteoporosis.

10. ***JC would like to directly target her lumbar vertebrae in her exercise plan. Ways to specifically target lumbar vertebrae include:***
    A. Running.
    B. Jumping.
    C. Cyclic.
    D. Any of the above.
    E. None of the above.

    Correct answer: E

    Comment:

    While research is limited regarding site-specific increases, a mixture of aerobic and resistance exercises is recommended to help increase bone mineral density.[9]

Key points

- A mixture of aerobic and resistive exercises is recommended for patients with osteoporosis.
- Physical therapists can develop an individualized plan of care for the patient in question focusing on his/her specific needs and goals.
- Exercises to avoid in patients with osteoporosis include those that increase pressure on vertebrae, as they may cause a vertebral compression fracture.

References

1. Erhan B, Ataker Y. Rehabilitation of patients with osteoporotic fractures. *J Clin Densitom.* 2020;23(4):534–538. https://doi.org/10.1016/j.jocd.2020.06.006.
2. Lam FM, Lau RW, Chung RC, Pang MY. The effect of whole body vibration on balance, mobility and falls in older adults: a systematic review and meta-analysis. *Maturitas.* 2012;72(3):206–213. https://doi.org/10.1016/j.maturitas.2012.04.009.
3. Giangregorio LM, McGill S, Wark JD, et al. Too fit to fracture: outcomes of a Delphi consensus process on physical activity and exercise recommendations for adults with osteoporosis with or without vertebral fractures. *Osteoporos Int.* 2015;26(3):891–910. https://doi.org/10.1007/s00198-014-2881-4.
4. Sampath Kumar A, Maiya AG, Shastry BA, et al. Exercise and insulin resistance in type 2 diabetes mellitus: a systematic review and meta-analysis. *Ann Phys Rehabil Med.* 2019;62(2):98–103. https://doi.org/10.1016/j.rehab.2018.11.001.
5. Yoo SZ, No MH, Heo JW, et al. Role of exercise in age-related sarcopenia. *J Exerc Rehabil.* 2018;14(4):551–558. Published 2018 August 24 10.12965/jer.1836268.134.
6. Garatachea N, Pareja-Galeano H, Sanchis-Gomar F, et al. Exercise attenuates the major hallmarks of aging. *Rejuvenation Res.* 2015;18(1):57–89. https://doi.org/10.1089/rej.2014.1623.
7. Troy KL, Mancuso ME, Butler TA, Johnson JE. Exercise early and often: effects of physical activity and exercise on women's bone health. *Int J Environ Res Public Health.* 2018;15(5):878. Published 2018 April 28 https://doi.org/10.3390/ijerph15050878.
8. Katzman WB, Vittinghoff E, Lin F, et al. Targeted spine strengthening exercise and posture training program to reduce hyperkyphosis in older adults: results from the study of hyperkyphosis, exercise, and function (SHEAF) randomized controlled trial. *Osteoporos Int.* 2017;28(10):2831–2841. https://doi.org/10.1007/s00198-017-4109-x.
9. Winters-Stone KM, Snow CM. Site-specific response of bone to exercise in premenopausal women. *Bone.* 2006;39(6):1203–1209. https://doi.org/10.1016/j.bone.2006.06.005.

CHAPTER 34

Falls—Part I—Endogenous causes☆

Learning objectives

- Recognize endogenous causes of repeated falls.
- Alcohol and over-the-counter medications that increase the fall risk.

The case study

Reason for seeking medical help

- AB was referred to the office after having sustained six falls in the last 6months. His wife is concerned that he is at risk of sustaining fractures. He has osteopenia, as evidenced by a T-score of −1.6 in his left femoral neck. His FRAX scores are 15% and 3.5% for the risks of sustaining a major or hip/femoral neck fracture. He is being treated with alendronate 70mg weekly.

Past medical/surgical history

- Benign prostatic hyperplasia.
- History of basal cell skin cancer.
- Right knee replacement 2008.
- Arthritis left hip.
- Seasonal allergies.

Personal habits

- No cigarette smoking.
- No excessive sodium.
- Drinks two cups of coffee a day and an occasional glass of sweet tea.
- Drinks one beer a couple days of week.
- Enjoys milk daily.
- Walks most days for about half an hour with his wife and dog.

☆ Mr. AB, 82-year-old Caucasian man, osteopenia, multiple falls.

Diagnosis and Treatment of Osteoporosis. https://doi.org/10.1016/B978-0-323-99550-4.00020-4
Copyright © 2024 Elsevier Inc. All rights are reserved, including those for text and data mining, AI training, and similar technologies.

Medication(s)

- Flomax 0.4 mg daily.
- Atorvastatin 10 mg daily.
- Vitamin D3 1000 units daily.
- Multivitamin daily.
- Melatonin 3 mg at bedtime as needed.
- Tylenol arthritis as needed.

Family history

- Positive for osteoporosis, older sister has no fractures.
- Positive for cardiovascular disease, father and brother have coronary artery disease.

Clinical examination

- Weight: 148 lbs., height: 71″.
- Mild kyphosis, mostly postural.
- Clinical examination does not reveal any significant clinical finding.

Laboratory results

- CMP: WNL, except GFR 59 mL/min.
- Serum 25-hydroxy-vitamin D: 46 ng/mL.

Multiple choice questions

Multiple disease processes can increase the risk of falls in the elderly. Arthropathies can cause gait imbalance due to pain. AB has a history of a knee replacement and has arthritis in his left hip that can cause a shift in his center of gravity as he ambulates and subsequently changes his overall gait.

His cognitive status is important to ascertain as confusion can lead to risky behavior, such as climbing ladders, walking up and down the stairs, without paying due attention to the stairs or activities he would normally avoid as they may increase the risk of sustaining a fall.

Cardiovascular disorders, such as orthostatic hypotension or arrhythmias, can also cause the patient to have dizziness upon standing. About 40% of older adults with cardiovascular disease experience orthostatic hypotension.[1]

Frequent urination as with BPH or a UTI can make the patient hurry to reach the bathroom in time and may trip over various objects.

1. ***Other endogenous factors to consider include:***
   A. Medications.
   B. Visual impairment.
   C. Sedentary lifestyle.
   D. Vestibular diseases.
   E. All of the above.

   Correct answer: E

   Comment:

   In older people repeated falls often have a multifactorial etiology. Preventing them is aimed at decreasing as many of the modifiable risk factors as possible.[2] Medications, such as hypnotics, sedatives, hypotensives, and diuretics, can all contribute and increase the risk for falls. Visual impairment, especially cataracts and bifocal eyeglasses, can add to the decreased or distorted perception of the environment and may lead to multiple falls. Sedentary lifestyles decrease muscular strength and can lead to muscle wasting. Vestibular diseases make patients dizzy and unstable, increasing their risk of falls.[3]

2. ***His last fall occurred in the middle of the night as he was going to the bathroom. He remembers heading to the bathroom to micturate and the next thing he knew he was lying on the floor. Luckily his wife was able to help him up and he did not sustain any serious injuries. Aside from environmental factors, AB can decrease the risk of sustaining another fall by:***
   A. Discontinuing melatonin use.
   B. Gait and strength evaluation to determine if physical therapy is needed.
   C. Limiting his fluid intake late in the evening and at night to decrease the number of times he needs to use the bathroom at night.
   D. Consider the use of a urinal at night.
   E. All of the above.

   Correct answer: E

   Comment:

   If AB has decreased strength or pain in the legs and/or an abnormal gait, these can contribute to his likelihood of having another fall. Limiting his fluid intake could potentially decrease the need for urination during the night. It is nevertheless important to balance this by making sure he is properly hydrated during the day to prevent dehydration. If AB is having a marked decrease in blood pressure, i.e. a drop of 20 mm or more in the systolic and/or diastolic blood pressure upon rising from the bed associated with dizziness, this increases the fall risk.

   Research regarding melatonin is limited. Discontinuing it may be appropriate if AB feels groggier or sedated when he takes it.

3. ***AB states that he experiences nocturia and typically needs to urinate 3–4 times per night. He usually goes to bed around 10 pm and wakes up at about 3 am but has difficulties***

falling back asleep after he urinates. An additional concern regarding his frequent urination is:

A. Disrupted circadian rhythm that may potentially increase the risk of falls.
B. He probably will need to nap during the day, as his sleep is less restful.
C. He may have a urinary tract infection.
D. A and B.
E. All of the above.

Correct answer: E

Comment:

A dysregulated sleep cycle can lead to orthostatic intolerance and further lead to falls. It can also lead to cognitive decline.[2] Melatonin plays an important role in the sleep/wake cycle which tends to decrease with age. Decreases in melatonin also may be linked with bone loss and subsequent osteoporosis.[2]

4. ***The following is/are true:***

A. A number of home-based exercise programs are available.
B. Home-based strength and retraining programs significantly reduce the rate of subsequent falls.
C. Adverse events included falls, injuries, and muscle soreness related to the exercise intervention.
D. All of the above.
E. None of the above

Correct answer: D

Comment:

All the above are true.[4] Their success is probably dependent on a number of factors including expertise and availability of staff to man such home-based strength and retraining programs.

5. ***During his visit AB reveals that he often drinks a beer on the nights he has more trouble sleeping. His normal routine is to get up and drink at least another beer before going back to bed. Important points to remember:***

A. Older adults are affected more rapidly and to a larger extent by alcohol than women.
B. Melatonin may interfere with the sleep/wake periods.
C. Beer increases the risk of nocturia.
D. A and C.
E. All of the above.

Correct answer: E

Comment:

AB is having at least one beer on nights he is unable to sleep but may be having up to three beers on some nights. This will affect his coordination and gait, making him at increased risk for falls.[5] The alcohol will also increase his nocturia. Adding a dose of melatonin with the alcohol may compound the problem by further impairing his cognition, gait, and reaction time, making his walk to the bathroom more dangerous. Melatonin research with regard to falls is somewhat limited at this time.

6. ***Interventions to decrease the fall risk for AB include:***
   A. Develop a sleep routine.
   B. Limit alcohol intake before going to bed.
   C. Limit/discontinue melatonin use.
   D. Physical exercise.
   E. All of the above.

   Correct answer: E

   Comment:

   As previously discussed, alcohol is harder to process in older adults. Limiting AB's intake to 1 beer and disassociating it from being considered a sleep aid will help with his cognition and balance, especially if he has polyuria at night. Creating an environment conducive to sleep, blackout curtains, cooler temperatures in his bedroom, consistent bedtimes, and limiting blue light exposure at nighttime should help with his ability to drift off to sleep. Melatonin use, while it can help reset his sleep/wake cycle, may impair his coordination and leave him more susceptible to sustaining repeated falls.

   Then, lastly, AB should be encouraged to remain awake during the day and to exercise as much as possible. Several exercises can be done while seated. Walking along the corridors during the day may help. The more he is able to move, within his abilities, the better he will sleep. Slowly increasing the distance walked will help strengthen the skeleton and increasing muscle mass. Also, exposure to sunlight will naturally help his circadian rhythm, which diminishes as age increases. AB, however, needs to be cautious about the amount of sun exposure as he has a history of skin cancer.

7. ***AB also reveals he occasionally takes Benadryl for sleep. He states at least once a week he will have a dose of Benadryl, usually after a particularly bad night. Adverse effects of antihistamines include:***
   A. Increased fall risk.
   B. Aggravated prostatic hypertrophy.
   C. Dizziness and impaired coordination.
   D. Blurred vision.
   E. All of the above.

   Correct answer: E

   Comment:

   Anticholinergic medications can increase the risk of falls by all of the above.[6] In addition, anticholinergic use, greater than 3 months, increases the risk of dementia in older individuals.[7] Given AB's recurrent falls, benign prostatic hypertrophy, nocturia, and age, he should discontinue any further Benadryl use. It is also important to avoid analgesics with sedative effects as these can also contribute to an increased risk of falls.

8. ***AB's evaluation reveals he has orthostatic hypotension: His supine blood pressure is 130/72, dropping to on standing of 95/65 standing up. Standing up induces dizziness and unsteadiness. The following is appropriate:***
   A. Stop tamsulosin (Flomax).
   B. Continue Flomax and monitor his orthostatic hypotension.
   C. Caution him of the use of Flomax because of his orthostatic hypotension.
   D. Evaluate his need for Flomax, his symptom relief, and his degree of orthostatic hypotension and subsequent fall/fracture risk.
   E. B and C.

   Correct answer: D

   Comment:

   The best option for AB is to evaluate the effectiveness of Flomax. If there is an appropriate alternative for him that does not have the same risk factors, then discontinuing it and starting a new medication is preferable. If Flomax is not relieving his symptoms, he can discontinue it and then be reevaluated for orthostatic hypotension. Given his recurrent falls, it is important to decrease any dizziness or unsteadiness related to medication use if possible.

9. ***AB is found to have peripheral neuropathy after a thorough history, laboratory studies, and clinical exam. Peripheral neuropathy:***
   A. Increases AB's fall risk.
   B. Can impair AB's dynamic balance.
   C. Can be addressed with physical therapy.
   D. A and B.
   E. All of the above.

   Correct answer: E

   Comment:

   Peripheral neuropathy results in muscle weakness and balance and gait disturbance. Physical therapy can be used to address the effects of peripheral neuropathy in the lower limbs.[8]

Key points

- Intrinsic risk factors of falls include cardiovascular disease, metabolic disease, dementia, and frequent urination.
- Additional risk factors for falls: orthostatic hypotension, certain medications, OTC medications, and alcohol.
- Sleep routines can help decrease fall risks.

References

1. Setters B, Holmes HM. Hypertension in the older adult. *Prim Care*. 2017;44(3):529–539. https://doi.org/10.1016/j.pop.2017.05.002.
2. Goswami N, Abulafia C, Vigo D, Moser M, Cornelissen G, Cardinali D. Falls risk, circadian rhythms and melatonin: current perspectives. *Clin Interv Aging*. 2020;15:2165–2174. Published 2020 November 11. https://doi.org/10.2147/CIA.S283342.
3. Carender WJ, Grzesiak M, Telian SA. Vestibular physical therapy and fall risk assessment. *Otolaryngol Clin North Am*. 2021;54(5):1015–1036. https://doi.org/10.1016/j.otc.2021.05.018.
4. Rinonapoli G, Ruggiero C, Meccariello L, Bisaccia M, Ceccarini P, Caraffa A. Osteoporosis in men: a review of an underestimated bone condition. *Int J Mol Sci*. 2021;22(4):2105. Published 2021 February 20. https://doi.org/10.3390/ijms22042105.
5. National Institute on Alcohol Abuse and Alcoholism. Older adults. https://www.niaaa.nih.gov/alcohols-effects-health/special-populations-co-occurring-disorders/older-adults.
6. Tan MP, Tan GJ, Mat S, et al. Use of medications with anticholinergic properties and the long-term risk of hospitalization for falls and fractures in the EPIC-Norfolk longitudinal cohort study. *Drugs Aging*. 2020;37(2):105–114. https://doi.org/10.1007/s40266-019-00731-3.
7. Dmochowski RR, Thai S, Iglay K, et al. Increased risk of incident dementia following use of anticholinergic agents: a systematic literature review and meta-analysis. *NeurourolUrodyn*. 2021;40(1):28–37. https://doi.org/10.1002/nau.24536.
8. Caronni A, Picardi M, Pintavalle G, et al. Responsiveness to rehabilitation of balance and gait impairment in elderly with peripheral neuropathy. *J Biomech*. 2019;94:31–38. https://doi.org/10.1016/j.jbiomech.2019.07.007.

CHAPTER 35

Falls—Part II—Environmental hazards☆

Learning objectives

- Recognize common environmental hazards increasing the risk of falls.
- Identify modifiable risk factors that increase the risk of repeated falls and fractures.

The case study

Reason for seeking medical help

TC is a 76-year-old Caucasian woman referred because she had 3 accidental falls about 4weeks ago while visiting her daughter, son-in-law, and grandchildren. She sustained extensive superficial injuries but did not fracture any bone. She is now back home and is concerned about these falls, especially as she is known to have osteoporosis. Her lowest T-score was −2.8 in the left femoral neck and she is being treated for osteoporosis. Otherwise, she is known to be in good health. She is receiving zoledronic acid (Reclast) yearly infusions since her diagnosis of osteoporosis just over 2 years ago. She is tolerating it well, but is concerned about the repeated falls she sustained.

Past medical/surgical history

- Surgical menopause age 48, 2years of hormonal replacement therapy.
- Fractured right wrist in her 30s doing step aerobics class.

Lifestyle

- Sedentary lifestyle. She does not exercise regularly.
- Works in her house, including cleaning and cooking.
- Babysits her 3-year-old grandson five days a week.
- She does not drink milk: she thinks she has lactose intolerance.
- She has one cup of coffee every day.

☆ TC, 76-year-old Caucasian woman, osteoporosis, history of repeated falls.

Diagnosis and Treatment of Osteoporosis. https://doi.org/10.1016/B978-0-323-99550-4.00019-8
Copyright © 2024 Elsevier Inc. All rights are reserved, including those for text and data mining, AI training, and similar technologies.

Medication(s)

- Vitamin D3 1000 IU daily.
- Calcium carbonate 1200 mg daily.
- Multivitamin daily.
- Reclast IV yearly; she has received two infusions. The next one is scheduled in about 9 months.
- Atorvastatin 10 mg daily.

Family history

- Positive for osteoporosis, mother sustained a distal radius fracture after minimal trauma: sliding on the wet floor in her bathroom.

Clinical examination

- Weight: 132 lbs; height: 64″, mild kyphosis.
- Mild osteoarthritic changes in both hands and knees. No pain. No limitation in the range of motion.

Laboratory results

- CMP and CBC: within normal limits.
- Serum 25-hydroxy-vitamin D: 45 ng/mL.

Multiple choice questions

1. **TC's most recent fall was about two weeks ago. She was wearing her slippers, carrying a laundry basket, and fell down three steps in her basement. She did not sustain a fracture but was badly bruised and is afraid of sustaining more falls. Recommendations for TC should include:**
   A. Avoid carrying large objects while going downstairs, if possible.
   B. Wear appropriate footwear when going down the stairs to the basement.
   C. Referral for a physical therapy evaluation to improve strength and balance.
   D. Make sure lighting is adequate before going downstairs.
   E. All of the above.

   Correct answer: E

   Comment:

   It is important to assess extrinsic factors that can cause a hazardous environment for patients such as TC. The stairs to her basement, especially if she cannot see them clearly, are an obvious risk factor, along with her loose ill-fitting slippers. In addition, she was carrying something so large that she could not see clearly the areas immediately surrounding her feet when she fell. Recommending her to use rubber-soled footwear for going up and down to the basement or any slippery surface will improve her traction on the steps. Having someone to help her carry laundry up and down or if she uses smaller baskets to transfer clothes can also decrease her risk factors.

Given TC's bruising, it is important to keep in mind that abuse could be a contributing factor to falls.

2. ***TC states that this is her fourth fall in a year. She is now fearful she will fall again. Risk factors for falls include:***
   A. Balance and gait issues, joint disorders, muscle weakness.
   B. Poor vision.
   C. Impaired cognition.
   D. Environmental causes.
   E. All of the above.

   Correct answer: E

   Comment:

   Balance and gait issues, poor vision, impaired cognition, and environmental causes are all risk factors for falls in older people. In TC's case, environmental causes seem to be the main cause of her most recent falls. However, impaired balance, localized muscle weakness, impaired vision and cognition should all be assessed to ascertain if they also contributed to her fall.[1]

   Patients can get easily in a vicious cycle with repeated falls: by decreasing their physical activity, their muscle strength and coordination are decreased, they feel unsteady, limit the amount of physical exercise performed, which in turn causes their muscles waste and they end up further increasing the risk of falling.[1] TC needs to break the fall cycle as soon as possible before muscular atrophy starts to develop.

   Several additional risk factors include loose rugs, pets, and especially clutter.[2] Rugs, especially small ones, that are not properly secured to the floor can also cause tripping or sliding, leading to a fall.

   Small pets, such as cats and dogs, can get underfoot or larger dogs can jump and knock an individual over. Lighting is often a big issue as older individuals often have trouble with cataracts. Bright lights, however, can also cause glare. Low lighting creates a dark environment, making it difficult to see items in their pathway.[2] In addition, clutter can also create an environmental hazard, increasing the fall risk.

3. ***Fracture Risk Assessment can be performed to determine a patient's risk of sustaining a fracture in the next 10 years. Risk factors included in the FRAX score are as follows:***
   A. BMD of femoral neck.
   B. Age.
   C. Previous fracture.
   D. Current smoker.

E. All of the above.

Correct answer: E

Comment:

Given that most fractures are preceded by falls, and that most falls are not followed by fractures, clinicians have an ideal opportunity of identifying and quantifying the risk of falls. Once a fall has occurred, the patient's fracture risk is elevated. Several algorithms are available to identify and quantify the risk of falls. The FRAX instrument incorporates multiple factors to determine a patient's 10-year probability of sustaining a major osteoporotic fracture and a hip fracture. It can be calculated with or without the bone mineral density and is typically used to determine if a patient with osteopenia should receive pharmacologic treatment for osteopenia or if a nonpharmacologic treatment approach is best. The FRAX algorithm is best used in addition to a thorough clinical assessment and history and not a stand-alone tool, unless it is for screening purposes.

4. ***TC has sustained several falls in the past few months and is now fearful she will fall again. She is experiencing the postanxiety fall syndrome. The following is/are correct:***

A. Repeated falls may lead to a fear of falling: the patients decrease their physical activity, which causes a loss of muscle bulk, decreased strength, impaired balance, and poor coordination. This leads to decreased overall function and increases the risk of the patient sustaining another fall.

B. An anxiolytic is needed.

C. The use of a walking aid such as a cane or walker should be discussed with the patient.

D. Patients should be referred for physical therapy to improve their balance.

E. A, C, and D.

Correct answer: E

Comment:

The postfall anxiety syndrome: Multiple falls can create an anxiety/fear cycle: a fall also can lead to avoidance of activities perceived as activities that may increase the risk of falling, which in turn leads to loss of muscular strength, balance, and coordination and further decreases in physical functions.[1–3]

It is important to break this cycle. If TC continues to reduce her degree of physical activity due to fear, she may increase the rate of her bone and muscle mass loss. Patients need physical therapy to help improve their balance. Thoroughly assessing the causes and pattern of falls and modifying risks factors should help decrease the anxiety experienced about falls.

A walker or a three- or four-pronged cane may be appealing to the patient. Single-pronged canes are not recommended as they may increase rather than decrease the patient's stability. The risk with anxiolytics is clouding of consciousness and impaired coordination, which may in turn increase the risk of sustaining falls.

5. ***With any fall, it is important to obtain a complete account if possible. Important factors to determine include:***
   A. Symptoms developing immediately prior to the fall such as lightheaded, dizziness, and palpitations.
   B. Activity involved in when the fall occurred: walking, climbing a ladder, going down steps.
   C. Location of the fall: where do the fall tend to occur and how the patients land.
   D. Injuries associated with the fall.
   E. All of the above.

   Correct answer: E

   Comment:

   A thorough assessment of events occurring immediately prior to the fall, during the fall, and postfall will help identify many risk factors for repeated falls.[1] If any factor is modifiable, it can be addressed immediately in order to help prevent a recurrence. Also, if someone witnesses the fall, the witness can help add details as the patient does not always have a clear memory of the events leading up to, during, and after the fall. TC did not experience any endogenous factor related to her fall. These are discussed in another case in this series.
6. ***Recommendations to increase muscular strength and balance following a fall include:***
   A. Home-based exercise program with a physical therapist.
   B. Gym-based exercise program with a personal trainer.
   C. In-office exercise classes.
   D. No exercises are recommended.
   E. A, B, and C.

   Correct answer: E

   Comment:

   Following a fall, a home-based exercise program led by a physical therapist is the best intervention to improve strength.[4] Patients can graduate to a gym-based program with a personal trainer if they so desire and have the financial means to accommodate this.
   A more accessible option is an in-home program with the goal of continuing the exercises even after the sessions have ended. Strength and balance training should continue for fall prevention.
7. ***Modifiable risk factors in relation to osteoporosis that increase the fracture risk:***
   A. Malnutrition.
   B. Alcohol abuse.
   C. Regular intake of over-the-counter hypnotics.
   D. Bifocal eyeglasses.
   E. All of the above.

   Correct answer: E

Comment:

Malnutrition can contribute to an increased fall risk and osteoporosis. A well-balanced diet is essential. Similarly, excessive salt, caffeine, and phosphoric acid induce a negative calcium balance and cause bone demineralization. It is important to address these modifiable risk factors with TC to help improve her osteoporosis and hopefully prevent a fracture should she sustain another fall in the future. Alcohol is better avoided, although one drink daily for women and two drinks for men appear to have a protective effect on the skeleton. It is, however, not clear whether it is the alcohol itself or the lifestyle associated with moderate alcohol intake that is beneficial. An excessive alcohol intake, however, has a negative effect.

Over-the-counter hypnotics increase the risk of falls and fractures as many hypnotics cloud the sensorium and interfere with neuromuscular coordination.

Bifocal eyeglasses increase the risk of fall and fractures. Patients, for instance, may experience difficulties finding the switch of the bedside lights, and selecting the correct eyeglasses at a time when a number of neural signals originating in the distended urinary bladder and retinas are streaming to the cerebral cortex.

8. ***Tools to assess the fall/fracture risk include:***
   A. Falls efficacy scale.
   B. Vulnerable elder survey.
   C. Get-up-and-Go test.
   D. STEADI initiative (stopping elderly accidents, death, and injuries).
   E. All of the above.

Correct answer: E

Comment:

According to the CDC, more than 95% of hip fractures in older adults are caused by falls.[5] Given this substantial risk, it is important to know what tools are available to help guide a fall risk assessment on a patient to hopefully avoid further falls and potential for hip fracture.

The Falls Efficacy Scale (FES) is one way to assess the fall risk, based on a self-assessment focused on ADLs, such as dressing, bathing, and walking around the house, and asks patients to rate their confidence level in performing these activities.[6] The Vulnerable Elder Survey (VES) also addresses ADLs but asks if the patients are unable to perform the task, if it is due to health or another reason entirely. VES also includes questions regarding needing help managing money, walking, bathing, lifting items, and crouching.[7]

The Timed Get-up-and-Go (TUG) test is an in-office test to see how long it takes the patient to go from the seated position to standing without using arm rests, walking 3m or 10ft before returning to sitting down. An older adult who takes 12 or more seconds to complete this task is at an increased risk of falling. Patients may use a waking aid during the task. TUG test should be used in conjunction with other testing or clinical exam as a predictor of falls.[8] This test is objective versus the previous surveys that rely more on patients' self-assessments.

The STEADI initiative developed by CDC focuses on screening, assessing, and intervening for fall risk in adults 65 and older. The TUG test is included in the assessment as well as polypharmacy, home hazards, and orthostatic blood pressure.[9] The STEADI initiative considers multiple factors including intrinsic and extrinsic factors, clinical data, and clinical assessment to help the provider develop an individualized plan for fall intervention.

9. ***Elderly patients who fall typically fall:***
   A. Backwards.
   B. Sideways.
   C. Forward.
   D. A and B.
   E. A, B, and C.

   Correct answer: D

   Comment:

   Elderly patients typically fall backwards or sideways versus younger people who tend to fall forward and therefore may catch themselves with their hands to reduce the impact of the fall.[2] This is a reason why hip fractures are more common in the elderly population.

   Also, as individuals age their proprioception decreases and they tend to have more problems with stability.[2] According to a study on adapted Utilitarian Judo, teaching patients how to fall backwards and sideways and get back decreased their fear of falling.[3] This study, however, included a very limited number of participants and needs further exploration, but is a good starting point in improving outcomes with falls and overcoming the fear of falling.

10. ***Assistive technology that helps prevent falls includes:***
    A. Motion-activated lighting.
    B. Walking aids: 4- or 3-pronged canes, walkers, rollators.
    C. Reaching aids.
    D. Virtual reality games.
    E. All of the above.

    Correct answer: E

    Comment:

    Motion-activated lighting will illuminate the space to decrease the chances of falls. Walking aids provide stability if patients are unsteady when walking. "Reachers" or "grabbers" help patients reach objects without having to overstretch and increase the risk of falls. Virtual reality games can also help increase awareness about environmental hazards. Falls Sensei is a 3D virtual reality game that educates older adults about environmental hazards which can increase the risk of fall.[10]

Case summary

Analysis of data

Factors predisposing to bone demineralization/osteoporosis in Mrs. TC's case
- Surgical menopause age 48.
- Positive family history.
- No regular exercise.

Factors reducing to bone demineralization/osteoporosis
- Zoledronic acid (Reclast) yearly IV infusion.
- Daily calcium tablet.
- Involved in house activities.

Facts increasing risk of falls/fractures
- Several recent falls.

Diagnosis

- Osteoporosis.

Management recommendations

Treatment recommendations

- Continue annual zoledronic acid (Reclast) IV infusions, for at least 2years. Then reevaluate the patient to determine whether or not to continue with zoledronic acid (Reclast).

Diagnostic test(s)

- None needed at this stage.

Lifestyle

- Incorporate and develop a regular exercise program.

Rehabilitation

- Physical therapy to help with balance.

DXA and radiologic

- Repeat DXA scan in 2 years.

Key points

- A number of factors extrinsic to the individual patient may increase the risk of falls and hence fractures.
- Fall risk assessment tools include Falls Efficacy Scale, Vulnerable Elder Survey, Get-Up-and-Go test, STEADI initiative.
- Assistive technology to help with balance includes motion detector lighting, canes, walkers, reaching aids, and VR games.

References

1. Ang GC, Low SL, How CH. Approach to falls among the elderly in the community. *Singapore Med J*. 2020;61(3):116–121. https://doi.org/10.11622/smedj.2020029.
2. Hamdy R. Fractures and repeated falls. *J Clin Densitom*. 2017;20(3):425–431.
3. Toronjo-Hornillo L, Castañeda-Vázquez C, Campos-Mesa MDC, et al. Effects of the application of a program of adapted utilitarian judo (JUA) on the fear of falling syndrome (FOF) for the health sustainability of the elderly population. *Int J Environ Res Public Health*. 2018;15(11):2526. Published 2018 November 12 https://doi.org/10.3390/ijerph15112526.
4. Liu-Ambrose T, Davis JC, Best JR, et al. Effect of a home-based exercise program on subsequent falls among community-dwelling high-risk older adults after a fall: a randomized clinical trial [published correction appears in JAMA. 2019;322(2):174]. *JAMA*. 2019;321(21):2092–2100. https://doi.org/10.1001/jama.2019.5795.
5. Centers for Disease Control and Prevention. Facts About Falls; 2021. https://www.cdc.gov/falls/facts.html.
6. Tinetti Falls Efficacy Scale | RehabMeasures Database (sralab.org).
7. Saliba S, Elliott M, Rubenstein LA, et al. The vulnerable elders survey (VES-13): a tool for identifying vulnerable elders in the community. *J Am Geriatr Soc*. 2001;49:1691–1699.
8. Barry E, Galvin R, Keogh C, Horgan F, Fahey T. Is the Timed Up and Go test a useful predictor of risk of falls in community dwelling older adults: a systematic review and meta-analysis. *BMC Geriatr*. 2014;14:14. Published 2014 February 1 https://doi.org/10.1186/1471-2318-14-14.
9. Centers for Disease Control and Prevention. STEADI-Older Adult Fall Prevention. https://www.cdc.gov/steadi/index.html.
10. Money AG, Atwal A, Boyce E, Gaber S, Windeatt S, Alexandrou K. Falls Sensei: a serious 3D exploration game to enable the detection of extrinsic home fall hazards for older adults. *BMC Med Inform Decis Mak*. 2019;19(1):85. Published 2019 April 16 https://doi.org/10.1186/s12911-019-0808-x.

Index

Note: Page numbers followed by *f* indicate figures, *t* indicate tables, and *b* indicate boxes.

9780323995504